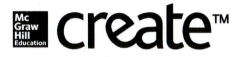

Taking Sides: Clashing Views
on Bioethical Issues, 17/e

Gregory E. Kaebnick

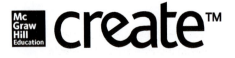

http://create.mheducation.com

ISBN-10: 1259873404   ISBN-13: 9781259873409

Contents

Detailed Table of Contents

Unit 3: Choices in Reproduction

Issue: Should Embryos Produced During IVF Be Considered Children?
YES: **Thomas Brejcha et al.,** from "Brief of Amici Curiae Missouri Right to Life, Lawyers for Life, and American Association of Pro-Life Obstetricians & Gynecologists," *Gadberry v. McQueen*, Missouri Court of Appeals Eastern District (2015)
NO: **Joseph J. Kodner and John M. Faust,** from "Brief of Amicus Curiae American Society for Reproductive Medicine in Support of Respondent," *Gadberry v. McQueen*, Missouri Court of Appeals Eastern District (2016)

In a friend-of-the-court brief submitted in a recent case in Missouri involving a dispute over embryos that a couple had put into storage, lawyers for the American Society for Reproductive Medicine argue that embryos are not persons and that treating them as such would have a profound negative effect on people who seek medical assistance in building their families. In a friend-of-the-court brief on the other side of the same case, lawyers representing several organizations that are opposed to abortion argue that science proves straightforwardly that embryos are persons, and that the embryos in the Missouri custody dispute should be given to the parent who seeks to take care of them.

Issue: Should a Pregnant Woman Be Punished for Exposing Her Fetus to Risk?
YES: **Liles Burke,** from *Hope Elisabeth Ankrom v. State of Alabama*, Circuit Court of Coffee County (2011)
NO: **Lynn M. Paltrow,** from "Punishment and Prejudice: Judging Drug-Using Pregnant Women," Beacon Press (1999)

Liles Burke sets out the majority opinion of the Alabama Court of Criminal Appeals in a case involving a pregnant woman who was found to have used cocaine while pregnant. Burke argues that Alabama law that forbids adults from exposing children to controlled substances applies in cases involving pregnant women and their fetuses. Attorney Lynn M. Paltrow argues that treating drug-using pregnant women as criminals targets poor, African American women while ignoring other drug usage and fails to provide the resources to assist them in recovery.

Unit 4: Professional Integrity

Issue: Should Physicians Be Allowed to Participate in Executions?
YES: **David Waisel,** from "Physician Participation in Capital Punishment," *Mayo Clinic Proceedings* (2007)
NO: **Atul Gawande,** from "When Law and Ethics Collide—Why Physicians Participate in Executions," *The New England Journal of Medicine* (2006)

David Waisel, a professor of medicine, argues that if the state is to administer capital punishment, then physicians may honorably seek to help the condemned die as painlessly as possible. Physician and journalist Atul Gawande supports capital punishment but believes physicians, as healers, should play no role in it.

Issue: Should Pharmacists Be Allowed to Deny Prescriptions on Grounds of Conscience?
YES: **Donald W. Herbe,** from "The Right to Refuse: A Call for Adequate Protection of a Pharmacist's Right to Refuse Facilitation of Abortion and Emergency Contraception," *Journal of Law and Health* (2002/2003)
NO: **Julie Cantor and Ken Baum,** from "The Limits of Conscientious Objection—May Pharmacists Refuse to Fill Prescriptions for Emergency Contraception?" *The New England Journal of Medicine* (2004)

Law student Donald W. Herbe asserts that pharmacists' moral beliefs concerning abortion and emergency contraception are genuinely fundamental and deserve respect. He proposes that professional pharmaceutical organizations lead the way to recognizing a true right of conscience, which would eventually result in universal legislation protecting against all potential ramifications of choosing conscience. Julie Cantor, a lawyer, and Ken Baum, a physician and lawyer, reject an absolute right to object, as well as no right to object, to these prescriptions but assert that pharmacists who cannot or will not dispense a drug have a professional obligation to meet the needs of their customers by referring them elsewhere.

Unit 5: The Development and Use of Biotechnology

Issue: Is the Use of Medical Tools to Enhance Human Beings Morally Troubling?
YES: **President's Council on Bioethics**, from *Beyond Therapy: Biotechnology and the Pursuit of Happiness*, U.S. Government Printing Office (2003)
NO: **Ronald Bailey,** from "The Case for Enhancing People," *The New Atlantis* (2011)

The President's Council on Bioethics, a presidential body formed by President Bush, argues that biotechnological interventions for making people better than normal raise profound concerns about the relationship between humans and nature, human identity, and human happiness. The libertarian science writer Ronald Bailey maintains that enhancements will only help people live better lives.

The Bush Administration's Domestic Policy Council argues that advances with adult stem cells and alternative sources of pluripotent stem cells make it unnecessary to conduct stem cell research that destroys human embryos, and that if the research is unnecessary, then it should not be done. Insoo Hyun, past chair of the Ethics and Public Policy Committee of the International Society for Stem Cell Research, argues that the alternatives present their own ethical questions and do not eliminate the need to conduct research on embryonic stem cells.

David H. Kaye and Michael E. Smith, professors of law, argue that a population-wide DNA database could not only help solve crimes but would be fairer than more limited databases. Mark A. Rothstein, also a professor of law and a prominent advocate for maintaining genetic privacy, and his coauthor Meghan K. Talbott argue that DNA databases should be more limited in size and use.

Nurse Sarah E. Shannon believes that ethically and legally parents have the right and duty to make decisions and to care for their family members who are unable to do so themselves and that we should not abandon parents of severely developmentally disabled children to the harsh social and economic realities that are barriers to good care. Nurse Teresa A. Savage believes that children like Ashley should have independent advocates, preferably persons with disabilities, to weigh the risks and benefits of proposed interventions.

The President's Commission for the Study of Bioethical Issues, a bioethics commission created by President Obama, calls for developing the field of synthetic biology, a branch of biological science that aims at genetically modifying organisms to carry out medical, industrial, and other tasks, with "prudent vigilance." Friends of the Earth, International Center for Technology Assessment, and the ETC Group, leading a group of civil society organizations, counter by recommending a "precautionary" approach and calling for a moratorium on the release and commercial use of synthetic organisms.

Kent H. Redford, William Adams, and Georgina M. Mace, who are consultants and researchers working on issues of biodiversity and conservation, propose that synthetic biology, though it is often thought of as providing tool for intervening into nature, can be used as well to protect nature, by aiding in the restoration and protection of species and ecosystems. Christopher J. Preston, professor of philosophy at University of Montana, counters that biotechnological restoration of a species will cut deeply into environmental values.

Unit 6: Access to Health Care

Philosopher James Stacey Taylor argues that the Affordable Care Act passed into law during President Obama' first term is unduly paternalistic, failing to pass muster even on the simple utilitarian grounds that could most easily support policies to require citizens to buy insurance. Timothy Stoltzfus Jost, a legal scholar, holds that the ACA is intended to create a national community of community aid, relying on the power of Congress to impose taxes.

Rajeev Raghavan and Ricardo Nuila, physicians who work with end-stage renal disease patients, argue that standardized coverage for dialysis treatments would alleviate the burden on taxpayers where the most undocumented residents live and would improve these patients' health, allowing them to return to work. David Stratas, a justice with the Federal Court of Appeals of Ontario, Canada, explains why Canada was justified in not providing health care benefits to an undocumented immigrant who lived in Toronto.

Physician Emil J. Freireich believes that patients with advanced cancer and limited life expectancy should have the same privilege as all individuals in a free society. Law professor George J. Annas argues that there is no constitutional right to demand experimental interventions, and that fully open access would undermine the FDA's ability to protect the public from unsafe drugs.

Law professor R. Alta Charo argues that vaccination against the human papillomavirus, which causes most cases of cervical cancer, should be mandatory except in cases of medical, religious, or philosophical objection. Law professors Gail Javitt and Lawrence O. Gostin and physician Deena Berkowitz believe that, given the limited data and experience, and the fact that HPV does not pose imminent and significant risk to others, mandating HPV vaccine is premature.

Psychiatrist Sally Satel contends that a regulated and legal system of rewarding organ donors will not only save lives but also stop the illegal trafficking that offers no protections for poor people around the world. The Institute of Medicine Committee on Increasing Rates of Organ Donation argues that a free market in organs is problematic because in live organ donation, both buyers and sellers may not have complete or accurate information, and selling organs of dead people raises concerns about commodification of human bodies.

Preface

This is a book about choices—hard and tragic choices. The choices are hard not only because they often involve life and death, but also because there are convincing arguments on both sides of the issues. An ethical dilemma, by definition, is one that poses a conflict not between good and evil but between one good principle and another that is equally good. The choices are hard because the decisions that are made—by individuals, groups, and public policymakers—will influence the kind of society we have today and the one we will have in the future. Although many of the views expressed in the selections in this volume are strong—even passionate—they are also subtle, concerned with the nuances of the particular debate. How one argues matters in bioethics; you will see and have to weigh the significance of varying rhetorical styles and appeals throughout this volume.

Although there are no easy answers to any of the issues in the book, the questions will be answered in some fashion—partly by individual choices and partly by decisions that are made by professionals and government. We must make them the best answers possible, and that can only be done by informed and thoughtful consideration. This book, then, can serve as a beginning for what ideally will become an ongoing process of examination and reflection. In approaching each new edition, the editor also must make some hard choices. In trying to keep the selections up to date, sometimes older ones must be replaced. In other instances, newer articles are just that—newer, but not necessarily better. Striking a balance between timeliness and timelessness is challenging. For each issue, additional points of view are noted in the follow-up section titled "Exploring the Issue," and readers are encouraged to pursue these references.

Gregory E. Kaebnick
The Hastings Center

Editor of This Volume

GREGORY E. KAEBNICK is a scholar at The Hastings Center and, since 2001, editor of the *Hastings Center Report*. His research interests have focused on emerging biotechnologies, including synthetic biology, genetic paternity testing, agricultural biotechnology, and behavioral genetics. He is the author of *Humans in Nature: The World As We Find It and the World As We Create It* (Oxford University Press, 2014) and editor of *The Ideal of Nature: Debates about Biotechnology and the Environment* (Johns Hopkins Press, 2011), co-editor with Lori Knowles of *Shaping Our Future: Law, Policy, and Ethics in an Era of Reproductive Genetics* (Johns Hopkins Press, 2007), and co-editor with Mark O. Rothstein, Thomas H. Murray, and Mary Anderlik Majumder of *Genetic Ties and the Family: The Impact of Paternity Testing on Parents and Children* (Johns Hopkins Press, 2005). He received his PhD (1998) and MS (1994) in philosophy from the University of Minnesota and his BA in religion from Swarthmore College (1986).

Dedication

For Hannah, Rebecca, and Gwen

Editors/Academic Advisory Board Members

Members of the Academic Advisory Board are instrumental in the final selection of articles for each edition of *Taking Sides*. Their review of articles for content, level, and appropriateness provides critical direction to the editors and staff. We think that you will find their careful consideration well reflected in this volume.

James Allison
Loveland Hurst High School

J.C. Andersen
University of Tampa

Barry Arnold
University of West Florida

Lawrence J. Berliner
University of Denver

Christine Bezotte
Elmira College

C. Anne Blakey
Ball State University

Barry Brock
Barry University

K. Joy Karnas
Cedar Crest College

Barbara Katz Rothman
Bernard M. Baruch College

Diane Kondratowicz
Elgin Community College

Neil Kugler
Boise State University

Andrew Marks
Texas Sate University, San Marcos

Heather McDivitt
Wingate University

Dave Miller
Clark State Community College

Wren Mills
Bowling Green Technical College

Jonathan Morris
Manchester Community College

Joseph B. Mosca
Monmouth University

Leelavati R. Murthy
Community College Allegheny County–Monroeville

Patricia E. Neff Claster
Edinboro University of Pennsylvania

Lawrence J. Nelson
Santa Clara University

Tracey Nicholls
Lewis College

Leonard Olson
California State University, Fresno

Mark Packard
Southeast Community College

Wendy Parker
Albany College of Pharmacy

Cindy Pavel
Ivy Tech Community College

Roberta L. Pohlman
Wright State University

Steve Reiter
Central Community College–Columbus

Robert L. Rhodes
Washtenaw Community College

Doug Rice
Sacramento State University

Ralph Rice
Wake Forest University School of Medicine

Christopher Robinson
Clarkson University

Jordy Rocheleau
Austin Peay State University

Michelle M. Rotert
Rock Valley College

Leon Schefers
Saint Mary's University of Minnesota

Nancy J. Schneider
University of Maine

Rafayel Seyranyan
Northern Virginia Community College

Mark Sheldon
Northwestern University

Sheryl Slaughter Ellis
Middle Tennessee State University

Richard Sneed
University of Central Oklahoma

Joseph A. Spadaro
Goodwin College

Aparna Sreenivasan
California State University

Llyod Steffen
Lehigh University

Suzette Stine
Lone Star College–Kingwood

Sharon Stratton
University of Tennessee

Julio F. Turrens
University of South Alabama

Lawrence Ulrich
University of Dayton

Mary Beth Van Ness
University of Toledo

Julia VanderMolen
Davenport University

Marisol White
Hartnell College

Betty Wolder Levin
Brooklyn College

Lissa Yogan
Valparaiso University

Introduction

Biology, Medicine, and Ethics

The term "bioethics" is usually attributed to the biologist Van Rensselaer Potter, who proposed it in a book in 1971 as a way of creating a bridge between the "two cultures" that had been identified a dozen years earlier by the British novelist C.P. Snow. The "two cultures" are the sciences and the humanities, which Snow lamented were growing increasingly far apart from each other, to the point that they seemed no longer to share a language. Bioethics, then, was supposed to provide that language. Potter's idea was that the broad set of scientific disciplines that go under the heading of "the biological sciences" or "the life sciences" was the scientific outcrop on which the bridge could be built.

Too, they were particularly in need of input from the humanities. The period in which Potter was developing these thoughts was a fertile period for biology, with scientific insights and biotechnologies that suggested a change in the human relationship with the natural world and certainly began to change medical practice. One of the most dramatic of these developments was the availability of kidney dialysis, which turned what had been a fatal diagnosis (kidney failure) into a potentially chronic condition. Because dialysis was exceedingly expensive and very scarce, not everybody who needed it could get it. In Seattle, as a 1962 story in *Life Magazine* explained to an amazed nation, a committee was formed to decide which patients would. The committee was making life-and-death decisions, of course, and it came to be known as the "God committee." In 1972, the national unease with these decisions led to a decision to provide coverage under Medicare for nearly any patient who needed it. Dialysis was not the only major new biomedical development in the 1960s and early 1970s, however. Organ transplantation became feasible thanks to the development of drugs to prevent the body's immune system from destroying a transplanted organ, the contraceptive pill was approved, and artificial respirators came into widespread use. Incrementally, doctors acquired tools that allowed them to actually help patients get well. Before antibiotics, of course, doctors mostly just presided over the sick.

Meanwhile, another revolution was also occurring on the other side of the bridge that bioethics was meant to be. The 1960s and 1970s were a period, famously, of intense cultural ferment, in which entrenched values were questioned and overturned. Authority and social inequality were widely challenged, and individual rights and social justice became prominent concerns both in popular culture and in academia, as illustrated in the civil rights movement, the protests against the Vietnam War, and Lyndon Johnson's Great Society. In medicine, the civil right movements generated a spin-off patients' rights movement, and the authority that had been granted physicians and the expectation of passivity from patients came under withering criticism. In health policy, a renewed effort was made to extend access to medical care, culminating in the creation of Medicaid in 1965.

In the late 1960s and early 1970s, bioethics emerged not just as a label but as the beginnings of a special area of scholarly research and writing. The Hastings Center, an independent research center known initially as the Institute for Society, Ethics, and the Life Sciences (later renamed after the town of Hastings-on-Hudson, New York, where it was originally located), and the Kennedy Institute of Ethics at Georgetown University launched this process. There is no one master discipline for bioethics: Instead, people come to it from many other disciplines—often from philosophy and from medicine, but also from other professions in the health sciences, from the law, from the social sciences, and from religion and literature among other disciplines in the humanities. Bioethics is seen as rigorously interdisciplinary—in this way, too, it is a kind of bridge. Today, it is possible to specialize in bioethics: A number of universities offer advanced degrees in bioethics, and some larger hospitals have "clinical ethicists" on staff, but even clinical ethicists usually have primary training in some other field. The scholarly work conducted in bioethics—on human subjects research, public health, health care policy, and the development and use of biotechnologies, in addition to clinical care issues that range from child-bearing to end-of-life decisions—reflects many professional, political, and disciplinary viewpoints.

Bioethics and Moral Philosophy

Because bioethics incorporates many fields, there are many ways of approaching bioethical problems. The challenge of how to increase the number of organs available for transplantation not only involves moral problems but also lends itself to sociological and economic analysis, for example. One possible way of increasing the number of organs would be to create a market for them, so that patients or their families would have some perhaps modest financial incentive to make organs available. But then sociological and economic questions arise: What would be the effect on society? Would the market work? Similarly, the question of whether to offer patients experimental drugs only in the context of clinical trials involves, in addition to a debate about individual rights versus public safety, some legal and regulatory concerns.

Often, in bioethical debates, discussion focuses on the relevant facts. How many people are infected with HPV and with what consequences, and which interventions are likely to have what consequences for this public health problem? Underneath all bioethical debates, however, are questions about the relative significance and implications of various moral values or principles. Particularly important are debates about individual freedom and responsibility versus the public good, equity, and responsibility for others. Given these foundational concerns, bioethics is often said to be a subset of ethics generally—the application to an interesting set of cases, all of which have to do with the life sciences, of moral philosophy.

A common account of how bioethics fits into academia is therefore that it is one kind of "applied ethics" or "professional ethics" (alongside, e.g., environmental ethics, business ethics, and journalism ethics), which itself fits under the broader heading of "moral philosophy." The other branches of moral philosophy are "normative ethics," which examines and clarifies the basic standards that govern action and character, and "metaethics," which examines the ultimate justifications and meaning of morality—asking, for example, where the basic standards come from and whether an answer to a moral question can be described as "true" or "false." (These branches are not always distinct from each other, however, and a single discussion in moral philosophy may delve into all of them. A defense of a fundamental moral standard may have metaethical implications and may lead to a discussion of applications.)

Moral Theories

Because bioethics draws heavily on moral philosophy, and is indeed sometimes seen as a kind of subfield of moral philosophy, books that explore a range of bioethical debates often include an outline of the most widely discussed theories of morality in the Western philosophical

canon. Just how moral theories can be legitimately used in moral deliberation is itself an interesting question, both for bioethics and for moral philosophy. It is a little odd, to say the least, to imagine a hospital ethicist who has been brought in to discuss a life-or-death decision launching into an explanation of what his chosen moral theory leads him to say. But even if moral theories are not invoked to reach specific judgments, they might still be useful in other ways. One might rely on general theories, for example, to reach mid-level moral rules—that lying is wrong, or that touching a person's body without that person's permission is wrong—that then lead to judgments in specific cases.

The oldest of the theoretic approaches that still has currency today is virtue theory, which has its roots in the writings of Aristotle. Virtue theory holds that the fundamental standards of morality are not standards of conduct, but standards of character. These standards, the virtues, are dispositions to behave in certain ways—to be honest, to be brave, and to be temperate. There is no one agreed-upon list of the virtues, nor can the virtues be articulated in such a way that one can develop an account of the virtues and straightforwardly deduce good judgments from that account. One must instead internalize these standards, through a process of long training. If one has gone through this process and acquired the virtues, then one will respond to new circumstances appropriately.

In bioethics, virtue theory has been used primarily to try to give an account of how doctors should treat patients. Virtue theory lends itself less well to discussions of public policy, although virtue-based discussions of policy issues can be found in the bioethics literature. Philippa Foote, one of the foremost twentieth-century philosophers in the virtue theory tradition, explored the ethics of euthanasia in an oft-discussed paper, but her goal there was to argue that in the context of a virtue theory, the moral distinction between "allowing someone to die" and "actively causing someone to die" can depend on the circumstances. One of the attractions of virtue theory is that it can allow for a certain flexibility and ambiguity that some find appropriate for moral reasoning. Aristotle famously drew a distinction between moral knowledge and scientific or mathematical knowledge; moral judgments hold "only for the most part." Also, an Aristotelian approach can embrace a rich and varied moral vocabulary.

In the thirteenth century, St. Thomas Aquinas drew on his reading of Aristotle to develop an account of morality known today as "natural law" theory. Aquinas held that the cosmos is divinely and rationally ordered, and that a moral law is part of the cosmic order. Further, it is part of God's plan that everyone can understand the moral law through the use of human reason. One can investigate the natural cosmic order and deduce right moral judgments. Natural law theorists often, therefore, hold that we can learn about morality partly by investigating human nature: What humans are designed (by God) to do can help us understand what they should do. Natural law theory may have influenced some of the scholars who are critical of using medical technology to change human nature. Although rarely explicitly invoked in secular bioethics, natural law theory has a considerable influence on Catholic bioethics.

The natural law account of how the moral law was apprehended by human reason has struck many later philosophers as obscure and unconvincing. The eighteenth-century Scottish Enlightenment philosopher David Hume was reacting partly against natural law theory when he argued that moral judgments are not a matter either of reason or of investigating the world, but instead are derived from what he called "the passions"—what today would be called emotions or attitudes. If you investigate a given case, he argued, you end up only with a set of facts, and it is impossible to derive a moral judgment purely from a set of facts. This point is often abbreviated in the dictum, "no ought from an is." The ought—the moral judgment—is a human response to the case, not part of the case itself.

Many philosophers have taken Hume to be making the metaethical claim that there are no true moral judgments, but only subjective opinions. This position is widely rejected in bioethics. However, Hume's skepticism that a moral judgment could be put on a rock-solid foundation—that one could give a proof of a position such that anyone who can reason and investigate the world would be rationally compelled to accept it—has been more influential (disappointing though it is to many). Also, Hume's view that moral claims cannot be derived purely from factual claims is invoked frequently (although some also reject it, on grounds that there are no purely factual descriptions of a case). A common view of moral reasoning in bioethics is that factual claims and value claims must be articulated more or less independently of each other, and that both are necessary to reach a conclusion.

The great German philosopher Immanuel Kant wrote that Hume "awakened" him from his "dogmatic slumbers." Much of Kant's work in philosophy, however, was devoted to trying to re-create, as best as possible, the foundations that Hume seemed to have destroyed. In moral philosophy, Kant proposed that there was indeed a moral law and that it could be derived from the nature of the

rational will itself. Roughly, the law Kant proposed is that one should act only on an intention that one could coherently will that every rational being would act on as well. To lie, for example, is to act on an intention to deceive others, but one could not (Kant wrote) coherently will that everybody would act on that intention, because if that happened, deception itself would be impossible. Deception requires trust, but if deception were universal, trust would be nonexistent. Kant called this law the "categorical imperative." He also offered what he believed was an alternative formulation of it, which was that one should never treat a rational being merely as a tool for achieving some other end; one should always treat a rational being also as an "end in itself"—that is, as having a value beyond any price, since to give something a price is always to see it as something one could sell in order to achieve some other end. From a careful application of these formulations of the categorical imperative, Kant thought, narrower moral rules and specific moral judgments could be derived.

Bioethics is deeply influenced by Kant, although very few bioethicists work by trying to apply the categorical imperative in quite the way Kant envisioned. What has caught on in bioethics is the idea that respect for autonomy provides a core, perhaps the core, moral guide. For Kant, autonomy meant the capacity of a rational being to rule itself and adhere to the categorical imperative. In bioethics, autonomy typically means something a little looser: the capacity of a person to make one's own life decisions (not necessarily always to choose the rational and right thing). Kant's idea that a rational will that has a value beyond price has also influenced bioethics. Human beings are often said to have a special dignity in virtue of being human, and both human beings and parts of human beings, such as organs, are sometimes said to be priceless—in the literal sense of being things that should not be bought and sold.

Kantian moral philosophy is described as deontological, meaning that it is about duties. (Deon means duty, in Greek.) It provides guidance for conduct, rather than character, and it identifies conduct that is required of a person regardless of outcome. A contrasting approach to guiding conduct is found in consequentialist moral theories, the most influential version of which is the utilitarian theory introduced by the British social reformer Jeremy Bentham and refined by the philosopher John Stuart Mill. Consequentialist theories hold that right actions are known by evaluating their outcomes. In utilitarian theory, the morally important outcome is happiness or well-being—"utility," in the parlance utilitarians sometimes adopt.

Mill also argued that happiness is typically best promoted by largely promoting individual liberty; individuals largely left to their own devices would discover for themselves the most effective ways of promoting their happiness, and their experimentation and creativity would help others promote their own happiness. The principle Mill set out, in his book *On Liberty*, is known as the harm principle: "the only purpose for which power can be rightfully exercised over any member of a civilized community, against his will, is to prevent harm to others."

Mill has been hugely influential in bioethics. Many accept that, even if good outcomes are not the sole criterion of good conduct, they are certainly very important, and the idea of respect for autonomy as understood in bioethics owes as much to Mill's discussion of liberty as to Kant's categorical imperative. The patients' rights movement is essentially an endorsement of the idea that people ought to be allowed to make decisions for themselves, even when they become patients, and even at the risk of harm to themselves. Physician paternalism is unacceptable. On the other hand, public health policy has often wrestled with the harm principle. Public health policy is often thought to require a kind of paternalism, insofar as the goal is not merely to prevent individuals from harming others but to encourage or require them to do things that are good for themselves.

Moral Reasoning in Bioethics

Bioethics is far from a straightforward application to cases of one or another moral theory, however. Just as the people come to bioethics from many different disciplines, the relevance of moral theory to bioethics is widely disputed. Many in the field who are not philosophers do not explicitly draw on a moral theory, and many also draw on multiple moral theories, according to what seems salient in a particular problem.

One of the most influential uses of theory in bioethics is what is sometimes called the "principlist" approach. In the early 1970s, news broke about a study, begun in 1932 and continued until 1972, in which poor, rural black men with syphilis were monitored by the Public Health Service but never treated, despite the discovery in the 1940s that penicillin was effective against the disease. The study was considered reminiscent of notorious Nazi experiments conducted on Jews and others in concentration camps during World War II, and the federal government responded to the scandal by creating the National Commission for the Protection of Human Subjects of Biomedical and Behavioral Research to lay out guidelines for the

ethically acceptable treatment of the subjects of medical research. The National Commission issued a number of recommendations, and then in 1978, in a document called simply the Belmont Report, outlined the underlying ethical principles that the commission members—scholars, religious leaders, and others—had been able to agree on. The three principles identified in the Report—respect for persons, beneficence, and justice—have turned into the basis for much of the work that has been done in bioethics.

The principle of respect for persons is derived from the Kantian idea that the capacity for autonomy, or self-determination, deserves great respect. The Belmont Report drew two conclusions from this principle—that people with autonomy should be allowed to make their own decisions (as long as those decisions do not harm others), and that people who because of age, illness, or other circumstances have less autonomy are entitled to protection. In order to ensure that people decide for themselves whether to participate in medical research, the report goes on to argue, they must be given adequate information about the research and their consent to participate must be explicitly sought. Thus the Report argued for truth-telling about medical research and for obtaining subjects' informed consent to participate in research.

The principle of beneficence is the guidance that, before the patients' rights movement, most doctors regarded as the overriding medical ethical principle. The principle is sometimes said to have two components, first that the doctor should do no harm to the patient (an idea expressed in Latin as *Primum non nocere*), and second that the doctor should act so as to benefit the patient. Both components are often said to be expressed in the Greek Hippocratic Oath: "I will apply dietetic measures for the benefit of the sick according to my ability and judgment; I will keep them from injustice and harm. . . . Whatever houses I may visit, I will comfort and benefit the sick, remaining free of all intentional injustice."

The National Commission also concluded that medical research should be guided by a principle of justice, which it understood as bearing on the question, "Who ought to receive the benefits of research and bear its burdens?" Arguably, the commission did less well in deciding precisely what justice requires. Instead of going on to identify rules that follow from the principle, it identified five different ways of guiding the allocation of benefits and burdens, ranging from "to each person an equal share" to "to each person according to merit."

The principlist approach was picked up and developed in a highly influential book, now in its sixth edition, titled *Principles of Biomedical Ethics*, by Tom L. Beauchamp and James F. Childress, which has been widely used to discuss moral dilemmas arising in clinical care, extending to medicine generally a framework originally developed to address issues in medical research. An assortment of other ways of thinking about clinical care dilemmas has also been proposed; however, some of them are in deliberate opposition to principlism. The casuistic approach proposed by Albert Jonsen and Stephen Toulmin, for example, argues that ethical guidance starts not with abstract principles but with well-accepted judgments in specific cases, which must then be extended to new cases through analogical reasoning. Clinical ethicists sometimes employ casuistic methodologies designed to encourage people struggling with a specific case to identify a wide range of facts and values that are relevant to a case. Feminist approaches sometimes embrace an ethic of caring, focusing on relationships instead of on individual autonomy.

Bioethical issues outside the contexts of decision making for specific people in medical research and clinical care usually draw on an even wider range of moral philosophical work. For example, in a series of books about the overall goals of medicine and the use of societal resources in medical research, Daniel Callahan, a co-founder of The Hastings Center, has drawn on "communitarianism," a view of moral values that has roots in Aristotelian philosophy, to argue that there should be limits to the use of medicine and the advance of medical research. Communitarianism emphasizes that the well-being of individuals is rooted in the well-being of the community, rather than in unlimited self-determination or the maximization of individual happiness. Debates about public health programs and about health policy—about access to health care and the distribution of health care resources—may deploy either communitarian or broadly utilitarian frameworks. Concerns about selfhood—about agency, authenticity, and dignity, for example—sometimes animate discussions of whether medical science should be used to alter human bodies or behaviors. Yet another way of thinking about the limits of the life sciences could be drawn from environmental ethics (which arguably falls within the ambit of "bioethics" as that term was initially proposed by Van Rensselaer Potter). Environmental ethicists often endorse the idea that not just human autonomy and happiness

have value but also nature has value, and that the value of nature ought to constrain what humans can do, using biotechnology or other methods, to naturally occurring species and ecosystems.

Answers and Insights

This book is organized so as to introduce readers to the full range of concerns that have been taken up in bioethics, from clinical dilemmas to questions about the use of biotechnology and just access to health care. It is also intended to canvass both fundamental and philosophical questions about the nature of medical decision making and the values relevant to the development and use of biotechnology, and more practical questions about, for example, the mechanisms for making good decisions at the end of life and for increasing the supply of organs available for transplantation.

Many of these societal problems do not admit of easy answers, and in fact, the title of this book notwithstanding, taking sides on these problems should not always be the goal. Careful exploration of contrasting positions, articulating differences of opinion, and recognizing that both sides may offer important moral insights, are at least the first step in taking sides, and sometimes it may be as far as one can realistically go. Of course, in many bioethical problems, both at the bedside and at the societal level, there is a dilemma that requires answering, one way or another, if only because doing nothing is still to make a decision of sorts. However far we go toward settling on answers, we ought to look for consensus wherever it is available. On some of the issues discussed in this book, some consensus is possible. The legacy of the National Commission for the Protection of Human Subjects of Biomedical and Behavioral Research is that people of different backgrounds can sometimes agree, both on specific recommendations and on the values that inform them. As later presidential bioethics commissions have occasionally discovered, however, the moral questions that led to the emergence of bioethics may uncover intractable controversies.

Gregory E. Kaebnick
The Hastings Center

Unit 1

UNIT

Medical Decision Making

*A*s *recently as 50 years ago, medical decision making was of concern only to physicians. With their presumed greater knowledge and with patients' best interests at heart, they were entrusted with making life-and-death decisions, as well as ordinary decisions. Ironically, although physicians had greater authority to make treatment decisions than they do today, they had less ability to treat. As the scientific understanding of the human body has advanced, and as the ability to intervene in the body surgically and pharmacologically has grown more sophisticated, the range of people who have an interest in making decisions—and in some cases, a right to do so—among the medical options has grown.*

Law and ethics have reaffirmed the status of the patient as the primary decision maker. Nevertheless, many ambiguous and troubling situations remain in implementing patients' wishes. The patient's preferences do not always settle a decision, especially when their preferences impinge on the rights of others, such as family members, physicians, and other patients. Patients also sometimes lack the cognitive ability to make important decisions, in which case the decision must be made by a surrogate acting on the patient's behalf. Cases that require surrogate decision makers can be among the most pressing imaginable; they are often about seriously ill or dying patients, and they can bring up all sorts of complexities about relationships among family members, loved ones, health care providers. And of course, deciding which patients lack decision-making ability—or when a given patient lacks decision-making ability—is very difficult. This unit explores the value given to the patient's decision-making ability and some of the issues that then arise when making medical decisions.

Selected, Edited, and with Issue Framing Material by:
Gregory E. Kaebnick, *The Hastings Center*

ISSUE

Is Patient Self-Determination the Central Value in Making Medical Decisions?

YES: Dan W. Brock and Steven A. Wartman, from "When Competent Patients Make Irrational Choices," *The New England Journal of Medicine* (1990)

NO: Gordon M. Stirrat and Robin Gill, from "Autonomy in Medical Ethics after O'Neill," *Journal of Medical Ethics* (2005)

Learning Outcomes
After reading this issue, you will be able to:
• Discuss the concepts of autonomy and informed consent, the relationship between them, and how they have been understood and employed in bioethics.

ISSUE SUMMARY

YES: Philosopher Dan Brock and physician Steven Wartman explicate the concept of "shared decision-making," in which decisions about the patient's medical care are reached through collaboration between the patient and the physician. Physicians should sometimes provide guidance to patients, argue Brock and Wartman, but decisions depend fundamentally on the patient's choices.

NO: British bioethicists Gordon Stirrat and Robin Gill, building on influential work by the moral philosopher Onora O'Neill, argue that the core moral value of medical decision-making is mutual trust in the covenantal relationship between patient and caregiver.

Informed consent is undoubtedly one of the best-known and, arguably, one of the least-implemented concepts in modern medicine. Although much of modern medical ethics has ancient roots, the idea of informed consent is relatively recent. Until the mid-twentieth century most medical ethics were firmly based on the obligations of physicians to act for the benefit of their patients. Information was supposed to be managed carefully in order to protect patients from bad news and to keep them hopeful.

The first "Code of Medical Ethics" of the American Medical Association relied heavily on the work of Thomas Percival, a British physician whose book *Medical Ethics* (1803) played a crucial role in the field for more than a century. Percival believed that the patient's right to the truth was less important than the physician's obligation to benefit the patient. Deception, in the interest of doing good, was thus justified. The patient's consent to treatment, informed or otherwise, is not mentioned in early codes of medical ethics, although on a practical level doctors had to have a patient's permission to perform most procedures.

The modern concept of informed consent came to medical ethics through the courts. The earliest influential decision was *Schloendorff v. New York Hospital* (1914), in which the court ruled that a patient's right to "self-determination" obligated a physician to obtain consent. This case laid the basis for further litigation. The most influential series of decisions occurred in the 1950s and 1960s, when rulings went beyond the obligation to obtain consent to include an explicit duty to disclose information relevant to the patient who is making a decision about consent.

While the earlier cases had been based on the patient's right to be free from unwanted bodily intrusion (legally, "battery"), the court in *Natanson v. Kline* (1960) held that physicians who withheld information while obtaining consent were guilty of negligence. Imposing a legal duty on physicians to inform their patients of the risks, benefits, and alternatives to treatment exposed them to the risk of malpractice suits. Another factor that influenced the ascendance of informed consent in medical treatment was parallel discussions about the ethics of research involving human subjects. Voluntary consent to participate in research was a cornerstone of the Nuremberg Code of 1947, which was issued after the trials of Nazi physicians who had performed lethal experiments on nonconsenting prisoners.

Nevertheless, traditions die hard, and little change was seen in actual practice until the resurgence of interest in medical ethics in the 1970s. In 1972 the case of *Canterbury v. Spence* established a far-reaching, patient-centered disclosure standard. The ruling stated, "The patient's right of self-decision can be effectively exercised only if the patient possesses enough information to enable an intelligent choice. . . . Social policy does not accept the paternalistic view that the physician may remain silent because

divulgence might prompt the patient to forego needed therapy." In the 1980s and 1990s court cases focused on individuals who lacked the competence to provide informed consent, such as comatose patients, children, and mentally ill persons.

Although the physician's duty to obtain informed consent and the patient's right to information are now firmly established in law and grounded in the ethical principle of respect for persons, medical practice varies considerably. In Stephen G. Post, ed., *Encyclopedia of Bioethics* (2003), Tom L. Beauchamp and Ruth R. Faden, philosophers who have studied informed consent extensively, assert, "The overwhelming impression from the empirical literature and from reported clinical experience is that the actual process of soliciting informed consent often falls short of a serious show of respect for the decisional authority of patients." The following selections illustrate two moderately but importantly contrasting views of patient autonomy. Dan Brock and Steven Wartman advance a modern version of the traditional view, according to which respect for patient autonomy remains the most important moral consideration in health care decision-making. Gordon Stirrat and Robin Gill argue for a more equal relationship between patients and physicians, with patient self-determination still important but balanced against respect for the moral agency of physicians. Patients and physicians should work to build trust in each other.

YES ↵

Dan W. Brock and Steven A. Wartman

When Competent Patients Make Irrational Choices

In recent years, physicians and patients have tended to move toward shared decision making. Although it sounds reasonable on the surface that patients and physicians should collaborate in making decisions about medical care, surprisingly little attention has been given to the complex and troubling issues that can arise. In particular, what does shared decision making imply for a physician's responsibilities when an apparently competent patient's choice appears to be irrational? A discussion of this issue requires a taxonomy of the different sources and forms of irrational decision making. We believe such a taxonomy should include the bias toward the present and near future, the belief that "it won't happen to me," the fear of pain or the medical experience, patients' values or wants that make no sense, framing effects, and conflicts between individual and social rationality. Our main aim here is to develop this taxonomy and thus to bring out some of the theoretical and practical obstacles involved in distinguishing between a patient's irrational choices, which the physician may seek to change, and merely unusual choices that should be respected. To avoid any misunderstanding, we emphasize at the outset that even the irrational choices of a competent patient must be respected if the patient cannot be persuaded to change them.

Shared Decision Making Between Physician and Patient

Historically, the professional ideal of the physician–patient relationship held that the physician directed care and made decisions about treatment; the patient's principal role was to comply with "doctor's orders." Although this paternalistic approach often took account of the patient's general preferences and attitudes toward treatment, it gave the patient only a minimal role in making decisions. When faced with what appeared to be a patient's irrational choices or preferences, physicians were encouraged by this approach to overlook or override them as not being in the patient's true interests.

Challenged by a number of forces within and outside the medical profession during the past two or three decades, the paternalistic approach has generally been replaced by the concept of shared decision making, in which both physicians and patients make active and essential contributions.[1] Physicians bring their medical training, knowledge, and expertise—including an understanding of the available treatment alternatives—to the diagnosis and management of patients' conditions. Patients bring a knowledge of their own subjective aims and values, through which the risks and benefits of various treatment options can be evaluated. With this approach, selecting the best treatment for a particular patient requires the contributions of both parties.[2]

This description of the division of labor oversimplifies the complexities of the roles and contributions of physicians and patients when real decisions about treatment are made, but it does highlight the patient's new, active part in that process. Some have concluded that in shared decision making, proper respect for patient autonomy and self-determination means accepting the patient's treatment preferences however they are arrived at. We believe that such a conclusion is unwarranted, because it fails to recognize the trade-off between the sometimes conflicting values that underlie shared decision making and that are involved in respecting or seeking to change patients' choices. The first value is the well-being of patients, which can require the physician to attempt to protect them from the harmful consequences of their choices when their judgment is irrational. The second value is respecting the right of patients to make decisions about their own lives when they are able. Whenever competent patients appear to be making irrational choices about treatment that are contrary to their own well-being, the two values will be in conflict.

From *The New England Journal of Medicine*, 322(22), May 31, 1990, pp. 1353–1355. Copyright © 1990 by the Massachusetts Medica'

Distinguishing choices that are truly irrational from those that are merely unusual often requires complex, difficult, and controversial judgments. When the physician properly judges a patient's treatment choice to be irrational, attempts to change that choice through persuasion are common and proper. Noncoercive and nonmanipulative attempts to persuade patients of the irrational and harmful nature of their choices do not violate their right of self-determination. Instead, they reflect an appropriate responsibility and concern for the patients' well-being.

Sometimes, however, attempts to persuade will fail. Physicians lack both ethical and legal authority to override patients' treatment choices unilaterally. Nevertheless, in a few cases an irrational choice that cannot be changed by persuasion may reflect a sufficiently serious impairment in decision making—and the consequences of that choice may be sufficiently harmful to the patient—to call the patient's competence into question. In such cases, the physician may begin an investigation of the patient's competence that can ultimately involve recourse to the courts. Since the vast majority of irrational decisions are made by apparently competent patients, we shall not address the determination of incompetence here.[3] Our concern is with the more usual cases, in which the patient's competence does not come into question. The responsibility to try to change their competent patients' irrational choices requires that physicians gain a better understanding of the different forms of irrational treatment choices and of the theoretical and practical difficulties involved in distinguishing truly irrational from merely unusual choices.

The Standard of Rational Decision Making

Any discussion of irrational decision making must rely on a description of rational decision making.[4] We believe it will be helpful to make that description explicit, if only in brief outline. Specifically, what is the norm of rationality that underlies the ideal of shared decision making between patients and physicians? Essentially, shared decision making entitles patients (or their surrogates if they are incompetent) to weigh the benefits and risks of alternative treatments, including the alternative of no treatment, according to their own values and to select the alternative that best promotes those values. In the language of decision theory, each patient's values will determine his or her utility function, and the rational choice will be the one that maximizes expected utility. Since treatment decisions always involve some degree of uncertainty about the beneficial and harmful effects of alternative treatments, these effects should be discounted by their probabilities (to the extent that they are known) in calculating the expected utility of various treatment alternatives. If the probabilities are not known, each patient's attitude toward risk will determine the weight given to uncertain beneficial or adverse effects.

Snared decision making requires that physicians ensure that their patients are well informed.[5] Thus, another aspect of rational decision making is that each patient has and uses correct information about relevant alternatives. This sketch of rational decision making relies ultimately on the patient's own aims and values, unless they are irrationally distorted in the ways discussed below, as the ends that guide decision making. An irrational choice is one that satisfies those aims and values less completely than another available choice.

There is a second notion of irrational decision making that deems a patient's choice irrational if it fails to promote a set of basic aims and values that belong to the physician or to standard guidelines of medical practice. Physicians who criticize a patient's choice as irrational in this sense are disagreeing with the basic aims and values by which the patient defines his or her own good, rather than arguing that the patient's choice will fail to promote those aims and values best. Since this second notion ignores the patient's own aims and values and thus fails to respect the right of self-determination, we rely here on the first account of rational and irrational choices.

Forms of Irrational Decision Making

We now turn to common forms of irrational decision making by patients or their surrogates (and sometimes by physicians). In many treatment decisions, more than one form of irrationality affects a single choice, but we separate them here for analytical clarity.

Bias toward the Present and Near Future

The ideal of rational decision making gives equal weight to a beneficial or harmful effect whenever it occurs in a person's life, with differences determined only by the size and probability of the effect. In the case of money it is rational to apply a discount rate, because a dollar received today can earn interest and is thus worth more than a dollar received 10 years from now. Some effects of health care are similar: it is rational to prefer a restoration of function now rather than later and to prefer that a loss of function occur as far in the future as possible, so as to minimize the period of disability. Similarly, it is rational to prefer that the loss of one's life be postponed for as long as possible, at least while it remains a life worth living. For other effects of medical care—especially pain and suffering—rational choice would seem to require indifference to their timing. In particular, it is irrational to refuse to undergo a painful experience now, if by undergoing it one can avoid a much worse experience in the future. Such a refusal would amount to preferring more rather than less pain or suffering in one's life.

Yet, as doctors know, medical practice is replete with such irrational choices by patients. Some patients who continue to smoke or drink heavily or who fail to follow relatively simple steps to control moderate hypertension may not be irrational, but are simply willing to gamble that they will beat the odds. Others, however, have given inadequate weight in their present decision making to the harm they are likely to suffer in the relatively distant future. We call this a bias to the present and near future, because people commonly give disproportionate weight to securing benefits and avoiding harm in the present and near future as opposed to the more distant future.[6] The physician's task in such cases is to help the patient fully appreciate the size and seriousness of the more distant harm or benefit, so that it can play an appropriate part in the patient's decision making.

"It Won't Happen to Me"

Patients may view the nature of the risk or harm of not following medical advice differently. This is especially true for events that have a low probability of occurring.[7] However, what constitutes low probability may vary considerably from patient to patient. Furthermore, since some patients are more willing to take risks than others, it is often difficult to determine whether a patient is more of a risk taker than most or whether the patient has simply failed to give adequate weight to a low probability or a distant event. This situation is complicated by the difficulty of distinguishing among patients who, for example, ignore a risk (that is, acknowledge the risk but decide to accept it), irrationally deny the possibility that an untoward event could happen to them, have "magical" or illusory beliefs about their vulnerability to harm, or simply have a different way of viewing the medical problem.[8] Adolescents, for example, are commonly subject to feelings of invulnerability to certain harms disproportionate to the real risk of those harms.

Physicians often need to gain some understanding of their patients' general attitudes toward risk and the extent to which they are risk averse, perhaps as evidenced by their past behavior. Physicians should attempt to distinguish among the possibilities noted above. Sometimes a physician can help a patient appreciate a risk more vividly

and relate it to the patient's life. However, for patients who deny a risk or have magical beliefs, a more detailed medical and scientific explanation is not likely to be helpful. In these cases, formal counseling or psychiatric evaluation may be more fruitful.

Fear of Pain or the Medical Experience

Many patients delay or will not even consider a particular treatment for fear of the perceived nature of the experience, although they may acknowledge that the treatment is clearly in their best interests. Sometimes their decision is coupled with some form of rationalization—"there's no need to do it yet," or "I'm too busy now with other things," for example. In other cases, when a dreaded experience draws near, a patient may be almost paralyzed with fear. Sometimes the fear may be focused not on pain or suffering but on other dreaded experiences, such as being "cut open" or being "put to sleep" in surgery. In still other cases, the fear of a disease such as cancer or the acquired immunodeficiency syndrome can prevent a person from making informed decisions about its treatment.

Determining when this form of irrational decision making is present is considerably complicated by the fact that no single, correct weight can be given to pain or a particular medical experience as measured against the beneficial outcomes for which the experience may be necessary. Patients differ, for example, in the degree to which they are prepared to tolerate painful treatments or conditions for the sake of other ends,[9] but these reasonable differences are difficult to distinguish from the undue weight some patients give to certain aspects of treatment because of irrational fear. Physicians may have seen patients who in the end were grateful that they had been pressured or even forced to undergo painful or dreaded treatments. The responsibility of the physician in these cases is a difficult one—to respect the different weights people give to avoiding pain and suffering, while helping patients overcome the irrational fear that prevents them from pursuing promising treatment plans. The physician's task will often involve helping patients to distinguish whether they are experiencing a fear that they want to overcome or whether they have made a choice with which they are comfortable.

What the Patient Wants Does Not Make Sense

When competent patients decline a recommended course of treatment because of an obvious and understandable, albeit unusual, belief—Jehovah's Witnesses, for example, who refuse blood transfusions—physicians (and the courts) commonly yield to that belief. When patients request treatment that physicians believe to be ineffective—Asian patients who request "coining," for example—physicians are not obliged to provide it, but they may respect the patients' right to pursue it when medically acceptable treatment is also provided. Special difficulties arise when a seemingly competent patient wants something that does not make sense and is not attributable to a clearly recognizable religious belief or cultural preference. It can be extremely difficult in these situations for the physician to determine the basis of the patient's preference. However unusual, the more the preference seems to reflect a deeply held, enduring value that is important in the patient's life, the stronger the case for respecting it, as long as it does not require that the physician participate in useless or medically unacceptable treatment.

In other cases, what the patient does not care about makes no sense. For example, patients may state that they understand but simply do not care that death or serious disability will result from a refusal of treatment. It may be difficult to determine whether this is an authentic, although unusual, choice, or the result of a distortion of values caused by a treatable condition such as depression.

Framing Effects

It is well known that the way choices are formulated and presented, or framed, can have major effects on decisions.[10] A simple example is the presentation of a surgical treatment as "substantially extending the lives of 70 percent of the patients who select it" or as "potentially killing on the operating table 30 percent of the patients who select it." Both characterizations may be true, but which is used, or emphasized, may have a substantial effect on the rate of selection of the surgery. There is a variety of different and more subtle framing effects, one of which we illustrate below.

Studies in the psychology of choice show that losses tend to loom larger than gains in most people's decision making. Of course, whether a particular outcome is viewed as a gain or loss depends on the reference point against which the outcome is compared. Many choices in medicine can be framed in either way. For example, lowering moderate hypertension can be presented as adding months to the patient's expected life span or as a way to avoid shortening the life span because of untreated hypertension. Neither framing of the choice before the patient is wrong; each simply relies on different characterizations of the patient's present situation. Tversky and Kahneman[10] have compared the framing effects in decision making to changes in perspective in visual judgments. Which of two mountains appears to be higher, for example, depends on the position from which one views them. There is, of

course, an objective standard by which the height of the mountains can be determined, but there appears to be no objectively correct way to frame many medical choices, such as that facing the patient with moderate hypertension. There are simply two different but correct ways to frame the choice, and the one that is used will influence whether some patients choose treatment. Sometimes, the best that physicians can do is present the choice in alternative ways in the hope of minimizing framing effects.

Individual versus Social Rationality

The Irrational Use of Resources

The circumstances that make individual choices rational can sometimes make the outcome of those choices irrational when viewed from a different perspective.[11] One factor fueling the intense pressure to control rapidly rising health care costs is the perception that resources are often used in circumstances in which their expected benefits do not justify their true costs. An insured patient has little or no economic incentive to weigh the true costs of medical care against its expected benefits. When patients have no out-of-pocket costs, it is rational for them to choose all the care that has any expected medical benefit, no matter how small or costly. If physicians accept the common professional norm that their obligation is to do whatever may benefit their patients, without regard to cost, then it is also rational for them to ignore the cost of care in making recommendations and decisions about treatment. The result will be the overuse of health care as compared with other goods and services whose benefits are weighed against their true costs. From the perspective of those who pay the insurance premiums (employers or the government, for example), the result is an irrational overallocation of resources to health care.

The issues raised by this form of irrational social choice involving the use of resources are very different from those involved in the forms of irrational patient choice previously discussed. It would be a mistake for physicians to seek to persuade insured patients that choosing care that is not cost effective is irrational. On the contrary, an insured patient's choice of such care is rational, but it leads to an irrational overallocation of resources to health care. Since the irrationality is not at the level of the insured patient's choice of treatment, the principal response to it cannot be at that level. A physician's failure to respect an insured patient's choice of such care on the grounds that it is irrational is not justifiable. Instead, the irrationality must be addressed where it exists—in the social and economic system of health care financing.

Public Health versus Individual Benefit

Often, physicians are concerned about the public health benefits of medical interventions, whereas their patients are not. For example, national campaigns to reduce serum cholesterol levels will clearly benefit the health of the country as a whole. However, the chance of a substantial benefit in a given patient may be very small. Consequently, some people may rationally decide that for them the benefits of the intervention do not outweigh its burdens. This distinction between community-wide and individual benefits has been called the "prevention paradox"; in it, a treatment that brings large benefits to the community may not seem worth the trouble to individual participants.[12] There is no true paradox, however. The existence of a society-wide benefit constitutes no reason to view as irrational an individual's choice to decline an intervention.

For some infectious diseases, preventing infection through the vaccination of one person (or shortening the period of transmissibility through treatment) lessens the risk of disease for others. A patient's or parent's refusal to accept immunization may be rational if the patient or parent is not concerned about the risks for others or believes that because enough of the population is immunized, the threat of the disease is minimal and the risks of immunization outweigh the benefits. In this case, for the protection of others, society may adopt mandatory immunization programs or physicians may seek to change the patient's mind. Patients do not have an unqualified right to make even rational individual choices that risk serious harm to others.

What Should Physicians Do?

Shared decision making respects the patient's right of self-determination but does not require that the patient's preferences be simply accepted when they are irrational. In most cases, it is appropriate for physicians to attempt to persuade competent patients to reconsider their irrational choices. However, distinguishing irrational preferences from those that simply express different attitudes, values, and beliefs can be difficult in both theory and practice. Physicians need to be sensitive to the complexity of these judgments in helping patients to make sound treatment choices. They must also bear in mind that even truly irrational choices are not sufficient to establish a patient's in-competence and to justify overriding them. The taxonomy of irrational treatment choices we have presented here (and expand on elsewhere[13]) is meant to be a beginning guide for further consideration of the issue. More research is needed on the frequency of irrational treatment choices and their different forms, as well as on how physicians and patients can work together to overcome them.

References

1. President's Commission for the Study of Ethical Problems in Medicine and Biomedical and Behavioral Research. Making health care decisions: the ethical and legal implications of informed consent in the patient-practitioner relationship. Vol. 1. Washington, D.C.: Government Printing Office, 1982.
2. Forrow L, Wartman SA, Brock DW. Science, ethics, and the making of clinical decisions. JAMA 1988; 259:3161–7.
3. Buchanan AE, Brock DW. Deciding for others: the ethics of surrogate decisionmaking. Cambridge: Cambridge University Press, 1989.
4. Pauker SG, Kassirer JP. Decision analysis. N Engl J Med 1987; 316:250–8.
5. Katz J. Why doctors don't disclose uncertainty. Hastings Cent Rep 1984; 14(l):35–44.
6. Parflt D. Reasons and persons. Oxford: Oxford University Press, 1984.
7. Tversky A, Kahneman D. Judgment under uncertainty: heuristics and biases. Science 1974; 185:1124–31.
8. GillickMR. Talking with patients about risk. J Gen Intern Med 1988; 3:166–70.
9. Cassell EJ, The relief of suffering. Arch Intern Med 1983; 143:522–3.
10. Tversky A, Kahneman D. The framing of decisions and the psychology of choice. Science 1981; 211:453–8.
11. Menzel PT. Medical costs, moral choices: a philosophy of health care economics in America. New Haven, Conn.: Yale University Press, 1983.
12. Rose G. Strategy of prevention: lessons from cardiovascular disease. BMJ 1981; 282:1847–51.
13. Kassirer JP, ed. Current therapy in internal medicine. 3rd ed. Philadelphia: B.C. Decker, 1990.

Dan W. Brock is a professor of medical ethics in the Department of Social Medicine at Harvard University, director of the Division of Medical Ethics at the Harvard Medical School, and director of the Harvard University Program in Ethics and Health.

Steven A. Wartman is a president of the Association of Academic Health Centers.

Gordon M. Stirrat and Robin Gill   ⟶ **NO**

Autonomy in Medical Ethics after O'Neill

We live in the "time of the triumph of autonomy in bioethics" in which "the law and ethics of medicine are dominated by one paradigm—the autonomy of the patient."[1] This is, perhaps, not surprising given that "from the outset, the conceptual framework of bioethics has accorded paramount status to the value-complex of individualism, underscoring the principles of individual rights, autonomy, self-determination and their legal expression in the jurisprudential notion of privacy."[2] These were the weapons required to attack and breach the citadel of medical paternalism that dominated the patient-doctor relationship until at least the middle of the twentieth century. One influential medical sociologist has argued that there is an important link between the "triumph of autonomy in American bioethics" and American individualistic culture more generally.[3] However, there are growing indications that a number of bioethicists are becoming less than comfortable with this individualism.[4] In this article we wish to argue that the individualistic paradigm of "autonomy" is an aberrant application and we wish to address the question, "How are we to understand 'autonomy' in medical ethics after Onora O'Neill's challenging Gifford[5] and Reith lectures?"[6]

Much writing on the subject of autonomy fails to define the term and the way the authors are using it.[7] Understood literally "autonomy" is self-governance or self-determination. Although originally applied by the ancient Greeks to city-states, philosophers extended the concept to people from the eighteenth century onwards. Kant, in particular, gave autonomy a central place and there it has remained. What has changed is the interpretation of "autonomy." O'Neill[5] believes that it has now become too individualistic. She reminds us that John Stuart Mill "hardly ever uses the word, autonomy" and when he does so refers to states rather than individuals. "Mill's version of autonomy," she asserts, "sees individuals not merely as choosing to implement whatever desires they

happen to have at a given moment, but as taking charge of those desires, as reflecting on and selecting among them in distinctive ways."[5] She also maintains that Kant never speaks of autonomous people or individuals and "he does not equate it with any distinctive form of personal independence or self-expression." She continues, "Kantian autonomy is manifested in a life in which duties are met, in which there is a respect for others and their rights." Kant's view of autonomy is not "a form of self expression," but "rather a matter of acting on certain sorts of principles, and specifically on principles of obligation." Thus in Kant's account of moral autonomy "there can be no possibility of freedom for any one individual if that person acts without reference to all other moral agents."[8] O'Neill entitles this "principled autonomy" (which we will contrast with "individualistic autonomy"). According to Jennings,[9] Kant and others established that "morality requires a person to assume responsibility for his or her choices, actions and decisions and to act on the basis of informed reason and autonomously held, principled commitments. Others in turn must respect the moral agency and reasonable commitments of the person in this sense."

Individualism has, of course, honourable origins in the humanism of the Renaissance, the rationality of the Enlightenment and the struggle for personal and political freedom out of which our Western democracies sprang. However, in the late twentieth century, this led to the operational concept that each of us carries our own "quantum" of ethics—"I have my ethics; you have yours and neither should impinge on the other." It also means that "rights" now tend to be claimed without any sense of reciprocal obligations and that "rights are multiplied, assumed or attributed where they do not exist, replacing the language of duties which oblige even where there are no rights."[10] In the opinion of Schneider,[1] "The overwhelming weight of bioethical opinion endorses not just the autonomy principle, but a potent version of it." He considers that this paradigm is sustained by the "assumption that autonomy is what primarily and pervasively want and need." Thus the dominant view of individualistic autonomy in much recent liberal bioethics (and more generally in Western society) is that it confers a "right to act on one's own judgment about matters affecting one's life, *without interference by others*"[10] (our italics). Following O'Neill, we believe that this individualistic version of autonomous choice is fundamentally flawed. We believe that medical ethics should always be set in the context of relationships and community. We believe that, if patient individualistic autonomy is to be the *sole* criterion for decision making, the patient–doctor relationship is reduced to that of client and technician. O'Neill[11] considers that "conceptions of individual autonomy cannot provide a sufficient and convincing starting point for bioethics, or even for medical ethics." She concludes, "The supposed triumph of individual autonomy over other principles—is an unsustainable illusion."

It might be argued that O'Neill's critique of individualistic autonomy has already triumphed in medical ethics and that there is now no need for us to critique it further. John Harris provides a striking illustration that this is not so. In a recent issue of the *Journal of Medical Ethics* (in which O'Neill five pages earlier argues that "contemporary accounts of autonomy have lost touch with their Kantian origins, in which the links between autonomy and respect for persons are well argued"[12]) Harris claims that[13]: "Autonomy, the values expressed as the ability to choose and have the freedom to choose between competing conceptions of how to live and indeed of why we do so, is connected to individuality in that *it is only by the exercise of autonomy that our lives become in any sense our own*. By shaping our lives for ourselves we assert our own values and our individuality" (our italics).

Schneider[1] suggests that there are two current models of autonomy—optional and mandatory. Brock[14] defines the former as entitling but not requiring a patient to take an active role in decision making regarding treatment. In the latter model (characteristically adopted by Hams) "it is practically unwise and morally objectionable for the patient to forswear making medical decisions personally."[1] Although this latter model seems to eliminate any residue of medical paternalism is it not in danger of replacing it with an equally (or possibly even more) unacceptable paternalism by bioethicists?

Building upon O'Neill, we recommend that a revision of the operational definition of patient autonomy is required for the twenty first century. We have been influenced by the following ideas: autonomy involving ethics as "the activity of—persons bound together in a common pursuit"[10]; patient autonomy as "the capacity to assess critically one's basic desires and values, and to act on those that one endorses on reflection"[15]; and also "those actions and decisions that tend to promote the settled goals of the individual."[16] In this model a patient is fully entitled, but not required, to take an active role in decision making regarding treatment. Adding these together, we suggest a principled version of patient autonomy that involves the provision of sufficient and understandable information and space for patients, who have the capacity to make a settled choice about medical interventions on themselves, to do so responsibly in a manner considerate to others. The extent to which they exercise their choices is an integral part of the process.

Trust and Autonomy

In her Reith Lectures for 2002 entitled "A Question of Trust," O'Neill[4] reminds us Confucius considered that the three things needed for government are weapons, food, and trust. If a ruler cannot hold on to all three they should give up weapons first and the food next. Trust should be guarded to the end because "without trust we cannot stand." This applies to us all whether as individuals or part of a community, institution or profession because "we have to be able to rely on others acting as they say that they will, and because we need others to accept that we will act as we say we will."[10] Trust and trustworthiness are two faces of the same coin. Without either there can be no valid currency. Trust is fundamental to a moral community" and arguably "the fundamental virtue at the heart of being a good doctor."[18] Illingworth describes trust as the scarcest of medical resources.[19]

In her influential book *Autonomy and Trust in Bioethics*[5] (based on her Gifford Lectures in the University of Edinburgh in 2001) O'Neill maintains that "trust is not a response to certainty about others' future actions." Indeed, "trust is needed precisely when and because we lack certainty about others' future actions." Thus, there is an inevitable element of risk in placing one's trust in someone or something that introduces a vulnerability to any relationship of trust. Thus "trust," by definition, requires faith that in this context is defined as "committing to that of which we can never be sure."[20] This does not mean that trust should be placed blindly. On the contrary, trust should only be placed in a person, object or organisation in the light of the best available evidence that he, she or it is trustworthy. Yancey reminds us, "a person who lives in faith must proceed on incomplete evidence, trusting in advance what will only make sense in reverse."[20]

On what does trustworthiness depend? To be trusted one must, first, show that one is trustworthy. The most immediately obvious criterion is "track record" or demonstration of competence. His England team mates trusted that Jonny Wilkinson would drop that goal in the last seconds of the Rugby World Cup Final because of their past experience of his prowess and despite the uncertainty caused by him having already missed two such kicks in the match. A second important criterion is the means by which competence is gained and attested. For healthcare professionals to be deemed trustworthy the public must trust that the bodies responsible for their training and regulation are fit for those purposes and that the individual practitioner has satisfied their requirements and will continue to do so.

Principled Autonomy and the Patient–Doctor Relationship

The patient–doctor relationship only works when each can trust the other. However, it can be argued that the imbalance of power usually heavily weighted in favour of the doctor means that he or she has the greater responsibility to be trustworthy. Schneider[1] has found autonomy to be striking by its absence in the concerns of people who are actually sick. He finds it interesting that autonomy should figure more in the thinking of people who are well and who are contemplating illness than it does in the thinking of those who are actually experiencing serious medical care. This might be part of a more or less conscious decision not to be involved in the making of decisions and that this is a way of giving meaning to what is happening in one's own life, including one's particular illness.[21] It is certainly interesting that the reaction of sick doctors can ironically be to prefer paternalism to personal autonomy.[22]

The patient–doctor relationship has traditionally been seen as covenantal rather than contractual. In the former there is a mutual, unspoken agreement between the parties that recognises the duties and obligations of each to the other.[23] Mutual trust is at the heart of this relationship and, unfortunately, trust has been eroded by a variety of high profile medical cases over recent years. As a result, it is now being suggested that the previous implicit compact among doctors, patients, and society has broken down. This is at a time when "managerial ethics" has become a powerful force in health care on both sides of the Atlantic backed by strong combination of government policy and commercial interest. As Jennings[9] points out, "Physician ethics tends to be patient-centred. . . . Managerial ethics, by contrast, has to do with setting the stage for formations of collective action by a large number of individuals." Thus, in this dominantly consequentialist model, it is not individuals (for example, doctors, nurses, dentists) but

systems that ultimately determine the care to be provided for patients. At one level this move is understandable. The product, "health care," costs far too much of a nation's gross national product for its delivery to be left to those (for example, the aforementioned doctors, nurses, dentists) who are both deemed to be self-interested and acting as the advocates for their patients without understanding "the greater good." On the other hand the final common pathway for the delivery of that care is the healthcare professional and it is at that level that trust is gained and bestowed. The ballot box and the "free-market" are hardly adequate systems of accountability for Granny's incontinence or daughter Liz's premature baby! This approach is surely antithetical to a proper view of patient principled autonomy and Illingworth[19] considers that trust within the doctor–patient relationship has been impaired by such managed care. Although the government of the day in the UK and the managed care organisations in the USA have great influence in determining the type, range, and quality of care provided they carry no ultimate responsibility for it in relation to the sick person. It is still the individual doctor or nurse who carries the responsibility for the delivery of substandard care even if that truly lies in the system within which they are trying to work to the best of their abilities. The conflict between these models requires much greater consideration than is currently occurring.

In the traditional "covenant relationship" the central obligations of the doctor are competence, compassion, caring, and good communication. Recognition of their autonomy means that patients must be treated with respect, be properly informed, be listened to, give their consent voluntarily and without coercion, and have their confidentiality fully respected. In short, people should be treated as people and not simply as "patients." Atkins[24] argues for consideration of the subjective character of experience to understand fully a patient's situation. This is more than empathy in which one tries to consider what it would be like if one were in the situation in which the patient finds him or herself. In Atkins's view we should go even further and try to understand what it is like for *that person* to be himself or herself.[24] Does the patient have any reciprocal obligations? Draper and Sorell[25] have considered patients' responsibilities in medical ethics. They argue, "medical ethics is one-sided" because "it dwells on the ethical obligations of doctors to the exclusion of those of patients." They continue: "Traditionally medical ethics has asserted that, as autonomous agents, competent patients must be allowed to decide for themselves the course of their medical treatment." "It is for the doctor to communicate effectively all the relevant information, assess the patient's competence, persuade without coercing, and abide by whatever decision the patient makes. Little or nothing is said about what kinds of decisions a patient ought to make." "Indeed mainstream medical ethics implies that a competent patient's decision is good simply by virtue of having been made by the patient." They suggest that taking responsibility for what is chosen is intrinsic to the exercise of autonomy. In practice this may be manifested in two very different ways. In the first, the very act of taking responsibility for an autonomous decision about one's health may make it more effective. For example, a freely reached decision to stop smoking is more likely to succeed than any external attempt to ban it. On the other hand, if one freely chooses and consents to an option with a specific risk of an adverse or unwanted outcome that has been fully explained, one can have no complaint if that adverse outcome occurs despite the procedure being performed competently. Thus, a woman with multiple fibroids who requests myomectomy and who is informed of a small risk that hysterectomy may be required and consents to the procedure on that basis, has no cause for complaint if it does actually occur even if the myomectomy were performed competently. Another very important issue falls within this second category, namely what is the responsibility of the individual for the effects of lifestyle on their health? This debate certainly needs more serious consideration than it is currently given.

Public health medicine poses other interesting dilemmas in the context of personal autonomy. Those who, for example, successfully oppose mass fluoridisation of water may be willing to trade the consequences for their own dental health against their perception of even a slight and, possibly, theoretical overall risk. How is this to be reconciled with the much greater good for the dental health of the whole population that would derive from mass fluoridisation of water? In considering public health versus individual benefit, Brock and Wartman[26] suggest that patients do not have an unqualified right to make even rational individual choices that risk serious harm to others.

Choice of Treatment

Properly understood in ethical terms choice/consent is typically a process rather than a single act. The term "informed choice" is often to be preferred over "informed consent." Choice implies offering options from which patients can indicate their preference (including none!). Properly informed choice and consent are very important in medical ethics. The best practice that expresses a proper patient–doctor relationship in which each fully respects the true autonomy of the other has several components.

There is, first, an unspoken covenant of trust between the doctor and patient that the latter's wishes expressed in the consent process will be honoured. It also typically involves a full and comprehensible explanation by the doctor of the problem(s) requiring intervention followed by an authoritative statement of the benefits and risks of the various options (including doing nothing). To reach a freely arrived at decision about their preferred choice (including no intervention and a wish *not* to make a decision), patients must understand the information provided and be given time to consider the options. (The appropriate length of time will vary depending on, for example, the urgency of the situation and a patient's state of mind, need for reflection and, perhaps discussion with family members.) This culminates in the gaining of valid consent to any procedure based intervention.

Unfortunately the very complexity of some areas of medical practice makes it difficult to make sure that patients have given their consent on the basis of properly informed choice. For example, some of the new developments in fertility treatment may require a basic knowledge of human biology beyond some patients. In addition their illness may render the patient even less able to consider these complexities. These, however, increase rather than lessen the doctor's responsibility to impart the information in a way patients are best able to understand in the context of their condition and status. Brock and Wartman[26] advocate shared decision making that "respects the patient's right of self-determination but does not require that the patient's preferences be simply accepted when they seem irrational." They note, however, that distinguishing irrational preferences from those that simply express different attitudes, values and beliefs can be "difficult in theory and practice."[26] To this dialogue doctors bring their medical training, knowledge, and expertise. Patients bring their narrative and knowledge of their own subjective aims and values. Selection of the best treatment for each patient requires the contribution of both parties.[26]

Baylis and Sherwin[27] suggest reasons why some women may reject the advice from obstetricians about their care during pregnancy. It may, for example, be due to the attitude of the doctors involved; or be because the advice runs contrary to the woman's values. An example of the latter would be if a woman has undergone fertility treatment and is now carrying three or more fetuses. She may be advised to undergo selective termination but, being adamantly opposed to abortion, she refuses. Among other suggested reasons is that there may be epistemological conflict leading to fundamental disagreement about the grounds on which medical knowledge is based. This can arise as a result of the intrinsic lack of certainty of medical knowledge, very different advice being given on the same clinical issue by different doctors, past tragic failures (for example, use of thalidomide in pregnancy) or past personal or family experience. She may distrust doctors, fail to understand the issues, or be afraid. There may be just too much advice "and it is simply not practical for anyone to follow it all"[27] or it may result from other concerns and constraints on her life (for example, demands of work, children, or social circumstances such as being a single parent, having an uncaring or abusive partner, and poverty). Of course, the reasons for rejecting the advice may not be fully understood even by the woman herself.

Brock and Wartman[26] remind us that even truly irrational choices are not sufficient to establish a patient's incompetence and to justify overriding them. A competent patient has the legal right to refuse medical treatment or intervention and doctors should not then intervene medically, however justified that intervention might be in medical terms. Among the areas in which this has at present been tested are performing a caesarean section against the wishes of the woman involved, sterilising a woman without her consent during an operation for other purposes, and removing healthy ovaries at hysterectomy without specific consent.

Requests for Treatment

A potential clash occurs between the (individualistic) autonomy of patient and doctor in those situations where a patient requests, or even demands, a particular form of treatment and the doctor considers it to be unjustified (or may currently be illegal, for example, euthanasia). This can, for example, be because:

- in his or her informed opinion the risk of the procedure outweighs the potential benefits
- it is medically inappropriate for that patient
- it would consume a scarce resource needed by other patients whose needs have a higher priority.

A patient does not have a right to any specific intervention if that would be detrimental to the rights of others. Among the possible examples giving rise to conflict are a request for the removal of a healthy limb because an otherwise competent person considers it to be diseased, or the more mainstream requests for elective caesarean section in the absence of any obstetric indication, and some novel forms of fertility treatment. It can also apply when the patient is requesting an intervention to which the doctor has a moral objection—for example, termination of pregnancy or female genital mutilation. In the former,

the doctor is considered to have a duty to refer the woman to another practitioner. This would not apply to the latter even if it were not illegal in the UK. The difference is justified in law but the ethics are less straightforward. Of the above criteria, the first two are more easily ethically justified than the third. In the first two, the doctor is acting on his or her informed view of the patient's best interests. The third is much more difficult to justify and enters the problematic area of rationing and priorities that is outside the scope of this paper.

Conclusion

We believe that the individualistic version of autonomous choice is fundamentally flawed and that medical ethics should always be set in the context of relationships and community.[5] We suggest a principled version of patient autonomy that involves the provision of sufficient and understandable information and space for patients, who has the capacity to make a settled choice about medical interventions on themselves, to do so responsibly in a manner considerate to others. We consider that this model best fits the optimal patient–doctor relationship in which there is a mutual, unspoken agreement between the parties that recognises the duties and obligations each to the other.[23] Bilateral trust is at the heart of this relationship.

Exercise by doctors of their clinical judgement is frequently attacked as "paternalism." In some instances this can be so, but it may also be the doctor fulfilling his or her duty to the patient by exercising his or her own autonomy and, as such, may be entirely justified. Indeed, there will be some occasions in which acquiescence to a requested intervention against one's clinical or ethical judgement will be abrogation of one's duty as a doctor.

References

1. Schneider CE. *The Practice of Autonomy: patients, doctors and medical decisions*. New York: Oxford University Press, 1998, 3, 9, 10, 226–31.

2. Fox R. The evolution of American bioethics: a sociological perspective. In: Weisz G, ed. *Social Science Perspectives on Medical Ethics*. Philadelphia; University of Pennsylvania Press, 1990:206.

3. Wolpe PR. The triumph of autonomy in American bioethics: a sociological view. In: Devries R, Subedi J, eds. *Bioethics and Society: Sociological Investigations of the Enterprise of Bioethics*. Englewood Cliff, NJ: Prentice Hall, 1998:38–59.

4. Tauber Al. Sick autonomy. *Perspect Biol Med* 2003;46:484–95.

5. O'Neill O. *Autonomy and Trust in Bioethics.* Cambridge: Cambridge University Press, 2002, 30, 83–5.

6. O'Neill O. A Question of Trust—Reith lectures 2002. bndon: BBC, 2002, www.BBC.co.uk/Radio4 (accessed 18 April 2002).

7. Dworkin G. *The Theory and Practice of Autonomy.* Cambridge: Cambridge University Press, 1988.

8. Campbell AV. *Health as Liberation.* Cleveland: The Pilgrim Press, 1995:14.

9. Jennings B. Good-bye to all that—autonomy. *J Clin Ethics* 2002;13:67–71.

10. Dunstan G. Should philosophy and medical ethics be left to the experts? In: Bewley S, Ward RH, eds. *Ethics in Obstetrics & Gynaecology.* London: RCOG Press, 1994:3.

11. O'Neill O. *Autonomy and Trust in Bioethics.* Cambridge: Cambridge University Press, 2002, 1–27, 73–95.

12. O'Neill O. Some limits of informed consent. *J Med Ethics* 2003;29:l, 5.

13. Harris J. Consent and end of life decisions. *J Med Ethics* 2003;29:1,10–11.

14. Brock D. Informed consent. In: McLean D, ed. *Life and Death: Philosophical Essays in Biomedical Ethics.* Cambridge: Cambridge University Press, 1993:33.

15. Reath A. Autonomy, ethical. In: *Concise Routledge Encyclopaedia of Philosophy.* London: Routledge, 2000:69.

16. Campbell AV. Personal communication.

17. Pellegrino E. Being a physician: does it make a moral difference? Advances in otolaryngology. *Head Neck Surg* 1992;6:l–10.

18. O'Donovan U. A profession of trust: reflections on a fundamental virtue, in: Thomasma DC, Kissell JL, eds. *The Health Care Professional as Friend and Healer.* Washington: Georgetown University Press, 2000:1–9.

19. Iliingworth P. Trust: the scarcest of medical resources. *J Med Philos* 2002;27:31–46.

20. Yancey P. *Reaching for the Invisible God.* Grand Rapids: Zondervan, 2000:95.

21. Dekkers W J M. Autonomy and dependence: chronic physical illness and decision-making capacity. *Med Healthcare Philos* 2001;4:185–92.

22. Spiro H M, Mandell HN. When doctors get sick. *Ann Intern Med* 1998,128:152–4.

23. May WF. The physician's covenant. In: McLean D, ed. *Images of the Healer in Medical Ethics.* Philadelphia: Westminster Press, 1983:106–44.

24. Atkins K. Autonomy and the subjective character of experience. *J Appl Philos* 2000; 17:71–9.

25. Draper H, Sorell T. Patient's responsibilities in medical ethics. *Bioethics* 2002;16:335–52.

26. Brock DW, Wartman SA. When competent patients make irrational choices. N *Engl J Med* 1990;322:1595–9.

27. Baylis F, Sherwin S. Judgements of non-compliance in pregnancy. In: Dickenson D, ed. *Ethical Issues in Maternal-Fetal Medicine.* Cambridge: Cambridge University Press, 2002:285–301.

GORDON M. STIRRAT is an emeritus professor of obstetrics and gynecology and a research fellow in ethics in medicine in the University of Bristol.

ROBIN GILL is the emeritus professor of applied theology at the University of Kent.

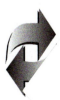

EXPLORING THE ISSUE

Is Patient Self-Determination the Central Value in Making Medical Decisions?

Critical Thinking and Reflection

1. How can one tell when a medical decision is made well? What, in your view, is the criterion for good medical decision-making?
2. Do all medical decisions involve autonomy and informed consent in the same way, or do different kinds of decisions involve them in different ways?
3. Both YES and NO selections register concerns with how informed consent has been put into practice and the effect it has had on medicine. Describe and compare their concerns.
4. What do you think is the most important attribute for a doctor who is closely involved with difficult medical decisions? What is that doctor's role?

Is There Common Ground?

A number of scholars have argued that although the concept of informed consent, and the principle underlying it of respect for patient autonomy, is undeniably central to Western values, informed consent cannot do quite the work that bioethicists have sometimes hoped. Eric Cassell argues, for example, that the experience of illness impairs patient's ability to make decisions, that the doctor's task is not merely to supply information to the patient but to support and guide the patient, and that the overriding consideration is the patient's well-being (*The Nature of Healing: The Modern Practice of Medicine* [Oxford University Press, 2012]). In a book on medical decision-making in the context of cancer, Rebecca Dresser and a group of other prominent medical ethicists discuss their own experiences as patients and the limits of seemingly central concepts like patient autonomy. Dresser notes, for example, that she needed her doctor to persuade her to accept an intervention that she, trying to act entirely autonomously, had been refusing (*Malignant: Medical Ethicists Confront Cancer* [Oxford University Press, 2012]). This general kind of approach to medical decision making is also sometimes known as "shared decision making."

Other constraints on informed consent are also accepted. If the patient lacks decision-making capacity, then the patient will not be able to give informed consent and other standards must be found. In addition, many commentators have pointed out that patient autonomy is also limited by the physician's autonomy. Patients have a

right not to be treated in ways they do not want, but they do not always have a right to get precisely the treatment they do want.

Additional Resources

The most comprehensive account of informed consent is *A History and Theory of Informed Consent* by Ruth L. Faden, Tom L. Beauchamp, and Nancy M. P. King (Oxford University Press, 1986). Another useful volume, particularly in terms of psychiatric treatment, is *Informed Consent: Legal Theory and Clinical Practice* by Paul S. Appelbaum, Charles W. Lidz, and Alan Meisel (Oxford University Press, 1987). Jay Katz's *The Silent World of Doctor and Patient* (Free Press, 1984; paper edition 2002, Johns Hopkins University Press) is an insightful discussion of the reasons physicians may be reluctant to disclose information to their patients. See also, Jessica W. Berg, Paul S. Appelbaum, Charles W. Lidz, and Lisa S. Parker, *Informed Consent: Legal Theory and Clinical Practice*, 2nd ed. (Oxford University Press, 2001), and Terrance C. McConnell, *Inalienable Rights: The Limits of Consent in Medicine and the Law* (Oxford University Press, 2000). Two articles in the *Journal of the American Medical Association* (September 13, 1995)—"Western Bioethics on the Navajo Reservation," by Joseph A. Carrese and Lorna A. Rhodes, and "Ethnicity and Attitudes

Toward Patient Autonomy," by Leslie J. Blackhall—suggest that disclosing negative information and involving patients in decision making may be contrary to the beliefs of certain ethnic populations. For further elaboration of Onora O'Neill's critique of informed consent, see Neil C. Manson and Onora O'Neill, *Rethinking Informed Consent in Bioethics* (Cambridge University Press, 2007). *The Ethics of Consent: Theory and Practice*, edited by Franklin Miller and Alan Wertheimer, brings together expert views on informed consent in many fields beyond bioethics (Oxford University Press, 2009).

Internet References . . .

The National Reference Center for Bioethics Literature

http://bioethics.georgetown.edu/

Bioethics Resources on the Web

http://bioethics.od.nih.gov/

Center for Adolescent Health and the Law

www.cahl.org

Selected, Edited, and with Issue Framing Material by:
Gregory E. Kaebnick, *The Hastings Center*

ISSUE

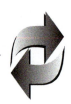

May Surrogate Decision Makers Terminate Care for a Person in a Persistent Vegetative State?

YES: Jay Wolfson, from "A Report to Governor Jeb Bush and the 6th Judicial Circuit in the Matter of Theresa Marie Schiavo" Sixth Judicial Circuit of Florida (2003)

NO: Tom Koch, from "The Challenge of Terri Schiavo: Lessons for Bioethics," *Journal of Medical Ethics* (2005)

Learning Outcomes
After reading this issue, you will be able to:
• Explain the concept of surrogate decision making and how it is related to patient autonomy.
• Explain artificial nutrition and hydration and its relationship to medical treatment.
• Discuss the concerns that those from a disability rights perspective have about surrogate decision making.

ISSUE SUMMARY

YES: Jay Wolfson, a lawyer and the special guardian ad litem appointed for Theresa Marie Schiavo, explains the clinical and legal considerations that justified removal of Ms. Schiavo's feeding tube, causing her to die.

NO: Tom Koch, an independent writer and researcher, holds that helping a person die cannot be said to benefit the person and that questions of personhood and sanctity of life gave reason to help her live.

Most medical decisions require the informed consent of the patient. Often, however, patients are incapable of giving informed consent, either because of an illness or an underlying condition like dementia, or because of the effects of treatment itself. In these cases, decisions must be made by a surrogate decision maker, that is, a person who makes decisions on behalf of the incapacitated person. A surrogate decision maker is either somebody designated by the patient to fill that role or a close family member or friend who knows the patient well and can be trusted to represent the patient's interests.

Some of the most difficult and controversial surrogate decision-making cases involve patients diagnosed as being in a persistent vegetative state, or PVS. Patients in a vegetative state show no evidence that they have any awareness of themselves or their surroundings. They do not respond to stimuli purposefully. To be diagnosed as being in a PVS, a patient must have been in a vegetative state for at least one month. In a 2010 study that used functional magnetic resonance imaging (fMRI) to study the brains of people in a PVS, some people who showed no outward signs of consciousness showed imaging findings associated with consciousness, but what these findings actually meant was not clear.

Unfortunately, it is possible to linger in a vegetative state for many years, even for decades. If that happens, and if the patient had never prepared a legal document known as an advance directive to explicitly identify his or her wishes for medical care in these circumstances, then a surrogate decision maker may have to decide what kind of medical care is appropriate, including whether to discontinue medical care altogether. When making these decisions, surrogate decision makers are supposed to follow a legal doctrine known as substituted judgment, which instructs them to try to determine what the patient would have wanted done. In Missouri and New York, surrogate decision makers must rely on the patient's own formal statements about his or her wishes, but in other states that accept substituted judgment, they can consider other evidence about the patient's wishes as well, such as conversations that they remember having with the patient.

One question that commonly arises about surrogate decision making has to do with what counts as "medical care." A patient in a PVS is incapable of swallowing and must therefore be given "artificial nutrition and hydration," typically through a tube placed into the stomach. Most legal and medical commentators hold that artificial nutrition and hydration is medical care, and that if the surrogate decision maker decides that stopping treatment is appropriate, then the feeding tube may be withdrawn. Some people believe, however, that artificial nutrition and hydration is just a matter of giving a person a meal, not of providing medical care.

Another common question is whether the medical diagnosis of PVS is reliable. An Internet search will quickly turn up stories of people who were thought to be in a PVS but turn out to be misdiagnosed. Indeed, some people who have been declared to be in a PVS are actually in what has been described as a "minimally conscious state": they demonstrate some awareness of self and surroundings, and magnetic resonance imaging (MRI) shows that their brains sometimes activate in response to stimuli, but their mental state fluctuates and can be very hard to distinguish from a vegetative state.

The difficulty of distinguishing PVS from a minimally conscious state complicates the medical decision making that must be made about them. First, of course, careful diagnostic work is needed to determine whether the patient is in a PVS or a minimally conscious state. The patient's prognosis will depend on the circumstances of the case. Recovery from a correctly diagnosed PVS is exceedingly rare, and after 12 months in a PVS, the condition is considered permanent. There are scattered cases of people in a minimally conscious state recovering, but many have no hope of meaningful recovery.

Once the patient's medical condition is established as well as possible, the surrogate must face the decisions about what treatments are appropriate. In the YES selection, legal scholar Jay Wolfson explains why medical care, including artificial nutrition and hydration, could be withdrawn from a patient in a PVS. Wolfson has wrestled with the decisions personally: In 2003, he was appointed guardian ad litem for Theresa Marie Schiavo, a woman who was in a PVS and whose husband believed that treatment should be withdrawn. In the NO selection, Tom Koch, an independent writer, lecturer, and researcher who has studied medical decision making concerning people with disabilities, explains why many people believed the decision to withdraw medical treatment from Schiavo was unacceptable.

YES ⤹

Jay Wolfson

A Report to Governor Jeb Bush and the 6th Judicial Circuit in the Matter of Theresa Marie Schiavo

Introduction

Sometimes good law is not enough, good medicine is not enough, and all too often, good intentions do not suffice. Sometimes, the answer is in the process, not the presumed outcome. We must be left with hope that the right thing will be done well.

We are, each of us, standing in Theresa Marie Schiavo's shoes. Each of us is profoundly affected by the decisions that have and will be made in this case. Advocates of privacy rights and death with dignity, and advocates of right to life and rights of the disabled provide the compelling definitional parameters of this matter.

On 31 October 2003, pursuant to the requirements of Florida H.B. 35-E (Chapter 2003-418, Laws of Florida) and the order of the Hon. David Demers, Chief Judge, Florida 6th Judicial Circuit, a Guardian Ad Litem was appointed for a period of thirty days with the following charge:

> "... make a report and recommendations to the Governor as to whether the Governor should lift the stay that he previously entered. The report will specifically address the feasibility and value of swallow tests for this ward and the feasibility and value of swallow therapy. Additionally, the report will include a thorough summary of everything that has taken place in the trial court and the appellate court concerning this case."

... The Guardian Ad Litem's efforts have been to deduce and represent the best wishes and best interests of Theresa Schiavo. In that no express, written advance directive existed, determining what Theresa's wishes might be require a combination of substituted judgment, reasonable person considerations, and an aggressive, objective assessment of the massive legal and clinical record that has been compiled over thirteen years. ...

Historical Facts in Theresa Marie Schiavo's Case

... On the tragic early morning of 25 February 1990, Theresa collapsed in the hallway of her apartment, waking [her husband] Michael, who called Theresa's family and 911. The lives of Theresa, Michael and the Schindlers were to change forever.

Theresa suffered a cardiac arrest. During the several minutes it took for paramedics to arrive, Theresa experienced loss of oxygen to the brain, or anoxia, for a period sufficiently long to cause permanent loss of brain function. Despite heroic efforts to resuscitate, Theresa remained unconscious and slipped into a coma. She was intubated, ventilated and trached, meaning that she was given life-saving medical technological interventions, without which she surely would have died that day. ...

Theresa spent two and a half months as an inpatient at Humana Northside Hospital, eventually emerging from her coma state, but not recovering consciousness. On 12 May 1990, following extensive testing, therapy and observation, she was discharged to the College Park skilled care and rehabilitation facility. Forty-nine days later, she was transferred again to Bayfront Hospital for additional, aggressive rehabilitation efforts. In September of 1990, she was brought home, but following only three weeks, she was returned to the College Park facility because the "family was overwhelmed by Terry's care needs."

On 18 June 1990, Michael was formally appointed by the court to serve as Theresa's legal guardian, because she was adjudicated to be incompetent by law. Michael's appointment was undisputed by the parties.

The clinical records within the massive case file indicate that Theresa was not responsive to neurological and swallowing tests. She received regular and intense physical, occupational and speech therapies.

From *A Report to Governor Jeb Bush and the 6th Judicial Circuit in the Matter of Theresa Marie Schiavo,* December 2003.

Theresa's husband, Michael Schiavo, and her mother, Mary Schindler, were virtual partners in their care of and dedication to Theresa. There is no question but that complete trust, mutual caring, explicit love and a common goal of caring for and rehabilitating Theresa, were the shared intentions of Michael Shiavo and the Schindlers. . . .

On 19 July 1991 Theresa was transferred to the Sable Palms skilled care facility. Periodic neurological exams, regular and aggressive physical, occupational and speech therapy continued through 1994.

Michael Schiavo, on Theresa's and his own behalf, initiated a medical malpractice lawsuit against the obstetrician who had been overseeing Theresa's fertility therapy. In 1993, the malpractice action concluded in Theresa and Michael's favor, resulting in a two element award: More than $750,000 in economic damages for Theresa, and a loss of consortium award (non economic damages) of $300,000 to Michael. The court established a trust fund for Theresa's financial award, with SouthTrust Bank as the Guardian and an independent trustee. This fund was meticulously managed and accounted for and Michael Schiavo had no control over its use. There is no evidence in the record of the trust administration documents of any mismanagement of Theresa's estate, and the records on this matter are excellently maintained.

After the malpractice case judgment, evidence of disaffection between the Schindlers and Michael Schiavo openly emerged for the first time. The Schindlers petitioned the court to remove Michael as Guardian. They made allegations that he was not caring for Theresa, and that his behavior was disruptive to Theresa's treatment and condition.

Proceedings concluded that there was no basis for the removal of Michael as Guardian. Further, it was determined that he had been very aggressive and attentive in his care of Theresa. . . .

By 1994, Michael's attitude and perspective about Theresa's condition changed. During the previous four years, he had insistently held to the premise that Theresa could recover and the evidence is incontrovertible that he gave his heart and soul to her treatment and care. This was in the face of consistent medical reports indicating that there was little or no likelihood for her improvement.

In early 1994 Theresa contracted a urinary tract infection and Michael, in consultation with Theresa's treating physician, elected not to treat the infection and simultaneously imposed a "do not resuscitate" order should Theresa experience cardiac arrest. When the nursing facility initiated an intervention to challenge this decision, Michael cancelled the orders. Following the incident involving the infection, Theresa was transferred to another skilled nursing facility.

Michael's decision not to treat was based upon discussions and consultation with Theresa's doctor, and was predicated on his reasoned belief that there was no longer any hope for Theresa's recovery. It had taken Michael more than three years to accommodate this reality and he was beginning to accept the idea of allowing Theresa to die naturally rather than remain in the non-cognitive, vegetative state. . . .

The Evolution of the Law about Dying and Nutrition in Florida

Our society is at a legal, political, biotechnological, bioethical and spiritual crossroad. Theresa Schiavo is alternately depicted as a living, loving person, capable of interacting at a level of cognition with her family and deserving of the right to continue to live—and as a tragically and profoundly brain damaged person, who earlier expressed a desire never to find herself in a circumstance analogous to waking up in a coffin—and being there forever. But she cannot speak to us now. So we must rely upon the auspices of good law and good medicine and the good intentions of those who marshal these arts in order to do our best to do the right thing well for Theresa Schiavo.

During the early 1970s the States began to revise their Probate Codes. There were many reasons for this, including a rapidly aging population, larger numbers of aged persons in the population, people living longer, new and advancing medical technologies that enhanced, extended and affected life, and changing values and orientations about death, dying and the medical-decision processes. These matters have been seriously addressed through a combination of inquiries and actions by church leaders, legislators, medical scientists, and the courts, as all have sought to respond to emerging issues such as those in the Quinlan, Cruzan, Browning, and now the Schiavo cases.

States cooperated with the federal Administration on Aging to address legislative and policy challenges surfacing around these matters. A particularly important topic related to medical technology and its use in the care, treatment and maintenance of patients, is when, who and by what means "artificial" life support and other medical interventions should or could be removed or never withheld in the first place.

Today, most states would afford an adult person the right to deny most health care treatments. But if the patient is a minor, unconscious, in a coma, in a vegetative state, or unable to communicate personal wishes and intentions, there are serious moral, ethical and legal questions that demanded attention. There had been inconsistencies, even within states, as to how decisions regarding termination or removal or withholding a procedure were made. There was also a long standing, well accepted recognition that the relationship between the patient and the physician—the sacred trust—served as the foundation for how and where and when many of these decisions would be made. Often, physicians, in consultation with family members and the patient have done what was deemed to be in best interests of the patient, given the physician's medical opinion and the express, known or believed intentions of the patient.

To reduce ambiguities, many states began to encourage and accept written advance directives as the basis for decisions regarding end of life treatment. Living wills, durable powers of attorney for health care and health care surrogate documents, stating a person's explicit intentions regarding end of life care, became increasingly accepted and even formalized into the statutory framework of most states. A written expression was deemed to be an important element in this process to avoid the possibility of confusion or uncertainty with respect to a person's intention regarding their health and medical care.

Throughout the 1980s and 1990s, Florida lawmakers struggled with how they would provide individuals with the prerogatives for establishing their wishes regarding end of life decisions, while at the same time, protecting against perceived and actual abuses and assisted suicides. Among the most sensitive of issues is this regard has been the withdrawal of artificial life support in the form of nutrition and hydration. The idea of withholding or withdrawing these has created significant debates within and across religious, philosophical and political groups and interests. But the topic has been addressed at great lengths by each of these groups, and there is surprising consensus in principle and even in practice.

The current, generally accepted applications to terminal illness or persistent vegetative state define artificial feeding as artificial life support that may be withheld or withdrawn. In 1989, the Florida Legislature permitted the withdrawal of artificial nutrition and hydration under very specific circumstances. In 1999, following extensive bipartisan efforts, life-prolonging procedures were redefined as "any medical procedure, treatment, or intervention, including artificially provided sustenance and hydration, which sustains, restores, or supplants a spontaneous vital function." It is noteworthy that the general principle of artificial nutrition as artificial life support that may be removed in terminal and even vegetative state conditions is reflected in nearly all state's laws and within the guidelines of end of life care enunciated by the American Conference of Catholic Bishops and other religious denominations.

These general principles are in no way intended to encourage or condone suicide or assisted suicide. But they reflect the acceptance of artificial nutrition as artificial life support that may be withdrawn or withheld as a matter of public policy, when these decisions capture the intentions of the person and with the premise that people should not be required to remain "artificially alive," or to have their natural peaceful deaths postponed and prolonged if they would otherwise choose not to, and that they should be allowed to die with dignity, and return, if their beliefs so accommodate, to God.

When written advance directives are not available, and the affected person is incompetent and unable to communicate, a decision to discontinue nutrition and hydration is especially challenging. But Florida law, as reflected in F.S. 765, and as interpreted through *In re Guardianship of Browning*, 568 So. 2d 4 (Fla. 1990), provides for a substituted judgment basis for such decisions and/or the presentation of clear and convincing evidence to demonstrate the intentions of the person.

It has been suggested that in the case of incapacitated persons, particularly those who have not expressed an advance directive, the "clear and convincing" evidence standard for establishing the intent to discontinue artificial life support is insufficient and incongruous. The insufficiency, it is argued, is because of the possibility of using information that is not accurate, complete or even honest. The incongruity is related to the "beyond a reasonable doubt" standard that serves as the basis for decisions to convict and then execute capitol felons.

If persons unable to speak for themselves have decisions made on their behalf by guardians or family members, the potential for abuse, barring clear protections, could lead to a "slippery slope" of actions to terminate the lives of disabled and incompetent persons. And it is not difficult to imagine bad decisions being made in order to make life easier for a family or to avoid spending funds remaining in the estate on the maintenance of a person.

There is, of course, the other side of that slippery slope, which would be to keep people in a situation they would never dream of: unable to die, unable to communicate, dependent for everything, and unaware, being maintained principally or entirely through state resources—and for reasons that may relate to guilt, fear, needs or wants of family members, rather than what the person's best wishes might otherwise have been.

And there is the chillingly practical, other public policy matter of the cost of maintaining persons diagnosed in persistent vegetative states and terminal conditions alive for potentially indefinite periods of time—at what inevitably becomes public expense. Here the "reasonable person" standard, with respect to how one would want to be treated were they in Theresa's shoes affects the discussion. This is not easy stuff, and should not be.

In withholding or withdrawing life support, or in keeping a person alive, there is the risk of transposing intentions and values. The reasoned, even substituted judgment decisions of guardians or loved ones may be based upon either a "quality of life determination," or the desires of family members. This remains a risk in a system that does not require an explicit, advance directive. . . .

Cruzan and the Role of States in Guidelines for Medical Decisions

. . . Not all states deploy the specific guidelines and measures adopted by Florida. Many states refuse to accept anything but advance, written directives of the person as a basis for removal of artificial life support. Florida has chosen to employ guidelines that include surrogate decisions by the bona fide legal guardian and/or clear and convincing evidence as to the intentions of the person.

In Theresa's case, evidence regarding her intentions consisted of admitted hearsay regarding conversations between Theresa and her spouse and spousal relatives. The context and nature of this hearsay were deemed sufficiently probative, competent and reliable to serve as a basis for admission, and was determined to be sufficiently clear and convincing. The court then served as proxy decision maker, essentially assuming the role of legal guardian. The privacy interests of the person, as established in the Florida Constitution, and as articulated with specificity in *Browning* . . . served as the legitimate legal bases for the court's conclusions to withdraw life support consistent with Florida Statute, 765.

Evidence regarding the persistent vegetative state consisted of highly credible medical testimony and documentation reflecting both early and recently performed neurological examinations and a case history that included early swallowing studies conducted multiple times nearly ten years ago.

The Swallowing Test and Neurological Function

The review of the medical and clinical evidence in the case goes directly to the issues of the feasibility and value of swallowing tests and swallowing therapy, and to the relationship between neurological function and swallowing food and liquid.

Three independent sets of swallowing tests were performed early in Theresa's medical treatment: 1991, 1992 and 1993. Each of these determined that Theresa was not able to swallow without risk of aspiration (and consequent infection).

Swallowing tests and swallowing therapy address many of the core issues in contention. If Theresa can swallow, then she can take nutrition and hydration orally, and it is argued that she would not elect to stop eating. But to orally eat and drink, Theresa must possess cognitive capacity beyond mere reflex, or she will not only fail to ingest, but could easily aspirate substances into her lungs and be subjected to infections and subsequent death. . . .

Early in Theresa's care, neurological examinations were performed to assess her cognitive capacity. Competent medical practitioners determined that Theresa was in what has been consistently defined as a persistent vegetative state—a finding that throughout the litigation was not disputed by either side. Quite recently, the Schindlers have disputed that Theresa is in a persistent vegetative state, and in the alternative, they have argued that even if she is, she deserves to live and be maintained via artificial nutrition and hydration. . . .

A particularly disarming aspect of persons diagnosed with persistent vegetative state is that they have waking and sleeping cycles. When awake, their eyes are often open, they make noises, they appear to track movement, they respond to deep pain, and appear startled by loud noises. Further, because the autonomic nervous system those brain related functions are not affected, they can often breathe (without a respirator) and swallow (saliva). But there is no purposeful, reproducible, interactive, awareness. There is some controversy within the scientific medical literature regarding the characterization and diagnosis of persons in a persistent vegetative state. Highly competent, scientifically based physicians using recognized measures and standards have deduced, within a high degree of medical certainty, that Theresa is in a persistent vegetative state. This evidence is compelling.

Terri is a living, breathing human being. When awake, she sometimes groans, makes noises that emulate laughter or crying, and may appear to track movement. But the scientific medical literature and the reports this GAL obtained from highly respected neuro-science researchers indicate that these activities are common and characteristic of persons in a persistent vegetative state.

In the month during which the GAL conducted research, interviews and compiled information, he sought to visit with Theresa as often as possible, sometimes daily, and sometimes, more than once each day. During that time, the GAL was not able to independently determine that there were consistent, repetitive, intentional, reproducible interactive and aware activities. When Theresa's mother and father were asked to join the GAL, there was no success in eliciting specific responses. Hours of observed videotape recordings of Theresa offer little objective insight about her awareness and interactive behaviors. There are instances where she appears to respond specifically to her mother. But these are not repetitive or consistent. There were instances during the GAL's visits, when responses seemed possible, but they were not consistent in any way.

This having been said, Theresa has a distinct presence about her. Being with Theresa, holding her hand, looking into her eyes and watching how she is lovingly treated by Michael, her parents and family and the clinical staff at hospice is an emotional experience. It would be easy to detach from her if she were comatose, asleep with her eyes closed and made no noises. This is the confusing thing for the lay person about persistent vegetative states.

Theresa's neurological tests and CT scans indicate objective measures of the persistent vegetative state. These data indicate that Theresa's cerebral cortex is principally liquid, having shrunken due to the severe anoxic trauma experienced thirteen years ago. The initial oxygen deprivation caused damage that could not be repaired, and the brain tissue in that area continued to devolve. It is noteworthy to recall that from the time of her collapse, and for more than three years, Theresa did receive active physical, occupational, speech and even recreational therapy. There is evidence early in her records of care that she said "no" during physical therapy session. That behavior did not recur and was not further referenced.

In recent months, individuals have come forward indicating that there are therapies and treatments and interventions that can literally regrow Theresa's functional, cerebral cortex brain tissue, restoring part or all of her functions. There is no scientifically valid, medically recognized evidence that this has been done or is possible, even in rats, according to the president of the American Society for Neuro-Transplantation. It is imaginable that some day such things may be possible; but holding out such promises to families of severely brain injured persons today may be a profound disservice.

In the observed circumstances, the behavior that Theresa manifests is attributable to brain stem and forebrain functions that are reflexive, rather than cognitive. And the substantive difference according to neurologists and neurosurgeons is that reflexive activities of this nature are neither conscious nor aware activities. And without cognition, there is no awareness. (Descartes addressed this in his proposition that it is our awareness, our consciousness that defines our being: "Cogito, ergo sum." This logic would imply that unless we are aware and conscious, we cease to be.)

By all measures in the literature, Theresa has beaten the odds in terms of surviving her persistent vegetative state condition. While younger persons fare better than older victims, life spans rarely, according to the American Academy of Neurology, exceed ten years following the onset of the condition. Persons who have been comatose have worse outcomes than those who have not. But Theresa has also far outlived any documented periods from which persons in persistent vegetative states have emerged in any functional capacity. The reasonable degree of medical certainty associated with her diagnosis and prognosis is very high. . . .

Summary of Guardian Ad Litem Recommendations

. . .

1. Should the Governor lift the stay that he previously entered relative to Theresa Schiavo's feeding tube?

   a. Yes. The Governor should lift the stay, if valid, independent scientific medical evidence clearly indicates that Theresa has no reasonable medical hope of regaining any swallowing function and/or if there is no evidence of cognitive function and no hope of improvement.

   b. No. The Governor should not lift the stay if valid, independent scientific medical evidence clearly indicates that Theresa has a reasonable medical hope of regaining any swallowing function and/or if there is evidence of cognitive function with or without hope of improvement.

2. Is there feasibility and value in swallowing tests and swallowing therapy given the totality of circumstances?

   a. Yes. There is feasibility and value in swallowing tests and swallowing therapy being administered if the parties agree in advance as to how the results of these tests will be used with respect to the decision about Theresa's future. If the parties do not agree in advance as to how the tests will be used, then the court must be prepared to once again make a final judgment on the matter. Given the history of the case, this would not, in and of itself, assure a resolution, and is not, therefore, deemed either feasible or of value to Theresa Schiavo without prior agreement.

The GAL concludes from the medical records and consultations with medical experts that the scope and weight of the medical information within the file concerning Theresa Schiavo consists of competent, well-documented information that she is in a persistent vegetative state with no likelihood of improvement, and that the neurological and speech pathology evidence in the file support the contention that she cannot take oral nutrition or hydration and cannot consciously interact with her environment.

The GAL concludes that the trier of fact and the evidence that served as the basis for the decisions regarding Theresa Schiavo were firmly grounded within Florida statutory and case law, which clearly and unequivocally provide for the removal of artificial nutrition in cases of persistent vegetative states, where there is no advance directive, through substituted/proxy judgment of the guardian and/or the court as guardian, and with the use of evidence regarding the medical condition and the intent of the parties that was deemed, by the trier of fact to be clear and convincing. . . .

We remain in Theresa Schiavo's shoes.

JAY WOLFSON is the distinguished service professor of public health and medicine, associate vice president for health law, policy and safety at the University of South Florida. In October 2003, he was appointed to serve as the special guardian ad litem for Theresa Marie Schiavo, reporting to the Florida governor and the courts.

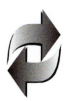

Tom Koch   **NO**

The Challenge of Terri Schiavo:
Lessons for Bioethics

Definitions

Since her collapse in 1990, Mrs Schiavo had been assumed to be in a "persistent vegetative state," legally defined in a Florida statute as a "permanent and irreversible condition of unconsciousness" from which no recovery is possible.[1] Withdrawal of nutrition and hydration permitting a "natural" death was therefore appropriate in a "terminal condition" like Mrs Schiavo's where end-of-life protocols are legally permitted in Florida statutes for "end-stage" cases.[2]

Those seeking Mrs Schiavo's continuance argued, however, her condition was only "end-stage" and "terminal" when hydration and nutrition were removed. Her life might have continued for years had her care continued. In this construction withdrawal of hydration and nutrition is active euthanasia neither warranted clinically nor to be accepted ethically. Simply, advocates of her continued care reject the argument that cessation of life support, prohibited in all other situations, is acceptable when physical or cognitive limits are defined as extreme.

More concretely, some challenge the diagnosis of persistent vegetative state itself as uncertain and open to challenge. This argument is given weight in a series of clinical studies published in recent years. Shewmon,[3] for example, argues that contrary to standard definitions we cannot state categorically that the vegetative state is defined by a total loss of cortical function. Others studying patients diagnosed as vegetative—a term many critiques reject as demeaning[4] have found that between 12% and 34% of patients diagnosed as persistently vegetative are at least minimally conscious and may respond to therapy.[5]

Suffering and "Quality of Life"

For some bioethicists the niceties of these distinctions are largely irrelevant. A person in Mrs Schiavo's obviously limited state is "suffering" from an unacceptably minimal "quality of life" that may be "naturally" ended by the withdrawal of hydration and nutrition. In such situations euthanasia is permissible, and in Helga Kuhse's words, "doctors should be permitted to give death a helping hand."[6]

If all cerebral function had ceased Mrs Schiavo could not have been suffering, however. And if she had been even minimally conscious then death by starvation and thirst would themselves have caused suffering that cannot, critics say, be supported. The doctor's "helping hand," encouraged by some bioethicists, seen from this perspective is malicious. To assume there is no "benefit" to continuation because treatment will be "futile"—with no curative value[7]—imposes upon the patient a doctor's frustration at being unable to do anything but maintain his or her patient in a limited state.

Further, arguing that Mrs Schiavo's quality of life was insupportable, and death therefore preferable to continuation, conjures for some the eugenic arguments famously argued by Binding and Hoche in 1920s Germany,[8] and more generally by US eugenicists from Haiselden to Mr Justice Oliver Wendell Holmes in the famous US Supreme Court decision *Buck v Bell* (for a comprehensive review of this history see Pernick, 1996[9]).

This critique empowers a radically different reading of not simply appropriate behaviour in the Schiavo case but in a range of situations—genetic, neurological, and post-traumatic injury—involving those with physical and cognitive limits. From this perspective the battle over Terri Schiavo's continuance was a special case within a far broader field of dispute over the legitimate rights of restricted persons and the broader duty for their continuing care. The importance of this challenge, and the strength of its argument, is signalled by US Congressional and state legislative involvement in this case. To the extent law reflects the ethics of a population, arguments in this case signal the rise of an ethical and moral construct strongly opposed to accepted standards of practice currently codified in law and the bioethics literature. For those who argue Mrs Schiavo's continuance, and by extension that of others in physically or cognitively limited

From *Journal of Medical Ethics*, Vol. 31, No. 7, July 1, 2005, pp. 376–378. Copyright © 2005 by Institute of Medical Ethics. Reprinted by permission of BMJ Publishing Group via Rightslink.

states, legislatures are the appropriate place to seek longer term relief, replacing codes informed by one ethical perspective with another.

Personhood

Perhaps the central issue in ethics and law is what we mean by personhood within the circle of protected life. Among Mrs Schiavo's supporters, and more generally within some disability communities, personhood is not an existential attribute based upon cognitive or physical abilities but a communal attribute whose meaning is grounded in one's relationship to others.[10] In this construction Mrs Schiavo was a person equal to others because her parents said she was and her continuance had been mandated by their historically anchored, unwavering commitment to that relationship's continuance.

The argument finds some support in the literature of medical ethics and bioethics. The enduring popularity of Oliver Sacks's work—from *Awakenings*[11] to *An Anthropologist on Mars*[12]—is based in large part on his insistence that even the most extreme neurological conditions deny neither personhood nor the duty to care. In this construct the sustaining relation need not be reciprocal to be respected. "I see how you love her," Sacks says to the father of an autistic artist.[13] "Does she love you, too?" The answer, one Sacks obviously accepts as sufficient, is: "She loves us as much as she can."

Stephen G Post implies a similar valuation when he considers a Cleveland man who lovingly maintains his persistently unconscious wife. "Even the PVS conditions does not disqualify a loved one from equal moral standing. . . . It further suggests that the concept of quality of life might be replaced by the quality of lives, including family members."[14] The result is a duty to care for the person the family member perceives as a person-in-relation.

The distance between this definition of the person and one of the person as a discrete, existential being lies at the heart of a now famous exchange between disability rights lawyer Harriet McBryde Johnson and Princeton University bioethicist Peter Singer.[15] She described a family's caring at home for a persistently unconscious teenager as "beautiful," an act that Singer thought somewhat "weird." The gulf between their ethical frames was sufficiently severe to prevent either from clearly arguing the primary values and resulting constructs that resulted in the apparently aesthetic judgements.[16]

It may be this sense of personhood as a shared rather than discrete quality that fuelled the extraordinary public demonstration of support for Terri Schiavo's survival. For those protesting the withdrawal of hydration and nutrition,

the act of demonstration served in itself as affirmation of Mrs Schiavo's personhood and thus her place within the protected circle of the state's "life interest" in its citizens. The unprecedented political involvement of the Florida State Legislature and the US Congress in the Schiavo case is, from this perspective, wholly appropriate. Where else in a democracy do citizens turn when they believe current policy and law are inappropriate, prejudicial, and unethical? When courts cannot offer redress the logical next step is to seek legislation that will alter the laws in a manner that permits future judicial support.

Sanctity of Life

The central concern of Mrs Schiavo's supporters appears to be that physical continuance is lexicographically a primary value violated by the discontinuation of her nutrition and hydration. That many who so argued in the Florida case did so from a religious perspective is neither surprising nor relevant. The operative law and ethic in North America, as it is in Europe, is at heart Judeo-Christian. The "sanctity of life" argument espoused by many in this case has deep roots in that tradition as well as a long secular tradition.

Peter Singer's famous declaration that "after ruling our thoughts and our decisions about life and death for nearly two thousand years, the traditional western ethic [of life sanctity] has collapsed" was clearly premature.[17] The Schiavo case signals a resurgence of this collapsed ethic as a lexicographically superior, primary value, one in which the default remains life sanctity irrespective of "quality." Whether those arguing a "culture of care," will do so uniformly and realistically—embracing the increased taxation a fully caring culture assuredly would require, for example—is a separate if important issue.

Conclusion

The story of the public debate surrounding Terri Schiavo should impress upon laypersons and professionals alike the uncertainty of the context in which issues of continuation and termination are argued ethically. Nobody knows what Mrs Schiavo would have wanted. She left no advance directive and in its absence her husband says one thing and her parents another. While the husband is the typical surrogate in this case his status has been challenged for a decade by her parents. Similarly, we do not know to an absolute certainty her cognitive status. Was she "minimally conscious" or permanently unconscious? In either case we do not know to an absolute certainty whether or not she sensed any discomfort from dehydration and starvation, or anything else. Our neurology is insufficient to make a definitive determination.

These uncertainties pale before the greater one: What is the ethical frame in which such cases should be judged? Bioethicists who assume the facts are clear and the frame for their application self-evident dismiss the concerns of those who coherently argue from a different ethical framework. The result will be to marginalise their own position, assuring their status as non-participants in the ethical, moral, legal, and political debates this case generally promotes.

Time to redefine the ethical principles of care for restricted people.

References

1. Florida Statute 765.101 s4; 12 a and b; 17.

2. Drager P. Terri Schiavo: Facts. manipulation . . . innuendo . . . bias . . . truth. American Society for Bioethics and the Humanities Annual Meeting, Montreal, PQ, 22–26 October 2003.

3. Shewmon AD. Critical analysis of conceptual domains of the vegetative state: sorting fact from fancy. Neurol Rehab 2004;19:343–7.

4. Koch T. The difference that difference makes: bioethics and the challenge—disability. J Med Philos 2004;29:703.

5. Schoenle PW, Witzke W. How vegetative is the vegetative state? Preserved semantic processing in VS patients—evidence from n 400 event-related potentials. Neurol Rehabil 2004;19:329–34 Andrews K, Murphy R, Littlewood C, Misdiagnosis of the vegetative state: retrospective study in a rehabilitation unit. BMJ 1996;313:13–16; Childs NL, Mercer WN, Childs HW. Accuracy of diagnosis of persistent vegetative state. Neurology 1993;43:1465–7.

6. Kuhse H. Voluntary euthanasia and other medical end-of-life decisions: doctors should be permitted to give death a helping hand. In: Thomasma DC, Kushner T, eds. Birth to Death: Science and Bioethics. New York: Cambridge University Press, 1996:247–58.

7. Jecker N, Schneiderman LJ. Stopping futile medical treatment: ethical issues. In: Thomasma DC, Kushner T, eds. Birth to Death: Science and Bioethics. New York: Cambridge University Press, 1996, 169–76; at 170.

8. Binding K, Hoche A. 1920. Permitting the destruction of unworthy life: its extent and form, In: Wright W, Deer P, Salmonon R, eds. Trans Issues in Law and Medicine 1992;8:231–68.

9. Pernick MS. The Black Stork: Eugenics and the death of "defective" babies in American medicine and motion pictures since 1915. New York: Oxford University Press, 1996.

10. Koch T, Singer P. Point counterpoint: the ideology of normalcy: the ethics of difference. J Disabil Policy Studies. 2005, in press.

11. Sacks O. Awakenings (1983) revised edn. New York: Harper Collins, 1990.

12. Sacks O. An Anthropologist on Mars. New York: Knopf, 1995.

13. See reference 17: p. 210.

14. Post SG. The moral challenge of Alzheimer disease. Baltimore, MD: Johns Hopkins Press, 1995:197–8.

15. Koch T. The difference that difference makes (see reference 3); Koch T. Disability and difference: balancing social and physical constructions, J Med Ethics. 2001;27:370–6; Koch T. Life quality vs. the "quality of life": Assumptions underlying prospective quality of life instruments in health care planning. Soc Sci Med 2000;51:419–28.

16. Lantos J. Johnson, Singer, Almodovar, and the aesthetics of bioethics. ASBH Exchange. 2003;6: 1, 2, 7.

17. Singer P. Rethinking Life and Death: The Collapse of Our Traditional Ethics. New York: St, Martin's Griffin 1005:1.

Tom Koch is the director of Information Outreach, Ltd., based in Vancouver, BC, where he conducts research on issues in bioethics and journalism.

EXPLORING THE ISSUE

May Surrogate Decision Makers Terminate Care for a Person in a Persistent Vegetative State?

Critical Thinking and Reflection

1. Would you want your surrogates to keep you alive if you were in a persistent vegetative state? What account of personhood and the value of life would you give as part of an explanation for that view?
2. If someone you love ended up in a PVS and you were asked to be the surrogate decision maker, what sort of evidence could you give to justify your views about what that person would have wanted done?
3. Express Tom Koch's concerns about the Schiavo case in your own words. Can you envision ways of responding constructively to Koch's concerns while still allowing surrogate decisions to withdraw medical treatment?

Is There Common Ground?

The case of Terri Schiavo garnered more media attention and political involvement than did the similar case of Nancy Cruzan, 30 years earlier. Cruzan's family was united in their effort to remove her feeding tube. In contrast, Schiavo's husband Michael began efforts to remove her feeding tube in 1998, declaring that this was his wife's wish should she be in a permanent nonresponsive condition, but her parents, Robert and Mary Schindler, vehemently opposed this action. The case was tried in the legal system and in the court of public opinion through extensive media coverage and political actions. In the end, Michael Schiavo prevailed and the feeding tube was removed.

Perhaps the best hope for reaching common ground in cases like that of Terri Schiavo is the realization that MRI might to some degree allow us to "see" into the brain of people with PVS and at least in some cases gain some confirmation of the diagnosis that otherwise must depend on close observation of the patient's behavior. At the same time, as some commentators have pointed out, it would be easy for family members and physicians to misinterpret the possible MRI results. An article in *New England Journal of Medicine* suggested that MRI might not only show that the brains of some patients now diagnosed as being in a PVS in fact respond to stimuli, but also even allow family and physicians to communicate with some of those minimally responsive patients—that we could

ask them to answer yes to a question by imagining that they are playing tennis, for example. But other commentators argue that we are a long way from knowing how to interpret the MRIs, and that meaningful communication with a patient would require much more than activation of different brain areas in response to yes–no questions.

Additional Resources

In March 2006, three books were published presenting different sides of the controversy: Michael Schiavo and Michael Hirsh published *Terri: The Truth* (Dutton); "Terri's Family" (her parents, brother, and sister) published *A Life That Matters: The Legacy of Terri Schiavo—A Lesson for Us All* (Warner Books); and Arthur L. Caplan, James J. McCartney, and Dominic A. Sisti published *The Case of Terri Schiavo: Ethics at the End of Life* (Prometheus).

For the ground-breaking work on the use of MRIs with patients in PVS, see M.M. Monti et al., "Willful Modulation of Brain Activity in Disorders of Consciousness," *New England Journal of Medicine* (vol. 362, 2010, pp. 579–589). For a critical discussion of this work, see J. Andrew Billings, Larry R. Churchill, and Richard Payne, "Severe Brain Injury and the Subjective Life," *Hastings Center Report* (vol. 40, no. 3, 2010, pp. 17–21).

Jay Wolfson has described his experience with Theresa Schiavo in a number of moving articles and essays. See Jay Wolfson, "Erring on the Side of Theresa Schiavo: Reflections of the Special Guardian ad Litem," *Hastings Center Report* (vol. 35, no. 3, 2005, pp. 16–19), and "The Basis for Decisions to End Life. The Schiavo Dilemma: An Essay by the Special Guardian Ad Litem," *Clinical Interventions in Aging* (vol. 1, no. 1, 2006, pp. 3–6).

Internet References . . .

Brain Injury Association of America

http://www.biausa.org/

National Disability Rights Network

www.napas.org/

The Brain Trauma Foundation

http://www.braintrauma.org/

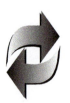

Unit 2

End-of-Life Dilemmas

*W*hat are physicians' ethical responsibilities associated with death and dying? Doctors are sworn "to do no harm," but this proscription is open to many different interpretations. Is it compatible with sometimes acting to bring about death? Society sometimes decides, through its legal processes, that a given individual deserves to die; can a physician be enlisted to help kill that individual? Should a physician be enlisted? And all people will eventually succumb to disease, injury, or mere aging, and on occasion, a person's death may appear to be natural and imminent, and perhaps the person may be suffering so greatly that he or she—or others who love that person—may want to hasten death in order to put an end to suffering. Is it ethically necessary to prolong life at all times under all circumstances? Medical personnel as well as families often face this agonizing question. The right of an individual to decide his or her own fate may conflict with society's interest in maintaining the value of human life. Even when doctors uphold the value of human life, however, they should surely strive to help their patients die with as little pain and suffering as possible. But what does that mean? How far may doctors go to bring about a "good" death? This unit examines some of these anguishing questions.

Selected, Edited, and with Issue Framing Material by:
Gregory E. Kaebnick, *The Hastings Center*

ISSUE

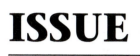

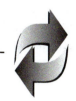

Is "Continuous Deep Sedation" a Valuable Treatment Option for Patients Who Are Close to Death?

YES: American Medical Association, from "Sedation to Unconsciousness in End-of-Life Care," *Report of the Council on Ethical and Judicial Affairs* (2008)

NO: Mohamed Y. Rady and Joseph L. Verheijde, from "Distress from Voluntary Refusal of Food and Fluids to Hasten Death: What Is the Role of Continuous Deep Sedation?" *Journal of Medical Ethics* (2012)

Learning Outcomes
After reading this issue, you will be able to:
• Describe the special challenges of caring for terminally ill patients in the late stages of their illness.
• Describe the concepts of euthanasia, palliative care, and the doctrine of double effect.

ISSUE SUMMARY

YES: The American Medical Association affirms that in cases of extreme suffering the physician's duty to relieve pain and suffering includes palliative sedation—using drugs that result in unconsciousness and may hasten death.

NO: Physicians Mohamed Rady and Joseph Verheijde argue that if sedation is used in conjunction with voluntary refusal of food and fluids to hasten death, then it is tantamount to assisted dying and may be bad for both the patient and the medical practitioner.

One persistent theme in bioethics is appropriate care and decision making at the end of life. Beginning with the case of Karen Ann Quinlan (see Introduction) and continuing through many highly publicized cases, philosophers, theologians, physicians, policymakers, and patients and family members have struggled with questions about what ethical standards should be used in determining how to use modern medical technology humanely and who should make those decisions. The most publicized cases have concerned young women—Karen Ann Quinlan, Nancy Cruzan, and Terry Schiavo. All suffered traumatic events that put them into long-term, nonresponsive states. But these situations arise even more frequently when individuals with chronic conditions, often frail and elderly, undergo a long period of debilitation before they reach the end of life.

Euthanasia—physician participation in administration of drugs that will result in death—is banned in all states. Only Oregon and Washington have laws that allow physicians under certain circumstances to prescribe but not administer lethal drugs to people at the end of life.

To respect individual autonomy—the right to choose what medical interventions one would or would not accept—many attempts have been made to encourage people to express their wishes through advance directives. Most people do not sign advance directives or in any way indicate their preferences for care at the end of life. Family members are often left to make these decisions based on what they think the patient would have wanted.

Beginning in the 1970s, hospices became an option for people who did not want aggressive medical care. The hospice movement started in Great Britain and emphasized comfort and spiritual care. Today there are over 5,000 hospices in the United States. Contrary to popular perception, which sees hospice as a place where people go to die, most hospice care is provided at home. There are, in addition, some freestanding hospices and hospice units in acute care hospitals and nursing homes. Medicare (the federal health insurance program for people over 65) has a special hospice benefit for people whose life expectancy is 6 months or less. Most people, however, come to hospice very late in the course of their disease, with a median length of stay of 26 days. They and their families fail to obtain the full benefit of the multidisciplinary hospice approach to care.

For many people, one of the drawbacks to hospice is the requirement to give up treatments that are intended to cure the disease. (Medications that ease pain and symptoms are permitted.) Palliative care has become an option in these situations. Palliative care has many of the same goals as hospice—relief of symptoms, multidisciplinary care of the whole person, family involvement—but also allows curative treatments. Importantly, it is available to individuals at any stage of disease. Most palliative care today is provided in hospitals, and there is no special insurance benefit for palliative care at home.

What then is "palliative" or "terminal" sedation and where does it fit in this array of options? Sedation—administering drugs that are to relieve pain or symptoms without causing loss of consciousness—is part of ordinary medical care (unless the patient objects). Depending on the severity of the patient's pain or symptoms, palliative care may include higher levels of medications, which may result in loss of consciousness but is not the intended result. The major controversy concerns the use of drugs in levels that are intended to cause loss of consciousness and are maintained at that level until the patient dies.

The following selections present clearly opposed positions. The American Medical Association's Council on Judicial and Ethical Affairs maintains that palliative sedation, within guidelines, is an acceptable extension of the physician's duty to relieve pain and suffering. Mohamed Rady and Joseph Verheijde argue that if a physician sedates a patient who is voluntarily refusing food and fluids to hasten death, then the physician has in effect participated in physician-assisted dying, which violates the ethical standards to which physicians should hold themselves.

YES ↵

American Medical Association

Sedation to Unconsciousness in End-of-Life Care

Introduction

The duty to relieve pain and suffering is central to the physician's role as healer and is an obligation physicians have to their patients. Palliative care is universally accepted as a multidisciplinary approach to prevent and relieve suffering of patients with life-limiting illnesses. In this setting, palliative sedation is an important technique for combating extreme suffering; however, there is much debate over the use of palliative sedation to unconsciousness because of its potential to be misconstrued as active euthanasia. Even when done properly, it may still provoke moral objection due to the mistaken perception of a risk of hastening death. . . .

This report examines the ethics of the palliative use of sedation to unconsciousness as an intervention of last resort for a terminally ill patient to reduce severe, refractory pain or other distressing clinical symptoms that have not been relieved by aggressive symptom-specific palliation. This report will not dwell on the specific ethics of withholding or withdrawing life-sustaining medical treatment, euthanasia, or physician-assisted suicide, all of which are addressed in the AMA's *Code of Medical Ethics,* but may differentiate palliative sedation to unconsciousness from such interventions for the purposes of clarification.

Background

. . . Palliative care is an integral part of the treatment regimen of terminally ill patients. However, even with the highest standards of care and attempts at palliation, it is estimated that between 5% and 35% of patients receiving palliative care in hospice programs experience severe pain and other intractable symptoms in the last week of life.[1] . . .

Clinical Issues

Palliative sedation to unconsciousness is only appropriate for terminally ill patients "as an intervention of last resort to reduce severe, refractory pain or other distressing

clinical symptoms that have not been relieved by aggressive symptom-specific palliation." Specifically, such clinical symptoms include pain, nausea and vomiting, shortness of breath, agitated delirium, and dyspnea. Additionally, palliative sedation to unconsciousness has been indicated for patients who exhibit urinary retention due to clot formation, gastrointestinal pain, uncontrolled bleeding, and myoclonus.[2] Severe psychological distress may also warrant palliative sedation to unconsciousness when potentially treatable mental health conditions have been excluded.[2] Purely existential suffering may be defined as the experience of agony and distress that results from living in an unbearable state of existence including, for example, death anxiety, isolation, and loss of control. Some have proposed that such suffering in and of itself should also be recognized as an appropriate indication for palliative sedation to unconsciousness, but this remains controversial.[3] However, the Council concurs with those who argue that existential suffering, distinct from previously listed clinical symptoms, is not an appropriate indication for treatment with palliative sedation to unconsciousness, because the causes of this type of suffering are better addressed by other interventions.[4] For example, palliative sedation to unconsciousness is not the way to address suffering created by social isolation and loneliness; rather such suffering should be addressed by providing the patient with needed social support. For patients whose suffering is existential, it is necessary to show compassion and enlist the support of the patient's broader social and spiritual network in order to address issues which are beyond the scope of clinical care.[5]

Ethical Considerations

As described above, a wide spectrum of actions can be taken to relieve the various forms of suffering a terminally ill patient may experience at the end of life. When the usual armamentarium of medical interventions has been exhausted, choices still remain; these range from letting the terminal illness take its course without further intervention to unacceptable choices, such as euthanasia. Actions that are solely intended to hasten the death of patients, such as physician-assisted suicide or euthanasia, are ethically and medically unacceptable (both are "fundamentally incompatible with the physician's role as healer"). In contrast, the withholding and withdrawing of life-sustaining treatment, when done based on the patient's autonomous refusal of unwanted care, and allowing the natural course of disease to take place, are ethically and medically appropriate. Palliative sedation to unconsciousness is intended to relieve patient suffering and, like withholding or withdrawing life support, may also allow the natural process of terminal disease to take place. A recent review of studies of opiate and sedative use in palliative care concluded that there is no evidence to support shortened survival of terminally ill patients who were sedated.[6,7]

Though evidence suggests that opiate and sedative use in the palliative care setting rarely if ever hastens patient death, ethical issues of "intention" and "proportionality" remain of concern. When exploring the ethics of palliative sedation and differentiating it from those of physician-assisted suicide and euthanasia, it is paramount to consider the primary intention of the measure being utilized. Although intended to relieve suffering, physician-assisted suicide and euthanasia achieve this by bringing about death, where palliative sedation is intended to relieve suffering by providing proportionate sedation. Death due to the course of a terminal illness is anticipated in a patient who receives palliative sedation to unconsciousness. However, bringing about the patient's death is not the intent of the sedation.[8] Although intent cannot be observed directly, it can be gauged in part by examining the medical record. Repeated doses or continuous infusions are indicators of proportionate palliative sedation, whereas one large dose or rapidly accelerating doses out of proportion to the level of immediate patient suffering may signify lack of knowledge or an inappropriate intention to hasten death.[3] These questions about intent demonstrate the importance of careful documentation in the medical record of purpose and strategy for patients receiving any palliative care including palliative sedation to unconsciousness.

The doctrine of double effect illuminates how intent makes some forms of end-of-life care morally permissible and others unacceptable. The principle of double effect is applied to situations where it is impossible to avoid all harmful actions. It requires that the good effect (relieving severe suffering) must outweigh the bad effect (potential to unintentionally hasten death), and that the bad effect (ending the patient's life) cannot be the means of achieving the good effect (relieving suffering).[9] Proportionality is also a central tenant of the principle of double effect; the level of sedation sought (and the associated risk of hastening death) must be in direct relationship with, and justified by,[10,11] the level of unacceptable suffering the patient is experiencing. The greater the patient's pain or suffering, the more a physician must be willing to sedate a patient in order to reduce and hopefully eliminate the unacceptable symptoms. The combination and amount of sedative must be just sufficient, but not more so, to relieve distressing clinical symptoms.[3] Furthermore, the concepts of proportionality and justification help to differentiate palliative sedation from physician-assisted suicide and euthanasia since in the case of palliative sedation the physician aims only to sedate to a level of unconsciousness and no further.[12]

It is also important to consider palliative sedation to unconsciousness from the perspectives of autonomy, beneficence, and non-maleficence. Similar to the ethical argument made for withholding or withdrawing life-sustaining medical treatment where the principle of patient autonomy requires that physicians respect the decision of a patient who possesses decision-making capacity to forgo life-sustaining treatment, autonomous decision-making dictates that a fully informed patient should also be able to choose palliative sedation. A designated surrogate decision-maker would also be able to choose palliative sedation for a patient who lacks decision-making capacity and meets the criteria for receiving sedation at the end of life. Requests for palliative sedation to unconsciousness (by patients or their surrogates) that do not fit within acceptable clinical parameters identified by the definition of palliative sedation are inappropriate. The principle of beneficence dictates taking necessary steps to relieve pain and suffering. When discussing the possibility of palliative sedation, it is necessary to fully inform the patient or surrogate about the various levels of sedation and whether intermittent sedation or continuous sedation to unconsciousness is an appropriate option. Patients and their surrogate decision-makers, with guidance from their physicians, should separately decide whether they will continue to receive any life-sustaining treatments and whether they want to maintain, withhold or withdraw life-sustaining interventions (including nutrition and hydration). . . .

Recommendation

The Council on Ethical and Judicial Affairs recommends that the following be adopted. . . .

> The duty to relieve pain and suffering is central to the physician's role as healer and is an obligation physicians have to their patients. Palliative sedation to unconsciousness is the administration of

sedative medication to the point of unconsciousness in a terminally ill patient. It is an intervention of last resort to reduce severe, refractory pain or other distressing clinical symptoms that do not respond to aggressive symptom-specific palliation. It is an accepted and appropriate component of end-of-life care under specific, relatively rare circumstances. When symptoms cannot be diminished through all other means of palliation, including symptom-specific treatments, it is the ethical obligation of a physician to offer palliative sedation to unconsciousness as an option for the relief of intractable symptoms. When considering the use of palliative sedation, the following ethical guidelines are recommended:

1. Patients may be offered palliative sedation when they are in the final stages of terminal illness. The rationale for all palliative care measures should be documented in the medical record.
2. Palliative sedation to unconsciousness may be considered for those terminally ill patients whose clinical symptoms have been unresponsive to aggressive, symptom-specific treatments.
3. Physicians should ensure that the patient and/or the patient's surrogate have given informed consent for palliative sedation to unconsciousness.
4. Physicians should consult with a multidisciplinary team, including an expert in the field of palliative care, to ensure that symptom-specific treatments have been sufficiently employed and that palliative sedation to unconsciousness is now the most appropriate course of treatment.
5. Physicians should discuss with their patients considering palliative sedation the care plan relative to degree and length (intermittent or constant) of sedation, and the specific expectations for continuing, withdrawing or withholding future life-sustaining treatments.
6. Once palliative sedation is begun, a process must be implemented to monitor for appropriate care.
7. Palliative sedation is not an appropriate response to suffering that is primarily existential, defined as the experience of agony and distress that may arise from such issues as death anxiety, isolation and loss of control. Existential suffering is better addressed by other interventions. For example, palliative sedation is not the way to address suffering created by social isolation and loneliness; such suffering should be addressed by providing the patient with needed social support.
8. Palliative sedation must never be used to intentionally cause a patient's death.

References

1. Quill, T. E., Byock, I. R., for the ACP-ASIM End-of-Life Care Consensus Panel. Responding to intractable terminal suffering: the role of terminal sedation and voluntary refusal of food and fluids. *Ann Intern Med.* 2000;132:408–414.
2. National Ethics Committee, Veterans Health Administration. The Ethics of palliative sedation as a therapy of last resort. *Am J Hosp Palliat Med.* 2007;23(6):483–491.
3. de Graeff A, Dean M. Palliative sedation therapy in the last weeks of life: a literature review and recommendations for standards. *J Palliat Med.* 2007 Feb;10(1):67–85.
4. Taylor BR, McCann RM. Controlled sedation for physical and existential suffering? *J of Palliat Med.* 2005;8(1):144–147.
5. Snyder L, Sulmasy DP, for the Etchis and Human Rights Committee, ACP-ASIM. Physician-assisted suicide—Position paper. *Ann Intern Med.* 2001;135:208–216.
6. Charter S, Viola R, Paterson J. Sedation for intractable distress in dying—A survey of experts. *Palliat Med.* 1998;12:255–296.
7. Morita T, Chinone Y, Ikenaga M, Miyoshi M, Nakaho T, Nishitateno K et al. Efficacy and safety of palliative sedation therapy: A multicenter, prospective, observational study conducted on specialized palliative care units in Japan. *J Pain Symptom Manage.* 2005;30(4):320–8.
8. Quill TE, Lo B, Brock DW. Palliative options of last resort: a comparison of voluntary stopping eating and drinking, terminal sedation, physician assisted suicide, and voluntary active euthanasia. *JAMA.* 1997;278(23):2099–2104.
9. Quill TE, Dresser R, Brock DW. The rule of double effect—a critique of its role in end-of-life decision making. *N Eng J Med.* 1997;337:1768–1771.
10. Cantor NL, Thomas GC. The legal bounds of physician conduct hastening death. *Buffalo L Rev.* 2000;48(1):83–173.
11. Kollas CD, Boyer-Kollas B, Kollas JW. Criminal prosecutions of physicians providing palliative or end-of-life care. *J Palliat Med.* 2008;11(3):233–241.
12. Emanuel E. Ethics in pain management: an introductory overview. *Pain Med.* 2001:2(2)112–6.

AMERICAN MEDICAL ASSOCIATION is a professional association for physicians.

Mohamed Y. Rady and Joseph L. Verheijde

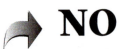

Distress from Voluntary Refusal of Food and Fluids to Hasten Death: What Is the Role of Continuous Deep Sedation?

Introduction

There is a growing trend to practise physician-assisted dying (death) (PAD) under the premise of providing quality palliative care in consensual and non-consensual life-ending situations.[1] The WHO envisages palliative care as a comprehensive system of managing pain and distressing symptoms without intending to shorten the end-of-life (EOL) trajectory.[1] In assisted dying, the EOL trajectory is shortened to relieve suffering.[1] Bundling PAD with palliative care is precarious because PAD: (1) contravenes the Hippocratic principle of "do not kill"; (2) transgresses cultural and religious values of some patients, families and healthcare professionals; and (3) violates basic human rights.[2]

Voluntary refusal of food and fluids (VRFF) is a legal method of PAD, although medical and societal acceptability is uncertain.[3] Etkind reported a patient with amyotrophic lateral sclerosis who desired to end life because of mental anguish and fear of unbearable future suffering.[4] The patient chose VRFF to hasten death after the onset of bulbar disease progression. In this paper we comment on: (1) unbearable suffering as an indication for PAD; (2) VRFF as a means to hasten death; (3) efficacy of continuous deep sedation (CDS) for optimal control of distress from VRFF; and (4) bundling assisted dying with palliative and hospice care.

Unbearable Suffering

When deciding on the use of CDS, severity of suffering is difficult to quantify objectively.[5] The interpretation of the adjectives "refractory" and "unbearable" is subjective. The Dutch Medical Society (KNMG) states that suffering must be lasting and unbearable to request euthanasia.[6] Persons ineligible for euthanasia but desiring to die can opt for VRFF and CDS.[6] Unbearable suffering is defined broadly enough to include cognitive (early dementia), psycho-social or existential distress.[6] It may also include various ". . . old-age afflictions that are neither life-threatening nor fatal in the vulnerable elderly" (p23)[6] such as diminished vision, hearing, mobility, fitness or independence:

> In the future, physicians will be confronted more than ever before with seniors in vulnerable positions, ever-more advanced in age and, moreover, keen to live independently for as long as possible (p22).[6] Many older people have various afflictions that are not actually life-threatening but do make them vulnerable . . . [I]t is wholly justifiable that vulnerability—extending to such dimensions as loss of function, loneliness and loss of autonomy—should be part of the equation physicians use to assess requests for euthanasia (p22).[6]

VRFF and Hastening of Death

Although VRFF may be legal, it can also result in a slow dying process. Etkind's case report illustrated the challenges of achieving optimal control of suffering from VRFF.[4] Nevertheless, VRFF is promoted as a legal and peaceful method of hastening death.[7] The KNMG even endorses VRFF for patients who are ineligible for euthanasia and whose ". . . suffering is not unbearable and lasting within the meaning of the Euthanasia Law" (p34).[6] "(A) patient with a strong wish to die may decide for himself to deny food and drink. In that case, the patient is making a conscious choice to hasten death" (p34).[6] The KNMG obligates physicians to provide due care with CDS or intermittent deep sedation regardless of agreement with the patient's decision. "When a patient dies due to not eating and drinking this constitutes a natural death, even if the patient was under continuous sedation according to accepted treatment" (p36).[6] However, the premise that death under CDS is "natural" has been refuted.[8] Hastening death by VRFF and CDS may even inflict additional harm and suffering.[9-11]

Efficacy of CDS in VRFF

Etkind's VRFF scenario compounded the patient's distress by the additional burden of physical manifestations of acute metabolic derangement from dehydration including agitation and bulbar weakness.[4] A vicious pathophysiological cycle was set in motion: worsening metabolic derangement from dehydration, uncontrollable agitation and escalating doses of sedatives.[3] It is a misconception that high doses of sedatives to obliterate consciousness always eradicate inner affective awareness of thirst and hunger. CDS may blunt the wakefulness component of human consciousness without abolishing internal awareness.[10,11] However, absent wakefulness prevents interacting with the environment. Scientific understanding of awareness of internal and external nociceptive stimuli under CDS is rudimentary.[11] Functional neuroimaging of the human brain in pharmacological and pathological states of coma heightens concerns that sedatives will not always abolish inner awareness of suffering.[11] Commentators have expressed reservations about whether CDS is the ideal method of achieving the goal of a rapid painless death[9-11] because the clinical efficacy of CDS remains unproven.

Assisted Dying and the Double-Effect Principle

Moral and professional obligations demand delivering optimal and comprehensive palliative care to the terminally ill patient. However, confusing the terminally ill patient with the imminently dying patient does not constitute a justification for hastening death. To differentiate assisted death from natural death, we objectively defined the term "imminently dying" by the onset of new lethal pathophysiology from acute life-threatening illness or fatal complications of the underlying disease.[12] For instance, the onset of bronchopneumonia secondary to bulbar palsy would constitute natural death in Etkind's case. On the other hand, VRFF and CDS introduce new lethal pathophysiology intended to hasten death.[3] The intent of VRFF (first act) is to consciously hasten death and the second act (use of sedatives) becomes a direct and predictable consequence of the first act. We have argued that administering sedatives and opioids in planned life-ending interventions based on the analysis of the double-effect principle—intention and causation of death—is not palliative care.[13] The use of sedatives with VRFF is commensurate with euthanasia.

Assisted Dying and Hospice Care

Deliberately hastening death by VRFF has unintended consequences. Patients suffer because of the slow dying process following dehydration and starvation. The difficulty of adequately controlling distress without bringing the dying process to a rapid conclusion by lethal pharmacological interventions can cause feelings of guilt among hospice and medical staff. We recommend that terminating life or assisted dying should not be conflated with palliative and hospice care. The Dutch KNMG arbitrarily defines VRFF with sedation to end life as 'natural death' and obligates physicians to participate in due care during this procedure.[6] Owing to the absence of empirical evidence for the efficacy of CDS in managing distress, it may be argued that VRFF with sedation may represent a cruel and inhumane method of terminating life. Narratives of physicians who have engaged in CDS have suggested that there is a real need to separate the practice of assisted dying from the practice of medicine.[13] Ultimately, the question that the medical profession and society must address is how to deal with patients requesting assistance with ending their lives. We urge that both the legal and societal debate should focus on sharpening the boundaries between assisted dying and palliative care. This separation is necessary (1) to uphold trust in the patient–physician relationship and (2) to preserve the integrity and ethics of the medical profession.

Conclusion

Although VRFF combined with CDS is a legal method of PAD for unbearable suffering, it can also result in a slow dying process. CDS may blunt the wakefulness component of human consciousness without eradicating inner affective awareness of thirst and hunger. Owing to the absence of empirical evidence on the efficacy of CDS in managing distress, it may be argued that VRFF with sedation represents a cruel and inhumane method of terminating life. Legal and societal debate should focus on sharpening the boundaries between assisted dying and palliative care.

References

1. Rady MY, Verheijde JL, Potts M. Quality palliative care or physician-assisted death: a comment on the French perspective of end-of-life care in neurological disorders. *J Clinic Res Bioeth* 2011;2:102e. http://www.omicsonline.org/2155-9627/2155-9627-2-102e.pdf (accessed 30 Sep 2011).

2. Pereira J. Legalizing euthanasia or assisted suicide: the illusion of safeguards and controls. *Curr Oncol* 2011;18:e38–45. http://www.current-oncology.com/index.php/oncology/article/view/883 (accessed 30 Sep 2011).

3. Rady MY, Verheijde JL. Continuous deep sedation until death: palliation or physician-assisted death? *Am J Hosp Palliat Care* 2010;27:205–14.

4. Etkind SN. Terminal sedation: an emotional decision in end of life care. *J Med Ethics* 2011. (In press).

5. Manzini JL. Palliative sedation: ethical perspectives from Latin America in comparison with European recommendations. *Curr Opin Support Palliat Care* 2011;5:279–84.

6. Koninklijke Nederlandsche Maatschappij tot bevordering der Geneeskunst (KNMG). *The Role of the Physician in the Voluntary Termination of Life*. (KNMG Position Paper). 2011. http://www.knmg.nl/voluntary-termination-of-life (accessed 30 Sep 2011).

7. Span P. Deciding to die, then shown the door. The New Old Age: Caring and Coping. *New York Times*. Published Online First: 24 August 2011. 1:59 pm. http://newoldage.blogs.nytimes.com/2011/08/24/deciding-to-die-then-shown-the-door/ (accessed 30 Sep 2011).

8. Raus K, Sterckx S, Mortier F. Continuous deep sedation at the end of life and the 'natural death' hypothesis. *Bioethics*. Published Online First: 17 January 2011. doi:2010.1111/j.1467-8519.2010.01861.x.

9. Raus K, Sterckx S, Mortier F. Is continuous sedation at the end of life an ethically preferable alternative to physician-assisted suicide? *Am J Bioeth* 2011;11:32–40.

10. Kon AA. Palliative sedation: it's not a panacea. *Am J Bioeth* 2011;11:41–2.

11. Carvalho TB, Rady MY, Verheijde JL. *et at.* Continuous deep sedation in end-of-life care: disentangling palliation from physician-assisted death. *Am J Bioeth* 2011;11:60–2.

12. Rady MY, Verheijde J. When is deactivating an implanted cardiac device physician-assisted death? Appraisal of the lethal pathophysiology and mode of death. *J Palliat Med* 2011;14:1086–8.

13. Douglas CD, Kerridge IH, Ankeny RA. Narratives of 'terminal sedation', and the importance of the intention-foresight distinction in palliative care practice. *Bioethics*. Published Online First: 4 July 2011. doi:2010.1111/j.1467-8519.2011.01895.x.

Mohamed Y. Rady is a professor of medicine in the Mayo Clinic's Department of Critical Care Medicine.

Joseph L. Verheijde is a manager of rehabilitation services with the Mayo Clinic.

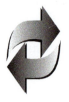

EXPLORING THE ISSUE

Is "Continuous Deep Sedation" a Valuable Treatment Option for Patients Who Are Close to Death?

Critical Thinking and Reflection

1. Do you agree with Rady and Verheijde that offering palliative sedation can be tantamount to killing a terminally ill person? If palliative sedation hastens death, is that morally wrong, in your view?
2. Do you accept the "doctrine of double effect" as an explanation for why it might hasten death yet be acceptable? Or do you think that if it hastens death, then whether hastening death is acceptable must be confronted head on?
3. The AMA's Council on Ethical and Judicial Affairs offers a number of recommendations intended to ensure that palliative sedation at the end of life is not misused. Do those recommendations seem adequate to you? Too restrictive?

Is There Common Ground?

Everyone agrees that patients in the last throes of a terminal illness should be made as comfortable as possible. There is also broad agreement among ethicists and palliative care specialists that this justifies palliation strong enough to make the patient unconscious.

How far to go with palliative sedation seems to depend, as Battin notes, on how much value one attaches to biological life as opposed to freedom from suffering and the ability to live out one's life in the manner one wishes. The debate about the value of biological life is often cast as a sharp contrast: Either we believe that life is sacred, or we reject that idea altogether. If we uphold it, then we think it should be preserved even at the cost of suffering and turmoil, and even if the person's life story has essentially ended. Some years ago, however, the legal theorist Ronald Dworkin argued in the book *Life's Dominion: An Argument about Abortion, Euthanasia, and Individual Freedom* that many people actually accept both sides of this contrast to some degree: They think that biological life has value in and of itself, and that suffering should be curtailed and the person's wishes honored. They just differ on exactly where they strike the balance.

Additional Resources

For a set of professional recommendations of the use of palliative sedation on patients very near death, see Timothy W. Kirk and Margaret M. Mahon, "National Hospice and Palliative Care Organization (NHPCO) Position Statement and Commentary on the Use of Palliative Sedation in Imminently Dying Terminally Ill Patients," *Journal of Pain and Symptom Management* (vol. 39, no. 5, 2010); www.nhpco.org/i4a/pages/index.cfm?pageid=4673. Also, see National Ethics Committee, Veterans Health Administration, "The Ethics of Palliative Sedation as a Therapy of Last Resort," *American Journal of Hospice and Palliative Care* (vol. 23, no. 6, 2007).

Palliative care is also discussed in Nancy Berlinger, Bruce Jennings, and Susan M. Wolf, *The Hastings Center Guidelines for Decisions on Life-Sustaining Treatment and Care Near the End of Life: Revised and Expanded Second Edition* (Oxford University Press, 2013).

In "Last-Resort Options for Palliative Sedation," Timothy E. Quill, Bernard Lo, Dan W. Brock, and Alan Meisel recommend that palliative care and hospice programs develop clear policies about various levels of palliative sedation, including mechanisms for training and ensuring clinician competency (*Annals of Internal Medicine*, September 15, 2009).

After reviewing organizational guidelines around palliative sedation, Jeffrey Berger concluded that "current guidelines treat palliative sedation to unconsciousness as an effective medical treatment for terminally ill patients who need relief from severe symptoms, yet also restrict its use in ways that are extraordinary for medical treatments." He proposes loosening the guidelines that require imminent death and the failure of other aggressive measures ("Rethinking Guidelines for the Use of Palliative Sedation," *Hastings Center Report*, May–June 2010).

In "Responding to Intractable Terminal Suffering: The Role of Terminal Sedation and Voluntary Refusal of Food and Fluids," Timothy E. Quill and Ira Byock, writing for the American College of Physicians–American Society of Internal Medicine End-of-Life Consensus Panel, assert that terminal sedation and voluntary refusal of hydration and nutrition are options that substantially increase patients' choices (*Annals of Internal Medicine*, March 7, 2000).

Erich H. Loewy, a physician, offers a personal commentary in "Terminal Sedation, Self-Starvation, and Orchestrating the End of Life," *Archives of Internal Medicine* (February 12, 2001). He believes that when end-of-life care is skillfully orchestrated by a well-trained and practiced team, "few persons will want to take refuge in these options of last resort." He says that there is an enormous difference between allowing people to end their lives in this way and encouraging it.

Internet References . . .

American Academy of Hospice and Palliative Medicine

http://aahpm.org/

National Hospice and Palliative Care Organization

www.nhpco.org

Selected, Edited, and with Issue Framing Material by:
Gregory E. Kaebnick, *The Hastings Center*

ISSUE

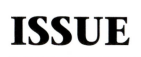

Should Physicians Be Allowed to Assist in Patient Suicide?

YES: Marcia Angell, from "The Supreme Court and Physician-Assisted Suicide—The Ultimate Right," *The New England Journal of Medicine* (1997)

NO: Kathleen M. Foley, from "Competent Care for the Dying Instead of Physician-Assisted Suicide," *The New England Journal of Medicine* (1997)

Learning Outcomes
After reading this issue, you will be able to:
• Discuss the ethical dilemma posed by physician-assisted suicide.
• Explain the differences between active and passive euthanasia and between voluntary and involuntary euthanasia.

ISSUE SUMMARY

YES: Physician Marcia Angell asserts that a physician's main duties are to respect patient autonomy and to relieve suffering, even if that sometimes means assisting in a patient's death.

NO: Physician Kathleen M. Foley counters that if physician-assisted suicide becomes legal, it will begin to substitute for interventions that otherwise might enhance the quality of life for dying patients.

Since the early 1980s, physicians, lawyers, philosophers, and judges have examined questions about withholding life-sustaining treatment. Their deliberations have resulted in a broad consensus that competent adults have the right to make decisions about their medical care, even if those decisions seem unjustifiable to others and even if they result in death. Furthermore, the right of individuals to name others to carry out their prior wishes or to make decisions if they should become incompetent is now well established. Thirty-eight states now have legislation allowing advance directives (commonly known as "living wills").

The debate in specific cases continues, but on the whole, patients' rights to self-determination have been bolstered by 80 or more legal cases, dozens of reports, and statements made by medical societies and other organizations.

As often occurs in bioethical debate, the resolution of one issue only highlights the lack of resolution about another. There is clearly no consensus about either euthanasia or physician-assisted suicide.

Like truth telling, euthanasia is an old problem given new dimensions by the ability of modern medical technology to prolong life. The word itself is Greek (literally, *happy death*) and the Greeks wrestled with the question of whether, in some cases, people would be better off dead. But the Hippocratic Oath in this instance was clear: "I will neither give a deadly drug to anybody if asked for it, nor will I make a suggestion to that effect." On the other hand, if the goal of medicine is not simply to prolong life but to reduce suffering, at some point the question of what measures should be taken or withdrawn will inevitably arise. The problem is: When death is inevitable, how far should one go in hastening it?

The majority of cases in which euthanasia is raised as a possibility are among the most difficult ethical issues to resolve, for they involve the conflict between a physician's duty to preserve life and the burden on the patient and the family that is created by fulfilling that duty. One common distinction is between *active* euthanasia (i.e., some positive act such as administering a lethal injection) and *passive* euthanasia (i.e., an inaction such as deciding not to administer antibiotics when the patient has a severe infection). Another common distinction is between *voluntary* euthanasia (i.e., the patient wishes to die and consents to the action that will make it happen) and *involuntary*—or better, *nonvoluntary*—euthanasia (i.e., the patient is unable to consent, perhaps because he or she is in a coma).

The YES and NO selections address a particularly controversial aspect of this issue. Is it ethical for a physician to assist in a hopelessly ill patient's suicide? Marcia Angell argues that sometimes hastening death should be an option for physicians although "reluctantly as a last resort." Angell states that a physician must consider patient autonomy and suffering when deciding upon care. Kathleen M. Foley contends that the medical profession should take the lead in developing guidelines for the end of life. This means that one must not confuse compassion for a patient's suffering with competence in care.

YES ←

Marcia Angell

The Supreme Court and Physician-Assisted Suicide—The Ultimate Right

The importance and contentious issue of physician-assisted suicide, now being argued before the U.S. Supreme Court, is the subject of the following two editorials. Writing in favor of permitting assisted suicide under certain circumstances is the Journal's executive editor, Dr. Marcia Angell. Arguing against it is Dr. Kathleen Foley, co-chief of the Pain and Palliative Care Service of Memorial Sloan-Kettering Cancer Center in New York. We hope these two editorials, which have in common the authors' view that care of the dying is too often inadequate, will help our readers in making their own judgments.

—Jerome P. Kassirer, M.D.

The U.S. Supreme Court will decide later this year whether to let stand decisions by two appeals courts permitting doctors to help terminally ill patients commit suicide.[1] The Ninth and Second Circuit Courts of Appeals last spring held that state laws in Washington and New York that ban assistance in suicide were unconstitutional as applied to doctors and their dying patients.[2,3] If the Supreme Court lets the decisions stand, physicians in 12 states, which include about half the population of the United States, would be allowed to provide the means for terminally ill patients to take their own lives, and the remaining states would rapidly follow suit. Not since *Roe v. Wade* has a Supreme Court decision been so fateful.

The decision will culminate several years of intense national debate, fueled by a number of highly publicized events. Perhaps most important among them is Dr. Jack Kevorkian's defiant assistance in some 44 suicides since 1990, to the dismay of many in the medical and legal establishments, but with substantial public support, as evidenced by the fact that three juries refused to convict him even in the face of a Michigan statute enacted for that purpose. Also since 1990, voters in three states have considered ballot initiatives that would legalize some form of physician-assisted dying, and in 1994 Oregon became the first state to approve such a measure.[4] (The Oregon law was stayed pending a court challenge.) Several surveys indicate that roughly two thirds of the American public now support physician-assisted suicide,[5,6] as do more than half the doctors in the United States,[6,7] despite the fact that influential physicians' organizations are opposed. It seems clear that many Americans are now so concerned about the possibility of a lingering, high-technology death that they are receptive to the idea of doctors' being allowed to help them die.

In this editorial I will explain why I believe the appeals courts were right and why I hope the Supreme Court will uphold their decisions. I am aware that this is a highly contentious issue, with good people and strong arguments on both sides. The American Medical Association (AMA) filed an amicus brief opposing the legalization of physician-assisted suicide,[8] and the Massachusetts Medical Society, which owns the *Journal*, was a signatory to it. But here I speak for myself, not the *Journal* or the Massachusetts Medical Society. The legal aspects of the case have been well discussed elsewhere, to me most compellingly in Ronald Dworkin's essay in the *New York Review of Books*.[9] I will focus primarily on the medical and ethical aspects.

I begin with the generally accepted premise that one of the most important ethical principles in medicine is respect for each patient's autonomy, and that when this principle conflicts with others, it should almost always take precedence. This premise is incorporated into our laws governing medical practice and research, including the requirement of informed consent to any treatment. In medicine, patients exercise their self-determination most dramatically when they ask that life-sustaining treatment be withdrawn. Although others may sometimes consider the request ill-founded, we are bound to honor it if the patient is mentally competent—that is, if the patient can understand the nature of the decision and its consequences.

A second starting point is the recognition that death is not fair and is often cruel. Some people die quickly, and others die slowly but peacefully. Some find personal or religious meaning in the process, as well as an opportunity for a final reconciliation with loved ones. But others, especially those with cancer, AIDS, or progressive neurologic disorders, may die by inches and in great anguish, despite every effort of their doctors and nurses. Although nearly all pain can be relieved, some cannot, and other symptoms, such as dyspnea, nausea, and weakness, are even more difficult to control. In addition, dying sometimes holds great indignities and existential suffering. Patients who happen to require some treatment to sustain their lives, such as assisted ventilation or dialysis, can hasten death by having the life-sustaining treatment withdrawn, but those who are not receiving life-sustaining treatment may desperately need help they cannot now get.

If the decisions of the appeals courts are upheld, states will not be able to prohibit doctors from helping such patients to die by prescribing a lethal dose of a drug and advising them on its use for suicide. State laws barring euthanasia (the administration of a lethal drug by a doctor) and assisted suicide for patients who are not terminally ill would not be affected. Furthermore, doctors would not be *required* to assist in suicide; they would simply have that option. Both appeals courts based their decisions on constitutional questions. This is important, because it shifted the focus of the debate from what the majority would approve through the political process, as exemplified by the Oregon initiative, to a matter of fundamental rights, which are largely immune from the political process. Indeed, the Ninth Circuit Court drew an explicit analogy between suicide and abortion, saying that both were personal choices protected by the Constitution and that forbidding doctors to assist would in effect nullify these rights. Although states could regulate assisted suicide, as they do abortion, they would not be permitted to regulate it out of existence.

It is hard to quarrel with the desire of a greatly suffering, dying patient for a quicker, more humane death or to disagree that it may be merciful to help bring that about. In those circumstances, loved ones are often relieved when death finally comes, as are the attending doctors and nurses. As the Second Circuit Court said (in the case of *Quill v. Vacco*), the state has no interest in prolonging such a life. Why, then, do so many people oppose legalizing physician-assisted suicide in these cases? There are a number of arguments against it, some stronger than others, but I believe none of them can offset the overriding duties of doctors to relieve suffering and to respect their patients' autonomy. Below I list several of the more important arguments against physician-assisted suicide and discuss why I believe they are in the last analysis unpersuasive.

Assisted suicide is a form of killing, which is always wrong. In contrast, withdrawing life-sustaining treatment simply allows the disease to take its course. There are three methods of hastening the death of a dying patient: withdrawing life-sustaining treatment, assisting suicide, and euthanasia. The right to stop treatment has been recognized repeatedly since the 1976 case of Karen Ann Quinlan[10] and was affirmed by the U.S. Supreme Court in the 1990 Cruzan decision[11] and the U.S. Congress in its 1990 Patient Self-Determination Act.[12] Although the legal underpinning is the right to be free of unwanted bodily invasion, the purpose of hastening death was explicitly acknowledged. In contrast, assisted suicide and euthanasia have not been accepted; euthanasia is illegal in all states, and assisted suicide is illegal in most of them.

Why the distinctions? Most would say they turn on the doctor's role: whether it is passive or active. When life-sustaining treatment is withdrawn, the doctor's role is considered passive and the cause of death is the underlying disease, despite the fact that switching off the ventilator of a patient dependent on it looks anything but passive and would be considered homicide if done without the consent of the patient or a proxy. In contrast, euthanasia by the injection of a lethal drug is active and directly causes the patient's death. Assisting suicide by supplying the necessary drugs is considered somewhere in between, more active than switching off a ventilator but less active than injecting drugs, hence morally and legally more ambiguous.

I believe, however, that these distinctions are too doctor-centered and not sufficiently patient-centered. We should ask ourselves not so much whether the doctor's role is passive or active but whether the *patient's* role is passive or active. From that perspective, the three methods of hastening death line up quite differently. When life-sustaining treatment is withdrawn from an incompetent patient at the request of a proxy or when euthanasia is performed, the patient may be utterly passive. Indeed, either act can be performed even if the patient is unaware of the decision. In sharp contrast, assisted suicide, by definition, cannot occur without the patient's knowledge and participation. Therefore, it must be active—that is to say, voluntary. That is a crucial distinction, because it provides an inherent safeguard against abuse that is not present with the other two methods of hastening death. If the loaded term "kill" is to be used, it is not the doctor who kills, but the patient. Primarily because euthanasia can be performed without the patient's participation, I oppose its legalization in this country.

Assisted suicide is not necessary. All suffering can be relieved if care givers are sufficiently skillful and compassionate, as illustrated by the hospice movement. I have no doubt that if expert palliative care were available to everyone who needed it, there would be few requests for assisted suicide. Even under the best of circumstances, however, there will always be a few patients whose suffering simply cannot be adequately alleviated. And there will be some who would prefer suicide to any other measures available, including the withdrawal of life-sustaining treatment or the use of heavy sedation. Surely, every effort should be made to improve palliative care, as I argued 15 years ago,[13] but when those efforts are unavailing and suffering patients desperately long to end their lives, physician-assisted suicide should be allowed. The argument that permitting it would divert us from redoubling our commitment to comfort care asks these patients to pay the penalty for our failings. It is also illogical. Good comfort care and the availability of physician-assisted suicide are no more mutually exclusive than good cardiologic care and the availability of heart transplantation.

Permitting assisted suicide would put us on a moral "slippery slope." Although in itself assisted suicide might be acceptable, it would lead inexorably to involuntary euthanasia. It is impossible to avoid slippery slopes in medicine (or in any aspect of life). The issue is how and where to find a purchase. For example, we accept the right of proxies to terminate life-sustaining treatment, despite the obvious potential for abuse, because the reasons for doing so outweigh the risks. We hope our procedures will safeguard patients. In the case of assisted suicide, its voluntary nature is the best protection against sliding down a slippery slope, but we also need to ensure that the request is thoughtful and freely made. Although it is possible that we may someday decide to legalize voluntary euthanasia under certain circumstances or assisted suicide for patients who are not terminally ill, legalizing assisted suicide for the dying does not in itself make these other decisions inevitable. Interestingly, recent reports from the Netherlands, where both euthanasia and physician-assisted suicide are permitted, indicate that fears about a slippery slope there have not been borne out.[14,15,16]

Assisted suicide would be a threat to the economically and socially vulnerable. The poor, disabled, and elderly might be coerced to request it. Admittedly, overburdened families or cost-conscious doctors might pressure vulnerable patients

to request suicide, but similar wrongdoing is at least as likely in the case of withdrawing life-sustaining treatment, since that decision can be made by proxy. Yet, there is no evidence of widespread abuse. The Ninth Circuit Court recalled that it was feared *Roe* v. *Wade* would lead to coercion of poor and uneducated women to request abortions, but that did not happen. The concern that coercion is more likely in this era of managed care, although understandable, would hold suffering patients hostage to the deficiencies of our health care system. Unfortunately, no human endeavor is immune to abuses. The question is not whether a perfect system can be devised, but whether abuses are likely to be sufficiently rare to be offset by the benefits to patients who otherwise would be condemned to face the end of their lives in protracted agony.

Depressed patients would seek physician-assisted suicide rather than help for their depression. Even in the terminally ill, a request for assisted suicide might signify treatable depression, not irreversible suffering. Patients suffering greatly at the end of life may also be depressed, but the depression does not necessarily explain their decision to commit suicide or make it irrational. Nor is it simple to diagnose depression in terminally ill patients. Sadness is to be expected, and some of the vegetative symptoms of depression are similar to the symptoms of terminal illness. The success of antidepressant treatment in these circumstances is also not ensured. Although there are anecdotes about patients who changed their minds about suicide after treatment,[17] we do not have good studies of how often that happens or the relation to antidepressant treatment. Dying patients who request assisted suicide and seem depressed should certainly be strongly encouraged to accept psychiatric treatment, but I do not believe that competent patients should be *required* to accept it as a condition of receiving assistance with suicide. On the other hand, doctors would not be required to comply with all requests; they would be expected to use their judgment, just as they do in so many other types of life-and-death decisions in medical practice.

Doctors should never participate in taking life. If there is to be assisted suicide, doctors must not be involved. Although most doctors favor permitting assisted suicide under certain circumstances, many who favor it believe that doctors should not provide the assistance.[6,7] To them, doctors should be unambiguously committed to life (although most doctors who hold this view would readily honor a patient's decision to have life-sustaining treatment withdrawn). The AMA, too, seems to object to physician-assisted suicide primarily because it violates the profession's mission. Like others, I find that position too abstract.[18] The highest ethical imperative of doctors should be to provide care in whatever way best serves patients' interests, in accord with each patient's wishes, not with a theoretical commitment to preserve life no matter what the cost in suffering.[19] If a patient requests help with suicide and the doctor believes the request is appropriate, requiring someone else to provide the assistance would be a form of abandonment. Doctors who are opposed in principle need not assist, but they should make their patients aware of their position early in the relationship so that a patient who chooses to select another doctor can do so. The greatest harm we can do is to consign a desperate patient to unbearable suffering—or force the patient to seek out a stranger like Dr. Kevorkian. Contrary to the frequent assertion that permitting physician-assisted suicide would lead patients to distrust their doctors, I believe distrust is more likely to arise from uncertainty about whether a doctor will honor a patient's wishes.

Physician-assisted suicide may occasionally be warranted, but it should remain illegal. If doctors risk prosecution, they will think twice before assisting with suicide. This argument wrongly shifts the focus from the patient to the doctor. Instead of reflecting the condition and wishes of patients, assisted suicide would reflect the courage and compassion of their doctors. Thus, patients with doctors like Timothy Quill, who described in a 1991 *Journal* article how he helped a patient take her life,[20] would get the help they need and want, but similar patients with less steadfast doctors would not. That makes no sense.

People do not need assistance to commit suicide. With enough determination, they can do it themselves. This is perhaps the cruelest of the arguments against physician-assisted suicide. Many patients at the end of life are, in fact, physically unable to commit suicide on their own. Others lack the resources to do so. It has sometimes been suggested that they can simply stop eating and drinking and kill themselves that way. Although this method has been described as peaceful under certain conditions,[21] no one should count on that. The fact is that this argument leaves most patients to their suffering. Some, usually men, manage to commit suicide using violent methods. Percy Bridgman, a Nobel laureate in physics who in 1961 shot himself rather than die of metastatic cancer, said in his suicide note, "It is not decent for Society to make a man do this to himself."[22]

My father, who knew nothing of Percy Bridgman, committed suicide under similar circumstances. He was 81 and had metastatic prostate cancer. The night before he was scheduled to be admitted to the hospital, he shot himself. Like Bridgman, he thought it might be his last chance. At the time, he was not in extreme pain, nor was he close to death (his life expectancy was probably longer than six months). But he was suffering nonetheless—from nausea and the side effects of antiemetic agents, weakness, incontinence, and hopelessness. Was he depressed? He would probably have freely admitted that he was, but he would have thought it beside the point. In any case, he was an intensely private man who would have refused psychiatric care. Was he overly concerned with maintaining control of the circumstances of his life and death? Many people would say so, but that was the way he was. It is the job of medicine to deal with patients as they are, not as we would like them to be.

I tell my father's story here because it makes an abstract issue very concrete. If physician-assisted suicide had been available, I have no doubt my father would have chosen it. He was protective of his family, and if he had felt he had the choice, he would have spared my mother the shock of finding his body. He did not tell her what he planned to do, because he knew she would stop him. I also believe my father would have waited if physician-assisted suicide had been available. If patients have access to drugs they can take when they choose, they will not feel they must commit suicide early, while they are still able to do it on their own. They would probably live longer and certainly more peacefully, and they might not even use the drugs.

Long before my father's death, I believed that physician-assisted suicide ought to be permissible under some circumstances, but his death strengthened my conviction that it is simply a part of good medical care—something to be done reluctantly and sadly, as a last resort, but done nonetheless. There should be safeguards to ensure that the decision is well considered and consistent, but they should not be so daunting or violative of privacy that they become obstacles instead of protections. In particular, they should be directed not toward reviewing the reasons for an autonomous decision, but only toward ensuring that the decision is indeed autonomous. If the Supreme Court upholds the decisions of the appeals courts, assisted suicide will not be forced on either patients or doctors, but it will be a choice for those patients who need it and those doctors willing to help. If, on the other hand, the Supreme Court overturns the lower courts' decisions, the issue will continue to be grappled with state by state, through the political process. But sooner or later, given the need and the widespread public support, physician-assisted suicide will be demanded of a compassionate profession.

References

1. Greenhouse L. High court to say if the dying have a right to suicide help. New York Times. October 2, 1996:A1.

2. Compassion in Dying v. Washington, 79 F.3d 790 (9th Cir. 1996).

3. Quill v. Vacco, 80 F.3d 716 (2d Cir. 1996).

4. Annas GJ. Death by prescription—the Oregon initiative. N Engl J Med 1994;331:1240–3.

5. Blendon RJ, Szalay US, Knox RA. Should physicians aid their patients in dying? The public perspective. JAMA 1992;267:2658–62.

6. Bachman JG, Alcser KH, Doukas DJ, Lichtenstein RL, Corning AD, Brody H. Attitudes of Michigan physicians and the public toward legalizing physician-assisted suicide and voluntary euthanasia. N Engl J Med 1996;334:303–9.

7. Lee MA, Nelson HD, Tilden VP, Ganzini L, Schmidt TA, Tolle SW. Legalizing assisted suicide—views of physicians in Oregon. N Engl J Med 1996;334: 310–5.

8. Gianelli DM. AMA to court: no suicide aid. American Medical News. November 25, 1996:1, 27, 28.

9. Dworkin R. Sex, death, and the courts. New York Review of Books. August 8, 1996.

10. In re: Quinlan, 70 N.J. 10, 355 A.2d 647 (1976).

11. Cruzan v. Director, Missouri Department of Health, 497 U.S. 261, 110 S.Ct. 2841 (1990).

12. Omnibus Budget Reconciliation Act of 1990, P.L. 101–508, sec. 4206 and 4751, 104 Stat. 1388, 1388–115, and 1388–204 (classified respectively at 42 U.S.C. 1395cc(f) (Medicare) and 1396a(w) (Medicaid) (1994)).

13. Angell M. The quality of mercy. N Engl J Med 1982; 306:98–9.

14. van der Maas PJ, van der Wal G, Haverkate I, et al. Euthanasia, physician-assisted suicide, and other medical practices involving the end of life in the Netherlands, 1990–1995. N Engl J Med 1996;335:1699–705.

15. van der Wal G, van der Maas PJ, Bosma JM, et al. Evaluation of the notification procedure for physician-assisted death in the Netherlands. N Engl J Med 1996;335:1706–11.

16. Angell M. Euthanasia in the Netherlands—good news or bad? N Engl J Med 1996;335:1676–8.

17. Chochinov HM, Wilson KG, Enns M, et al. Desire for death in the terminally ill. Am J Psychiatry 1995; 152:1185–91.

18. Cassel CK, Meier DE. Morals and moralism in the debate over euthanasia and assisted suicide. N Engl J Med 1990;323:750–2.

19. Angell M. Doctors and assisted suicide. Ann R Coll Physicians Surg Can 1991;24:493–4.

20. Quill TE. Death and dignity—a case of individualized decision making. N Engl J Med 1991;324:691–4.

21. Lynn J, Childress JF. Must patients always be given food and water? Hastings Cent Rep 1983;13(5):17–21.

22. Nuland SB. How we die. New York: Alfred A. Knopf, 1994:152.

MARCIA ANGELL is a senior lecturer in the Department of Social Medicine at Harvard Medical School and the former editor-in-chief of *The New England Journal of Medicine*.

Kathleen M. Foley 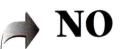 **NO**

Competent Care for the Dying Instead of Physician-Assisted Suicide

While the Supreme Court is reviewing the decisions by the Second and Ninth Circuit Courts of Appeals to reverse state bans on assisted suicide, there is a unique opportunity to engage the public, health care professionals, and the government in a national discussion of how American medicine and society should address the needs of dying patients and their families. Such a discussion is critical if we are to understand the process of dying from the point of view of patients and their families and to identify existing barriers to appropriate, humane, compassionate care at the end of life. Rational discourse must replace the polarized debate over physician-assisted suicide and euthanasia. Facts, not anecdotes, are necessary to establish a common ground and frame a system of health care for the terminally ill that provides the best possible quality of living while dying.

The biased language of the appeals courts evinces little respect for the vulnerability and dependency of the dying. Judge Stephen Reinhardt, writing for the Ninth Circuit Court, applied the liberty-interest clause of the Fourteenth Amendment, advocating a constitutional right to assisted suicide. He stated, "The competent terminally ill adult, having lived nearly the full measure of his life, has a strong interest in choosing a dignified and humane death, rather than being reduced to a state of helplessness, diapered, sedated, incompetent."[1] Judge Roger J. Miner, writing for the Second Circuit Court of Appeals, applied the equal-rights clause of the Fourteenth Amendment and went on to emphasize that the state "has no interest in prolonging a life that is ending."[2] This statement is more than legal jargon. It serves as a chilling reminder of the low priority given to the dying when it comes to state resources and protection.

The appeals courts' assertion of a constitutional right to assisted suicide is narrowly restricted to the terminally ill. The courts have decided that it is the patient's condition that justifies killing and that the terminally ill are special—so special that they deserve assistance in dying. This group alone can receive such assistance. The courts' response to the New York and Washington cases they reviewed is the

dangerous form of affirmative action in the name of compassion. It runs the risk of further devaluing the lives of terminally ill patients and may provide the excuse for society to abrogate its responsibility for their care.

Both circuit courts went even further in asserting that physicians are already assisting in patients' deaths when they withdraw life-sustaining treatments such as respirators or administer high doses of pain medication that hasten death. The appeals courts argued that providing a lethal prescription to allow a terminally ill patient to commit suicide is essentially the same as withdrawing life-sustaining treatment or aggressively treating pain. Judicial reasoning that eliminates the distinction between letting a person die and killing runs counter to physicians' standards of palliative care.[3] The courts' purported goal in blurring these distinctions was to bring society's legal rules more closely in line with the moral value it places on the relief of suffering.[4]

In the real world in which physicians care for dying patients, withdrawing treatment and aggressively treating pain are acts that respect patients' autonomous decisions not to be battered by medical technology and to be relieved of their suffering. The physician's intent is to provide care, not death. Physicians do struggle with doubts about their own intentions.[5] The courts' arguments fuel their ambivalence about withdrawing life-sustaining treatments or using opioid or sedative infusions to treat intractable symptoms in dying patients. Physicians are trained and socialized to preserve life. Yet saying that physicians struggle with doubts about their intentions in performing these acts is not the same as saying that their intention is to kill. In palliative care, the goal is to relieve suffering, and the quality of life, not the quantity, is of utmost importance.

Whatever the courts say, specialists in palliative care do not think that they practice physician-assisted suicide or euthanasia.[6] Palliative medicine has developed guidelines for aggressive pharmacologic management of intractable symptoms in dying patients, including sedation for those near death.[3,7,8] The World Health Organization has endorsed palliative care as an integral component of a national health care policy and has strongly recommended to its member countries that they not consider legalizing physician-assisted suicide and euthanasia until they have addressed the needs of their citizens for pain relief and palliative care.[9] The courts have disregarded this formidable recommendation and, in fact, are indirectly suggesting that the World Health Organization supports assisted suicide.

Yet the courts' support of assisted suicide reflects the requests of the physicians who initiated the suits and parallels the numerous surveys demonstrating that a large proportion of physicians support the legalization of physician-assisted suicide.[10,11,12,13,14,15] A smaller proportion of physicians are willing to provide such assistance, and an even smaller proportion are willing to inject a lethal dose of medication with the intent of killing a patient (active voluntary euthanasia). These survey data reveal a gap between the attitudes and behavior of physicians; 20 to 70 percent of physicians favor the legalization of physician-assisted suicide, but only 2 to 4 percent favor active voluntary euthanasia, and only approximately 2 to 13 percent have actually aided patients in dying, by either providing a prescription or administering a lethal injection. The limitations of these surveys, which are legion, include inconsistent definitions of physician-assisted suicide and euthanasia, lack of information about nonrespondents, and provisions for maintaining confidentiality that have led to inaccurate reporting.[13,16] Since physicians' attitudes toward alternatives to assisted suicide have not been studied, there is a void in our knowledge about the priority that physicians place on physician-assisted suicide.

The willingness of physicians to assist patients in dying appears to be determined by numerous complex factors, including religious beliefs, personal values, medical specialty, age, practice setting, and perspective on the use of financial resources.[13,16,17,18,19] Studies of patients' preferences for care at the end of life demonstrate that physicians' preferences strongly influence those of their patients.[13] Making physician-assisted suicide a medical treatment when it is so strongly dependent on these physician-related variables would result in a regulatory impossibility.[19] Physicians would have to disclose their values and attitudes to patients to avoid potential conflict.[13] A survey by Ganzini et al. demonstrated that psychiatrists' responses to requests to evaluate patients were highly determined by their attitudes.[13] In a study by Emanuel et al., depressed patients with cancer said they would view positively those physicians who acknowledged their willingness to assist in suicide. In contrast, patients with cancer who were suffering from pain would be suspicious of such physicians.[11]

In this controversy, physicians fall into one of three groups. Those who support physician-assisted suicide see it as a compassionate response to a medical need, a symbol of nonabandonment, and a means to reestablish patients' trust in doctors who have used technology excessively.[20] They argue that regulation of physician-assisted suicide is possible and, in fact, necessary to control the actions of physicians who are currently providing assistance surreptitiously.[21] The two remaining groups of physicians oppose legalization.[19, 22, 23, 24] One group is morally opposed to physician-assisted suicide and emphasizes the need to preserve the professionalism of medicine and the commitment to "do no harm." These physicians view aiding a patient in dying as a form of abandonment, because a physician needs to walk the last mile with the patient, as a witness, not as an executioner. Legalization would endorse justified killing, according to these physicians, and guidelines would not be followed, even if they could be developed. Furthermore, these physicians are concerned that the conflation of assisted suicide with the withdrawal of life support or adequate treatment of pain would make it even harder for dying patients, because there would be a backlash against existing policies. The other group is not ethically opposed to physician-assisted suicide and, in fact, sees it as acceptable in exceptional cases, but these physicians believe that one cannot regulate the unregulatable.[19] On this basis, the New York State Task Force on Life and the Law, a 24-member committee with broad public and professional representation, voted unanimously against the legalization of physician-assisted suicide.[24] All three groups of physicians agree that a national effort is needed to improve the care of the dying. Yet it does seem that those in favor of legalizing physician-assisted suicide are disingenuous in their use of this issue as a wedge. If this form of assistance with dying is legalized, the courts will be forced to broaden the assistance to include active voluntary euthanasia and, eventually, assistance in response to requests from proxies.

One cannot easily categorize the patients who request physician-assisted suicide or euthanasia. Some surveys of physicians have attempted to determine retrospectively the prevalence and nature of these requests.[10] Pain, AIDS, and neurodegenerative disorders are the most common conditions in patients requesting assistance in dying. There is a wide range in the age of such patients, but many are younger persons with AIDS.[10] From the limited data available, the factors most commonly involved in requests for assistance are concern about future loss of control, being or becoming a burden to others, or being unable to care for oneself and fear of severe pain.[10] A small number of recent studies have directly asked terminally ill patients with cancer or AIDS about their desire for death.[25,26,27] All these studies show that the desire for death is closely associated with depression and that pain and lack of social support are contributing factors.

Do we know enough, on the basis of several legal cases, to develop a public policy that will profoundly change medicine's role in society?[1,2] Approximately 2.4 million Americans die each year. We have almost no information on how they die and only general information on where they die. Sixty-one percent die in hospitals, 17 percent in nursing homes, and the remainder at home, with approximately 10 to 14 percent of those at home receiving hospice care.

The available data suggest that physicians are inadequately trained to assess and manage the multifactorial symptoms commonly associated with patients' requests for physician-assisted suicide. According to the American Medical Association's report on medical education, only 5 of 126 medical schools in the United States require a separate course in the care of the dying.[28] Of 7048 residency programs, only 26 percent offer a course on the medical and legal aspects of care at the end of life as a regular part of the curriculum. According to a survey of 1068 accredited residency programs in family medicine, internal medicine, and pediatrics and fellowship programs in geriatrics, each resident or fellow coordinates the care of 10 or fewer dying patients annually.[28] Almost 15 percent of the programs offer no formal training in terminal care. Despite the availability of hospice programs, only 17 percent of the training programs offer a hospice rotation, and the rotation is required in only half of those programs; 9 percent of the programs have residents or fellows serving as members of hospice teams. In a recent survey of 55 residency programs and over 1400 residents, conducted by the American Board of Internal Medicine, the residents were asked to rate their perception of adequate training in care at the end of life. Seventy-two percent reported that they had received adequate training in managing pain and other symptoms; 62 percent, that they had received adequate training in telling patients that they are dying; 38 percent, in describing what the process will be like; and 32 percent, in talking to patients who request assistance in dying or a hastened death (Blank L: personal communication).

The lack of training in the care of the dying is evident in practice. Several studies have concluded that poor communication between physicians and patients, physicians' lack of knowledge about national guidelines for such care, and their lack of knowledge about the control of symptoms are barriers to the provision of good care at the end of life.[23,29,30]

Yet there is now a large body of data on the components of suffering in patients with advanced terminal disease, and these data provide the basis for treatment algorithms.[3] There are three major factors in suffering:

pain and other physical symptoms, psychological distress, and existential distress (described as the experience of life without meaning). It is not only the patients who suffer but also their families and the health care professionals attending them. These experiences of suffering are often closely and inextricably related. Perceived distress in any one of the three groups amplifies distress in the others.[31,32]

Pain is the most common symptom in dying patients, and according to recent data from U.S. studies, 56 percent of outpatients with cancer, 82 percent of outpatients with AIDS, 50 percent of hospitalized patients with various diagnoses, and 36 percent of nursing home residents have inadequate management of pain during the course of their terminal illness.[33,34,35,36] Members of minority groups and women, both those with cancer and those with AIDS, as well as the elderly, receive less pain treatment than other groups of patients. In a survey of 1177 physicians who had treated a total of more than 70,000 patients with cancer in the previous six months, 76 percent of the respondents cited lack of knowledge as a barrier to their ability to control pain.[37] Severe pain that is not adequately controlled interferes with the quality of life, including the activities of daily living, sleep, and social interactions.[33,38]

Other physical symptoms are also prevalent among the dying. Studies of patients with advanced cancer and of the elderly in the year before death show that they have numerous symptoms that worsen the quality of life, such as fatigue, dyspnea, delirium, nausea, and vomiting.[36,38]

Along with these physical symptoms, dying patients have a variety of well-described psychological symptoms, with a high prevalence of anxiety and depression in patients with cancer or AIDS and the elderly.[27,39] For example, more than 60 percent of patients with advanced cancer have psychiatric problems, with adjustment disorders, depression, anxiety, and delirium reported most frequently. Various factors that contribute to the prevalence and severity of psychological distress in the terminally ill have been identified.[39] The diagnosis of depression is difficult to make in medically ill patients[3,26,40]; 94 percent of the Oregon psychiatrists surveyed by Ganzini et al. were not confident that they could determine, in a single evaluation, whether a psychiatric disorder was impairing the judgment of a patient who requested assistance with suicide.[13]

Attention has recently been focused on the interaction between uncontrolled symptoms and vulnerability to suicide in patients with cancer or AIDS.[41] Data from studies of both groups of patients suggest that uncontrolled pain contributes to depression and that persistent pain interferes with patients' ability to receive support from their families and others. Patients with AIDS have a high risk of suicide that is independent of physical symptoms.

Among New York City residents with AIDS, the relative risk of suicide in men between the ages of 20 and 59 years was 36 times higher than the risk among men without AIDS in the same age group and 66 times higher than the risk in the general population.[41] Patients with AIDS who committed suicide generally did so within nine months after receiving the diagnosis; 25 percent had made a previous suicide attempt, 50 percent had reported severe depression, and 40 percent had seen a psychiatrist within four days before committing suicide. As previously noted, the desire to die is most closely associated with the diagnosis of depression.[26,27] Suicide is the eighth leading cause of death in the United States, and the incidence of suicide is higher in patients with cancer or AIDS and in elderly men than in the general population. Conwell and Caine reported that depression was underdiagnosed by primary care physicians in a cohort of elderly patients who subsequently committed suicide; 75 percent of the patients had seen a primary care physician during the last month of life but had not received a diagnosis of depression.[22]

The relation between depression and the desire to hasten death may vary among subgroups of dying patients. We have no data, except for studies of a small number of patients with cancer or AIDS. The effect of treatment for depression on the desire to hasten death and on requests for assistance in doing so has not been examined in the medically ill population, except for a small study in which four of six patients who initially wished to hasten death changed their minds within two weeks.[26]

There is also the concern that certain patients, particularly members of minority groups that are estranged from the health care system, may be reluctant to receive treatment for their physical or psychological symptoms because of the fear that their physicians will, in fact, hasten death. There is now some evidence that the legalization of assisted suicide in the Northern Territory of Australia has undermined the Aborigines' trust in the medical care system[42]; this experience may serve as an example for the United States, with its multicultural population.

The multiple physical and psychological symptoms in the terminally ill and elderly are compounded by a substantial degree of existential distress. Reporting on their interviews with Washington State physicians whose patients had requested assistance in dying, Back et al. noted the physicians' lack of sophistication in assessing such nonphysical suffering.[10]

In summary, there are fundamental physician-related barriers to appropriate, humane, and compassionate care for the dying. These range from attitudinal and behavioral barriers to educational and economic barriers. Physicians do not know enough about their patients,

themselves, or suffering to provide assistance with dying as a medical treatment for the relief of suffering. Physicians need to explore their own perspectives on the meaning of suffering in order to develop their own approaches to the care of the dying. They need insight into how the nature of the doctor-patient relationship influences their own decision making. If legalized, physician-assisted suicide will be a substitute for rational therapeutic, psychological, and social interventions that might otherwise enhance the quality of life for patients who are dying. The medical profession needs to take the lead in developing guidelines for good care of dying patients. Identifying the factors related to physicians, patients, and the health care system that pose barriers to appropriate care at the end of life should be the first step in a national dialogue to educate health care professionals and the public on the topic of death and dying. Death is an issue that society as a whole faces, and it requires a compassionate response. But we should not confuse compassion with competence in the care of terminally ill patients.

References

1. Reinhardt, Compassion in Dying v. State of Washington, 79 F. 3d 790 9th Cir. 1996.
2. Miner, Quill v. Vacco 80 F. 3d 716 2nd Cir. 1996.
3. Doyle D, Hanks GWC, MacDonald N. The Oxford textbook of palliative medicine. New York: Oxford University Press, 1993.
4. Orentlicher D. The legalization of physician-assisted suicide. N Engl J Med 1996;335:663–7.
5. Wilson WC, Smedira NG, Fink C, McDowell JA, Luce JM. Ordering and administration of sedatives and analgesics during the withholding and withdrawal of life support from critically ill patients. JAMA 1992; 267:949–53.
6. Foley KM. The relationship of pain and symptom management to patient requests for physician-assisted suicide. J Pain Symptom Manage 1991;6:289–97.
7. Cherny NI, Coyle N, Foley KM. Guidelines in the care of the dying patient. Hematol Oncol Clin North Am 1996;10:261–86.
8. Cherny NI, Portenoy RK. Sedation in the management of refractory symptoms: guidelines for evaluation and treatment. J Palliat Care 1994;10(2): 31–8.
9. Cancer pain relief and palliative care. Geneva: World Health Organization, 1989.
10. Back AL, Wallace JI, Starks HE, Pearlman RA. Physician-assisted suicide and euthanasia in Washington State: patient requests and physician responses. JAMA 1996;275:919–25.

11. Emanuel EJ, Fairclough DL, Daniels ER, Clarridge BR. Euthanasia and physician-assisted suicide: attitudes and experiences of oncology patients, oncologists, and the public. Lancet 1996;347:1805–10.

12. Lee MA, Nelson HD, Tilden VP, Ganzini L, Schmidt TA, Tolle SW. Legalizing assisted suicide—views of physicians in Oregon. N Engl J Med 1996;334: 310–5.

13. Ganzini L, Fenn DS, Lee MA, Heintz RT, Bloom JD. Attitudes of Oregon psychiatrists toward physician-assisted suicide. Am J Psychiatry 1996; 153:1469–75.

14. Cohen JS, Fihn SD, Boyko EJ, Jonsen AR, Wood RW. Attitudes toward assisted suicide and euthanasia among physicians in Washington State. N Engl J Med 1994;331:89–94.

15. Doukas DJ, Waterhouse D, Gorenflo DW, Seid J. Attitudes and behaviors on physician-assisted death: a study of Michigan oncologists. J Clin Oncol 1995;13:1055–61.

16. Morrison S, Meier D. Physician-assisted dying: fashioning public policy with an absence of data. Generations. Winter 1994:48–53.

17. Portenoy RK, Coyle N, Kash K, et al. Determinants of the willingness to endorse assisted suicide: a survey of physicians, nurses, and social workers. Psychosomatics (in press).

18. Fins J. Physician-assisted suicide and the right to care. Cancer Control 1996;3:272–8.

19. Callahan D, White M. The legalization of physician-assisted suicide: creating a regulatory Potemkin Village. U Richmond Law Rev 1996;30:1–83.

20. Quill TE. Death and dignity—a case of individualized decision making. N Engl J Med 1991;324:691–4.

21. Quill TE, Cassel CK, Meier DE. Care of the hopelessly ill—proposed clinical criteria for physician-assisted suicide. N Engl J Med 1992;327:1380–4.

22. Conwell Y, Caine ED. Rational suicide and the right to die—reality and myth. N Engl J Med 1991;325:1100–3.

23. Foley KM. Pain, physician assisted suicide and euthanasia. Pain Forum 1995;4:163–78.

24. When death is sought: assisted suicide and euthanasia in the medical context. New York: New York State Task Force on Life and the Law, May 1994.

25. Brown JH, Henteleff P, Barakat S, Rowe CJ. Is it normal for terminally ill patients to desire death? Am J Psychiatry 1986;143:208–11.

26. Chochinov HM, Wilson KG, Enns M, et al. Desire for death in the terminally ill. Am J Psychiatry 1995;152:1185–91.

27. Breitbart W, Rosenfeld BD, Passik SD. Interest in physician-assisted suicide among ambulatory HIV-infected patients. Am J Psychiatry 1996;153:238–42.

28. Hill TP. Treating the dying patient: the challenge for medical education. Arch Intern Med 1995;155:1265–9.

29. Callahan D. Once again reality: now where do we go? Hastings Cent Rep 1995;25(6):Suppl:S33–S36.

30. Solomon MZ, O'Donnell L, Jennings B, et al. Decisions near the end of life: professional views on life-sustaining treatments. Am J Public Health 1993; 83:14–23.

31. Cherny NI, Coyle N, Foley KM. Suffering in the advanced cancer patient: definition and taxonomy. J Palliat Care 1994;10(2):57–70.

32. Cassel EJ. The nature of suffering and the goals of medicine. N Engl J Med 1982;306:639–45.

33. Cleeland CS, Gonin R, Hatfield AK, et al. Pain and its treatment in outpatients with metastatic cancer. N Engl J Med 1994;330:592–6.

34. Breitbart W, Rosenfeld BD, Passik SD, McDonald MV, Thaler H, Portenoy RK. The undertreatment of pain in ambulatory AIDS patients. Pain 1996; 65:243–9.

35. The SUPPORT Principal Investigators. A controlled trial to improve care for seriously ill hospitalized patients. JAMA 1995;274:1591–8.

36. Seale C, Cartwright A. The year before death. Hants, England: Avebury, 1994.

37. Von Roenn JH, Cleeland CS, Gonin R, Hatfield AK, Pandya KJ. Physician attitudes and practice in cancer pain management: a survey from the Eastern Cooperative Oncology Group. Ann Intern Med 1993;119:121–6.

38. Portenoy RK. Pain and quality of life: clinical issues and implications for research. Oncology 1990;4:172–8.

39. Breitbart W. Suicide risk and pain in cancer and AIDS patients. In: Chapman CR, Foley KM, eds. Current and emerging issues in cancer pain. New York: Raven Press, 1993.

40. Chochinov H, Wilson KG, Enns M, Lander S. Prevalence of depression in the terminally ill: effects of diagnostic criteria and symptom threshold judgments. Am J Psychiatry 1994;151:537–40.

41. Passik S, McDonald M, Rosenfeld B, Breitbart W. End of life issues in patients with AIDS: clinical and research considerations. J Pharm Care Pain Symptom Control 1995;3:91–111.

42. NT "success" in easing rural fear of euthanasia. The Age. August 31, 1996:A7.

KATHLEEN M. FOLEY holds The Society of Memorial Sloan-Kettering Cancer Center chair in pain research. She is a professor of neurology and pharmacology at the Weill Medical College of Cornell University and attending neurologist in the Pain and Palliative Care Service at Memorial Sloan-Kettering, New York City.

EXPLORING THE ISSUE

Should Physicians Be Allowed to Assist in Patient Suicide?

Critical Thinking and Reflection

1. In your view, does a person's autonomy ever encompass a right to end one's own life? If so, under what circumstances and with what safeguards?
2. What is the most compelling reason for permitting physician-assisted suicide—the curtailment of the patient's suffering or the completion of the patient's life plans?
3. If a patient who expresses a desire to die is diagnosed with depression, should the depression be treated before agreeing to help the patient die?
4. If physician-assisted death is permitted, would the physician's role as caregiver be undermined? Do you see physician-assisted death more as a case of commitment to patients or abandonment of patients? Why?

Is There Common Ground?

In 1997, Oregon became the first state to implement a law legalizing physician-assisted suicide. The Death with Dignity Act was originally passed in 1994, but its implementation was delayed until 1997, when it was upheld by a large majority of voters. Under this law, a person who is mentally competent and suffering from a terminal illness (likely to die within 6 months) may receive lethal drugs from a physician. The person has to consult two doctors and wait 15 days before obtaining the drugs. A similar law was enacted in Washington in 2008, and the Montana Supreme Court decision in the 2010 case *Baxter v. Montana* has made physician-assisted suicide permissible in Montana. Efforts to make physician-assisted suicide legal in other states have so far failed but have not stopped. The Death with Dignity Act was offered as a ballot measure in Massachusetts in 2012.

Very few patients in Oregon actually use the option of requesting physician-assisted suicide, and the number has remained stable since 2002. Fewer than 1,000 people have obtained prescriptions for drugs to end their lives, and about 600 have actually used the drugs, according to Oregon's Public Health Division. Those most likely to request drugs were married, white, more highly educated, and had cancer as a primary diagnosis. Physicians who wrote prescriptions have reported that patient requests stemmed from concerns related to loss of autonomy, decreasing ability to participate in enjoyable activities, and loss of dignity, rather than unbearable pain. Nearly all patients were enrolled in hospice and had health insurance.

Washington's experience with physician-assisted suicide has been similar so far to Oregon's.

In the Netherlands, euthanasia—defined as "the intentional termination of the life of a patient at his or her request by a physician"—was legalized in 2002. The practice had occurred before 2002 without repercussions for the physician. About 9,700 requests are made each year. Those who oppose the practice claim that not all requests are voluntary.

Additional Resources

Information about the experience in Oregon is available from the Oregon Department of Human Services and is available at http://public.health.oregon .gov/ProviderPartnerResources/EvaluationResearch/ DeathwithDignityAct/Pages/index.aspx.

Susan Tolle and colleagues have published research on how many people in Oregon consider physician-assisted suicide as compared to the number who follow through with it, and on the barriers to fulfilling their intentions (Susan W. Tolle et al., "Characteristics and Proportion of Dying Oregonians Who Personally Consider Physician-Assisted Suicide," *Journal of Clinical Ethics* [Summer 2004]).

In "Legal Regulation of Physician-Assisted Death—The Latest Report Cards," *The New England Journal of Medicine* (May 10, 2007), Timothy E. Quill concludes that legalization has resulted in more open conversation and careful evaluation of end-of-life options.

In November 2008, voters in the state of Washington approved a measure similar to Oregon's law. In 1991, voters rejected a bill that would allow doctors to administer the lethal medications; the 2008 version requires patients to take the medications on their own.

A review of the impact in Oregon and the Netherlands of physician-assisted suicide on "vulnerable" groups such as the elderly, women, people with low educational status, racial and ethnic minorities, and people with psychiatric illness found no evidence that these groups were disproportionately involved. The only people with a heightened risk were people with AIDS. Those who received physician-assisted suicide were more likely to be better educated, have more economic and social resources, and professional status (Margaret P. Battin et al., "Legal Physician-Assisted Dying in Oregon and the Netherlands: Evidence Concerning the Impact on Patients in 'Vulnerable' Groups," *Journal of Medical Ethics* [2007]).

Physician-Assisted Dying: The Case for Palliative Care and Patient Choice, edited by Timothy E. Quill and Margaret P. Battin, is a collection of articles that presents the case for the legalization of physician-assisted dying (Johns Hopkins University Press, 2004). Opposing the practice are the authors in *The Case Against Assisted Suicide*, edited by Kathleen E. Foley and Herbert Hendin (Johns Hopkins University Press, 2002). See also Arthur L. Caplan, Lois Snyder, and Kathy Feber-Langendoen, "The Role of Guidelines in the Practice of Physician-Assisted Suicide," *Annals of Internal Medicine* (March 21, 2000). The entire issue is devoted to this subject.

Internet References . . .

American Academy of Hospice and Palliative Medicine

http://aahpm.org/

Euthanasia and Physician-Assisted Suicide: All Sides of the Issues

http://www.religioustolerance.org/euthanas.htm

U.S. Catholic Conference of Bishops

http://www.usccb.org/issues-and-action/human-life -and-dignity/assisted-suicide/

Unit 3

UNIT

Choices in Reproduction

*F*ew bioethical issues are more hotly contested than questions concerning reproduction. The most polarized question remains the morality of abortion, where common ground has been elusive for many decades. Advances in medical technology, such as in vitro fertilization and egg donation, have opened up new fronts in the battle over abortion at the same time that they have opened new possibilities for infertile couples while challenging traditional notions of family. Another type of technological advance—the ability to see images of the developing fetus—has enhanced our understanding of normal fetal growth and of birth defects. How can we responsibly use these technologies to help people have families, giving adults greater powers to choose to have children—and perhaps to choose which child to have—while protecting our traditional understanding of what's morally important about children and about the parent-child relationship?

Medical advances have also given us greater insight into the circumstances that lead to normal fetal growth and those that cause fetal abnormalities. While many behaviors of pregnant women expose fetuses to risk, and while fathers' exposure to chemicals and other toxic substances also affects fetuses, attention has focused mainly on the mothers' use of illegal drugs. Preventing risk to fetuses raises troubling questions concerning the role of police and the courts in medical matters and the best way to assist drug-addicted women. The issues in this unit come to grips with some of the most perplexing and fundamental questions that confront medical practitioners, individual women and their partners, and society in general.

Selected, Edited, and with Issue Framing Material by:
Gregory E. Kaebnick, *The Hastings Center*

ISSUE

Should Embryos Produced During IVF Be Considered Children?

YES: Thomas Brejcha et al., from "Brief of Amici Curiae Missouri Right to Life, Lawyers for Life, and American Association of Pro-Life Obstetricians & Gynecologists," *Gadberry v. McQueen*, Missouri Court of Appeals Eastern District (2015)

NO: Joseph J. Kodner and John M. Faust, from "Brief of Amicus Curiae American Society for Reproductive Medicine in Support of Respondent," *Gadberry v. McQueen*, Missouri Court of Appeals Eastern District (2016)

Learning Outcomes

After reading this issue, you will be able to:

- Discuss the ethical dilemma posed by abortion.
- Discuss how different views of the embryo's status might affect reproductive medicine.
- Describe the concept of personhood and the connection to personhood of scientific information about embryonic development.

ISSUE SUMMARY

YES: In a friend-of-the-court brief submitted in a recent case in Missouri involving a dispute over embryos that a couple had put into storage, lawyers for the American Society for Reproductive Medicine argue that embryos are not persons and that treating them as such would have a profound negative effect on people who seek medical assistance in building their families.

NO: In a friend-of-the-court brief on the other side of the same case, lawyers representing several organizations that are opposed to abortion argue that science proves straightforwardly that embryos are persons, and that the embryos in the Missouri custody dispute should be given to the parent who seeks to take care of them.

Abortion has been one the most divisive bioethical issues of our time. The issue has been a persistent one in history, but in the past 40 years or so it has been particularly deeply polarized. One view—known as "pro-life"—sees abortion as the wanton slaughter of innocent life. The other view—"pro-choice"—considers abortion as an option that must be available to women if they are to control their own reproductive lives and therefore enjoy the same freedoms as men. According to the pro-life view, a human being is created at the moment of conception—at the moment that a human egg and sperm conjoin to form an embryo. Although that single cell undergoes constant division and development, it is impossible to identify (according to the pro-life view) any one moment at which an embryo can be said to have suddenly become a person. Moreover, a belief that we should protect the weakest among us and avoid making distinctions among human beings on the basis of their abilities should generate a moral commitment not to make any arbitrary distinctions.

According to the pro-choice view, women have the right to choose to have an abortion, especially if there are important issues at stake, such as preventing the birth of a child with a severe genetic defect or choosing not to become a parent as a result of rape or incest. In the pro-choice view, human organisms are not necessarily persons, and it is the killing of persons that is unacceptable.

Some pro-choice positions also incorporate some elements of pro-life positions. Gradualist positions, for instance, hold that early-stage embryos do not warrant protections but that late-stage fetuses, while not necessarily full persons, are close enough to being persons that should not be killed. Maggie Little holds that embryos and fetuses are not persons but that they are "burgeoning human life" and deserve respect; moreover, Little holds that a woman may become committed to a developing human life in a way that generates moral duties toward it. In his book *Life's Dominion*, Ronald Dworkin holds that both biological human life and personhood possess value but that an examination of personhood nonetheless supports a defense of the right to choose abortion; it is therefore possible to believe, he argues, that abortion is morally wicked yet that women must be given the right to choose abortion.

Behind the strongly held convictions about the moral status of the fetus, as political scientist Mary Segers has pointed out, are widely differing views about what determines value (for example, whether value is inherent in a thing, is determined by God, or is ascribed to things in the world by human beings), the relationship between morality and law, and the use and limits of political solutions to social problems. Those who condemn abortion as immoral generally follow a classical tradition in which abortion is a public matter because it involves our conception of how we should live together in an ideal society. Those who accept the idea of abortion on the other hand, generally the liberal, individualistic ethos of contemporary society. They believe that abortion is a private choice and that public policy should reflect how citizens behave, not some unattainable ideal.

In the past decade, the debate about abortion has generated a number of subsidiary debates, such as whether particular abortion methods (such as the so-called "partial-birth abortion" or "intact dilation and evacuation") may be prohibited, whether limits to abortion may be imposed based on fetal sentience (which occurs earlier than viability), whether special restrictions may be imposed on doctors who perform abortions in order to protect the health of pregnant women, and what kinds of counseling should be required for women who request an abortion. A movement has also emerged to attack *Roe v. Wade* by passing "personhood" measures, which would aim to change the legal definitions of the word "person" to explicitly include a fertilized egg, embryo, or fetus. Passing such a law in the form of a constitutional amendment would have the effect of outlawing abortion; most proposed personhood laws, however, are proposed at the state level. In 2008, some pro-life groups banded together to form a national group called Personhood USA to press for personhood measures across the country, sometimes by supporting citizen-initiated ballot measures and sometimes through state legislation. As of 2016, none of the personhood measures had yet become law, although according to data from NARAL, 20 personhood bills were introduced in 2015. Such laws would not be constitutional, since they would be in conflict with *Roe v. Wade.*

Given the difficulty so far of passing personhood measures and the constitutional bar that would invalidate them, those who are pro-life are deeply split about their political advisability. Some, advocating for a more patient and incremental approach, have cautioned against them, worrying that advocating for personhood measures may actually be counterproductive. A fallback position is adoption of a measure that incorporates explicit language recognizing that the law must be applied in a manner that accords with the rulings of the Supreme Court concerning abortion.

The readings below address a Missouri law passed in 1986 that takes this fallback position. It declares that every human being is a person from conception, but it also acknowledges that it is subject to the decisions of the Supreme Court, as indeed any law must be. The law nonetheless provides an interesting and important opportunity for thinking about the moral status of embryos, and perhaps introducing and advocating for the idea that embryos should be treated as human beings, because of the possibility that it can support constitutionally acceptable policy protecting embryos that have been created and are maintained outside a woman's body. The readings below are amicus briefs—friend-of-the-court briefs—submitted by pro-life and pro-choice groups, respectively, on opposite sides of a case that involves a dispute over embryos that a couple had put into storage. Representatives of a pro-life group of attorneys argue that, given Missouri law and the current state of the science on embryonic development, the embryos should be treated as persons and should therefore be given to the parent who will protect them. Lawyers for the American Society for Reproductive Medicine, a professional medical group whose members offer in vitro fertilization to help parents conceive, argue that the embryos are not persons and that treating them as such would have harmful effects on couples seeking medical aid in having children.

YES ↵

Thomas Brejcha et al.

Brief of Amici Curiae Missouri Right to Life, Lawyers for Life, and American Association of Pro-Life Obstetricians & Gynecologists

Introduction

In February, 2007, Justin Gadberry and Jalesia McQueen-Gadberry used in vitro fertilization (IVF) to produce four human embryos. Two of them were implanted in Jalesia immediately, were brought to birth, and are now eight-year-old boys named Tristan and Brevin. The other two were cryopreserved. They still remain unthawed and unborn, because Justin's and Jalesia's marriage broke down in 2010, and since then Justin and Jalesia have not agreed on how to treat them. In the divorce case that is now on appeal to this Court, the trial court treated the two cryopreserved embryos as property, not children. But current scientific knowledge has advanced since the early days of IVF and cryopreservation procedures. The advances demonstrate that the two frozen embryos are human beings.

Moreover, Missouri law protects the rights of human beings from their very beginning pursuant to Mo. Rev. Stat. § 1.205. The trial court did not mention § 1.205 in its judgment. . . .

The consequences of this appeal to these embryonic human beings are life and death. They are not lifeless property; they are living siblings of two boys who were conceived at the same time as they were. This brief will describe current science, analyze the key Missouri statute and case law on the subject, and recommend that this Court consider the best interests of these young human beings in determining this appeal. . . .

Statement of Facts

Petitioner, Jalesia McQueen-Gadberry, now Jalesia McQueen ("Jalesia"), and Justin Gadberry ("Justin") were married in September, 2005. (Transcript of trial, p. 4. Citations to the transcript will be abbreviated in the form, "Tr. 4," hereinafter.) At the time, Justin was on active duty

in the U.S. Army at Fort Bragg, North Carolina (Tr. 79, 152). Jalesia lived and worked in the St. Louis area (Tr. 78). Jalesia asked Justin to consider storing semen even before they were married (Tr. 77, 151–152), because she was older than Justin and they wanted to have children (Id). Also, when they were married, Justin was facing deployment in the Middle East (Tr. 77, 153).

At some point after the marriage, Justin provided a sperm specimen to Jalesia's physician, Dr. Ronald Wilbois in the St. Louis area (Tr. 80, 154–155). Justin met with Dr. Wilbois before his deployment overseas, gave him the sperm specimen to freeze, but never met with him again (Tr. 155). While Justin was overseas, Jalesia attempted to become pregnant by artificial insemination from the frozen sperm, but the attempts were not successful (Tr. 78, 153).

In February, 2007, after Justin returned to Fort Bragg from Iraq, Justin consented to the use of in vitro fertilization (Tr. 155). His intention was to have children (Id.) Four embryos were created using Jalesia's eggs and the sperm that Justin had provided in 2005 (Tr. 79, 154–155). Two of the embryos were transferred to Jalesia's womb and implanted, and as a result she gave birth to twin boys, Tristan and Brevin, in November, 2007 (Tr. 80, 155). The remaining two embryonic children were cryopreserved by Dr. Wilbois and stored by him in the St. Louis area (Tr. 80).

In May, 2010, Dr. Wilbois notified Jalesia and Justin that he was retiring, and arrangements would need to be made in respect to the two frozen embryonic children that he held in storage (Tr. 80, 160). . . . The parties separated in September, 2010 (Tr. 4). Although the parties' relations afterward were apparently quite acrimonious, by the time of trial in September, 2014, the parties had agreed on the disposition of certain property and upon conditions for joint custody and visitation of Tristan and Brevin, who were then six years old (Tr. 7–9, 13–14,

176–177). However, after they separated, the parties disagreed on what should happen with the two embryonic children at the Fairfax Cryobank facility in the event of divorce (Tr. 160, 168–169). At trial, Jalesia testified that she wanted to implant them and bring them to birth (Tr. 78). The guardian ad litem for these two children pressed her on her wishes, asking whether she would accept one and allow Justin to have one, or whether she would allow one or both to be donated to another couple (Tr. 131). Jalesia rejected the first alternative on the ground she knew Justin would destroy whichever one he received (Id.). She rejected the other alternative on the basis that these were her children and both were siblings of Tristan and Brevin (Id.). She said that personally she would agree not to hold Justin financially responsible for the two children, but she also opined that course of action may be against public policy (Tr. 122). She would be willing to discuss financial support with Justin (Id.).

Justin completely rejected ever allowing the two embryonic children to be turned over to Jalesia (Tr. 170). He suggested they could be donated to an infertile couple or to a scientific research laboratory, or they could be destroyed (Tr. 171). If the only choice were between himself and Jalesia, he would take them (Id.).

He testified that the environment between himself and Jalesia was too broken to bring more children into it; notwithstanding the agreement on custody and visitation previously submitted to the Court for approval, he asserted they could not co-parent Tristan and Brevin (Id.). He would find it "absurd" and "offensive" to bring more children into the broken environment between him and Jalesia (Tr. 171–172). The parties did not have the financial and emotional resources, he claimed, to deal with two more born children (Id.). . . .

The trial court declared that the embryonic children "are not minor children as defined in RSMo. 452" (Judgment, ¶ 39). It concluded that "Missouri Courts and Legislature provide no guidance concerning these issues" (Id., ¶ 46). It ruled that the embryonic children are marital property (Id., ¶ 40), but of a unique type, because what one party does with them in the future may impose unwanted obligations on the other, and the parties' intentions expressed in the courtroom did not bind them in the future (Id., ¶¶ 41, 44). Finding the approach taken in Iowa on this issue to be persuasive, the trial court awarded the embryonic children as marital property jointly to the parties with a restriction that "no transfer, release, or use of the frozen embryos shall occur without the signed authorization of both Husband and Wife" (Id., ¶ 58). However, either one could renew the storage contracts and pay the storage fees for them unilaterally (Id., 59).

Argument

. . . I. The trial court erred in concluding that the frozen embryos produced by in vitro fertilization were not children and in awarding them as marital property, because the court had a duty to make a determination of custody of the embryos according to their best interests, in that scientific research establishes that upon fertilization, unique human beings have been produced who cannot care for themselves.

The question as to when a human being comes into existence can and should be answered based on the most recent scientific evidence relating to the inception of human life. It is not a debate for ethicists, theologians, politicians, or journalists; it is a question of demonstrable scientific fact that must be answered as such, regardless of whatever ethical or legal consequences may flow from the fact. . . .

Justin's sperm and Jalesia's eggs (oocytes) were germ cells or gametes, each containing a haploid number (½ or 23) of the chromosomes that a somatic or body cell contains (46). This makeup permits the male and female germ cells to create a single cell that has a diploid or full set of chromosomes. Maureen L. Condic, When Does Human Life Begin: Scientific Evidence and Terminology Revisited, 8 Univ. of St. Thomas J. Law & Pub. Policy 44, 76–77 (2014) ("Human Life Scientific Evidence"). . . . At the instant of sperm–oocyte plasma binding in normal (and in vitro) human reproduction, a series of biochemical and molecular events occurs generating a one-cell embryo called a zygote, whose cell composition and behavior are immediately different from that of the sperm and oocyte (Id. at 47 and 79 fig. 1. The zygote's molecular composition is unique, with sperm and oocyte-derived components. The zygote immediately behaves as a new and unique human organism, using cell components to direct his or her own development, not just as a single cell, but towards "production of interacting groups of cells, tissues, and structures in a specific spatial and temporal sequence" (Id. at 48). In other words, the zygote immediately initiates a trajectory of development that ends only with the demise of the human organism. . . .

The scientific research is clear that from the time of fertilization as a one-cell zygote, an embryo is not a mere collection or aggregate of cells, but an internally directed, dynamic organism. . . .

An organism is distinguished by the interaction of its parts "in the context of a coordinated whole." Id. . . . Condic elaborates as follows:

> From the moment of sperm-egg fusion, a human zygote acts as a complete whole, with all the parts of the zygote interacting in an orchestrated

fashion to generate the structures and relationships required for the zygote to continue developing towards its state. . . . The zygote acts immediately and decisively to initiate a program of development that will, if uninterrupted by accident, disease, or external intervention, proceed seamlessly through formation of the definitive body, birth, childhood, adolescence, maturity, and aging, ending with death. This coordinated behavior is the very hallmark of an organism (Westchester Institute White Paper at 7. . . .)

Among the symbolic sculptures at an exit of the Supreme Court of the United States is a statue of a turtle, symbolizing that the law moves slowly behind society. In *Roe v. Wade*, 410 U.S. 113 (1973), the Supreme Court characterized unborn humans as "potential life," expressly citing the scientific knowledge at the time (Id. at 159, 160, 161, and n.62). That knowledge is now more than 40 years old. The foregoing outline of current human embryology establishes that while human development is indeed a process, lasting throughout prenatal and postnatal life, it begins with a particular event, fertilization. This Court should recognize, as the trial court did not, what science now unmistakably establishes and that the Missouri General Assembly has acknowledged in the law of this State—new human life is created at the instant of sperm–oocyte binding. The parents who contribute the sperm and oocyte for the express purpose of fertilization exercise their right to procreate at fertilization, when a new human being comes into existence and begins to direct his or her own development until death.

II. The trial court erred in concluding that the frozen embryos produced by in vitro fertilization were not children and in awarding them as marital property, because the court had a duty to make a determination of custody of the embryos according to their best interests, in that the laws of Missouri acknowledge that upon fertilization, unique human beings have been produced who have the rights of human beings but cannot care for themselves, and other states' jurisprudence beginning with *Davis v. Davis* have not assimilated current scientific research.

A. Missouri Law Acknowledges the Legal Rights of Human Embryos

Missouri has long acknowledged by statute that a human embryo is a person with protectable rights in life, health, and well-being from the moment of conception onward. The General Assembly has provided as follows:

1.205. 1. The general assembly of this state finds that:

(1) The life of each human being begins at conception;

(2) Unborn children have protectable interests in life, health, and well-being;

(3) The natural parents of unborn children have protectable interests in the life, health, and well-being of their unborn child . . .

Mo. Rev. Stat. § 1.205. . . .

The trial court's attention was directed to this statute and the cases that interpret it. Petitioner's Proposed Judgment and Law, pp. 4–6 (filed October 14, 2014). Inexplicably, the trial court simply ignored the statute and interpretive authorities. The judgment is bereft of any allusion to them. The trial court wrote, "Missouri Courts and Legislature provide no guidance concerning these issues" (Judgment, ¶ 46).

Whatever the reason for the Court's refusal to address § 1.205, the omission is quite startling. It is an essential part of the role of courts in a representative government to carry out the intent of the legislature. . . .

III. The trial court erred in concluding that a constitutional right "not to procreate" requires both parties' agreement in the future to allow the frozen embryos to live and also in failing to protect the best interests of the embryos, because the court had a duty to make a determination of custody of these human beings, in that such a right not to procreate is moot when procreation has already occurred, and the best interests of the embryonic children include fostering their care, growth, and relationships with their parents and siblings.

A. The "Right Not to Procreate" Is Moot Because Procreation Has Already Occurred.

The trial court opined that the parties' "fundamental rights to privacy and equal protection under the 14th Amendment to the U. S. Constitution will be violated if either is forced to procreate against his or her wishes." The trial court erred. The parties have already procreated; neither has to contribute any more gametes or take any similar action in order for new human beings to be created. . . .

B. The Cases Resting on Principles of Strict Contract, Balancing-of-Interests, and Contemporaneous Mutual Consent Fail to Recognize the Human Status of the Embryos and the General Assembly's Command to Interpret All Missouri Statutes Accordingly.

The trial court in the case at bar purported to adopt a balancing-of-interests approach but at the same time found the decisions of the courts of Iowa to be particularly persuasive (Judgment, ¶¶ 47–48). The leading Iowa case is In Re: Marriage of Witten, 672 N.W.2d 768 (Iowa 2003). . . . There is no indication in Witten that scientific knowledge regarding the creation of human beings was presented to the Iowa Supreme Court which could have informed such an overarching principle. When it turned to Iowa's divorce statute, therefore, the Court did not interpret it to include a duty to insure the best interests of "fertilized eggs that have not even resulted in a pregnancy" (Id. at 780).

Lacking the most current scientific research and guidance from the Iowa Legislature, the Witten Court failed to acknowledge that the progenitors had already made their reproductive choice when they created the human embryos that they placed in cryostorage. . . .

C. The Best Interests of the Human Embryos Begin with Continued Life

The most important interest of an embryo is his or her interest in continued life. No other right is of any avail if a human being is not around to invoke it. In accordance with the Legislature's command, all other laws of Missouri must be interpreted with the status of each human being at its earliest stages in mind. . . .

Conclusion

All humans are unique and irreplaceable. All face challenges in their family life as they grow up; there are no perfect families. Each one of the children of Jalesia and Justin has a place in their family and in the world to grow and flourish. Missouri law, particularly § 1.205, protects their right to be nurtured in their family and their opportunity to seek and find their place in the world.

MISSOURI RIGHT TO LIFE is a grassroots pro-life organization based in Jefferson City, Missouri. **LAWYERS FOR LIFE**, part of Americans United for Life, is a network of attorneys that addresses abortion and other issues that involve decisions about the preservation of human life. **THE AMERICAN ASSOCIATION OF PRO-LIFE OBSTETRICIANS AND GYNECOLOGISTS** is a pro-life advocacy group whose members are primarily obstetricians and gynecologists.

Joseph J. Kodner and John M. Faust

→ **NO**

Brief of Amicus Curiae American Society for Reproductive Medicine in Support of Respondent

Statement of Facts

During their marriage, Appellant Jalesia McQueen and Respondent Justin Gadberry created four embryos together through in vitro fertilization (LF71). Two of the embryos were implanted and, as a result, Appellant gave birth to two children (Id.). The remaining two embryos were cryopreserved (Id.). When the parties later divorced, a dispute arose concerning the custody and disposition of the cryopreserved embryos (LF77). Holding that the embryos are a "unique" type of marital property, the trial court awarded them jointly to the parties with a restriction that "no transfer, release, or use of the frozen embryos shall occur without the signed authorization of both Husband and Wife" (LF 76–78, 80. . . .)

Argument

I. Resolving Embryo Custody Disputes With A "Best Interests Of the Embryo" Approach Would Have Significant Adverse Implications for Fertility Care.

Appellant and her supporting amici argue that, because the Missouri legislature has deemed human life to begin at conception and required state laws to be construed consistently with that finding, disputes such as this one over the custody of unimplanted embryos must be resolved according to the "best interests" of the embryos, as if they were children subject to Missouri's child custody statute (RSMo. Chapter 452). See Appellant Br. at 28; Thomas More Law Center Br. ("TMLC Br.") at 2–4; Missouri Right to Life, et al. Br. ("MRL Br.") at 7–8. The practical implications of that position are profound, particularly because Appellant and her amici are arguing that "continued life" or "future life and development" is the most fundamental of the embryos' "best interests," compelled to be enforced under Missouri law. See Appellant Br. at 31–34; MRL Br. at 37–38. In assisted reproduction, there is no precise way to know, in advance, exactly how

many eggs can be successfully extracted and fertilized, or how many of the resulting embryos, assuming they prove suitable for implantation, should be implanted to achieve a successful pregnancy. As a result, it is very common—indeed, typical—for more embryos to be created than are transferred to the woman's uterus at any given time. Practice Committee of the ASRM, criteria for number of embryos to transfer: a committee opinion, 99 Fertility and Sterility 44 (January 2013). In consultation with her patient(s), the physician makes a professional judgment regarding implantation, attempting to maximize the chances of achieving pregnancy without unduly risking multiple births. In assessing the chromosomal soundness and other indications of each embryo's suitability for implantation, depending on the pertinent medical history and genetic makeup of the contributing adults, the physician may also recommend testing those embryos, since genetic predisposition to some very serious child-onset and even adult-onset health conditions can be revealed through such testing—Huntington disease, early onset Alzheimer disease, and breast cancer among them. Ethics Committee of the ASRM, Use of preimplantation genetic diagnosis for serious adult onset conditions: a committee opinion, 100 Fertility and Sterility 54 (July 2013).

If Appellant's "best interests" position were to prevail here, however, then in the event of a dispute between the man and woman who contributed their genetic material to the embryos, courts in such cases would be pressed to decide that, properly speaking, there is no such thing as an "excess" embryo. From that viewpoint, every embryo—not just the ones initially selected for implantation—must be considered a child from the moment of fertilization, with interests of its own that require it be implanted and given an opportunity to develop and be born, even if one or both of the adults who created them prefer otherwise. This could mean that excess embryos cannot be placed into long-term storage, much less ever discarded, nor even donated for stem cell research, despite the recognized importance of that work in developing revolutionary treatments for "a wide range of diseases and conditions, including Parkinson disease, Alzheimer disease, cancer, spinal cord injury, and juvenile-onset diabetes." Ethics Committee of the ASRM, Donating embryos for human embryonic stem cell (hESC) research: a committee opinion, 100 Fertility and Sterility 935, 936 (October 2013) (discussing federal Executive Order 13505, "permit[ting] embryos remaining after fertility treatment to be used in the creation of [human embryonic stem cell] lines").

Courts could be urged as well to enjoin testing embryos, on grounds that the embryo has a right to life regardless of the prospect of serious disease or that the testing procedure itself poses a risk to the embryo, regardless of the potentially countervailing opportunity to detect and prevent the transmission of genetic disorders to new generations, and to avoid the often crushing emotional and economic impact of managing these illnesses. See 100 Fertility and Sterility at 55; Ethics Committee of the ASRM, The moral and legal status of the preembryo, 62 Fertility and Sterility 32S (November 1994) . . .

Donating the excess embryos for parenting by others may not be a workable solution, either, because, if the embryos are deemed to be "children," then their donation to infertile recipients might be deemed an "adoption," and thus might entail the home visits, judicial review, and other rigorous procedural requirements that typically must precede the adoption of an existing child. Ethics Committee of the ASTM, Defining embryo donation: a committee opinion, 99 Fertility and Sterility 1846–47 (June 2013) . . .

One can expect serious questions, too, about whether and to what extent those adults who contribute their genetic material to the embryos are deemed to be financially responsible for them, even when brought to birth against the wishes of one or both of those adults as the result of a "best interests of the embryo" approach. It is difficult to overstate the adverse impact on fertility care from concerns like these. Infertility is a very significant medical problem, affecting about 7.3 million Americans, or about one out of every eight couples of reproductive age . . . . For the many people who consider addressing this problem with assisted reproductive technology, . . . the decision is deeply emotional, fraught with concerns about the intimate, personal nature of the process, its cost, its uncertainty, and the impact on the couple's relationship should the process not yield the hoped-for results . . . .

If Appellant were to prevail here, couples already facing those challenges would also have to accept that, by seeking this type of medical assistance, their individual choices about what happens to their own genetic contributions may cease to be theirs should they ever have a dispute over the handling of the embryos they create—every one of which, whether initially selected for implantation or not, would have to be treated as if it were already a fully-formed person, with all attendant rights, from the moment of conception. This is a tremendous burden to place on patients seeking fertility care, and one that may cause a significant number of them to just accept their infertility, and possibly abandon hopes for a family altogether, rather than commit to a process in which they may be deemed to have created more people than they ever intended.

If they seek fertility care at all, moreover, couples may face significant pressure to produce fewer embryos than they, in consultation with their doctors, would otherwise conclude are optimal for achieving a successful pregnancy. That is because, according to Appellant and her amici, couples who choose to contribute their genetic material to create embryos have already exercised their procreative choice in favor of making a child out of every one of them, irrevocably assuming the rights and responsibilities of becoming a parent and waiving any further individual right to choose not to develop any of those embryos into live children . . . . From a patient care perspective, these are all unacceptable results, . . . none of which, ASRM respectfully submits, is required by science or the law.

II. Embryos Are Not Individual "Persons" from the Moment of Fertilization.

Whatever other asserted basis there may have been for the Missouri legislature's 1986 enactment concerning when life begins, there is no biological basis for treating an embryo, from the moment of conception, as if it were a single human person . . . . It is true that an alive, human, genetically unique entity emerges at fertilization . . . . At this stage, however, this entity—a zygote—has only a limited chance for development into a living newborn, even under normal conditions, i.e., outside the context of assisted reproduction. Moreover, throughout the course of the next several cell divisions, the entity will lack the "developmental singleness of one person," that is, each cell in this cluster of cells retains the full developmental potential that the zygote had to produce a complete individual human being, and also, importantly, the potential that either more than one individual (in the case of twinning) or less than one individual (in the case of cell fragmentation, fusion, or regression to a nonviable entity) will result. Only sometime later, in an ongoing process that spans about 14 days postfertilization, do the entity's cells resolve into the differentiated layers of more specialized cells that characterize a developing organism, as opposed to a packet of identical cells.

An outer, "extraembryonic" layer forms, which is principally involved in placental interaction with the woman's uterus, and also a two-layer inner cell mass, with each of those internal regions themselves separated by a third layer called the "primitive streak." If it survives, this multilayered inner cell mass, called the "embryonic disc," is what will develop into a child, if and only if the embryo is successfully implanted and there is a pregnancy. Indeed, only now—at a time that corresponds roughly to the initiation of pregnancy-related physiological changes in the mother—is it possible to say that twinning or regression will not occur, such that we now have an entity that is biologically committed to forming a single human being. And only later, of course, will this entity undergo the functional, behavioral, psychic, and social development that many, in ordinary lay terms, would consider to be the hallmarks of human individuality and "personhood."

With these considerations in mind, ASRM has always steered a cautious middle course in defining the status of an embryo. That is, embryos are not mere property, but they are not "people," either. In particular:

> The preembryo is due greater respect than other human tissue because of its potential to become a person and because of its symbolic meaning for many people. Yet, it should not be treated as a person, because it has not yet developed the features of personhood, it is not yet established as developmentally individual, and it may never realize its biologic potential. Ethics Committee of the ASRM, The moral and legal status of the preembryo, 62 Fertility and Sterility 33S (November 1994) . . . .

ASRM recognizes that the Court has been asked to address the implications of a legislative enactment that defines when life begins and, with certain important exceptions discussed below, requires "acknowledge[ment]," on behalf of unborn children, of the rights possessed by "other persons, citizens, and residents" of Missouri (RSMo. § 1.205). Where it applies at all, however, this required "acknowledgement" is not necessarily the same thing as equating the status of the unborn with that of "persons" in every legal context. Because the implications of doing so are so sweeping and serious (see Part I above), and because there is no clear biological imperative to do so (as just discussed), ASRM urges the Court to assure itself that there is a legal imperative to doing so before taking such a dramatic step. In fact, as shown below, there is no such imperative applicable here.

III. Section 1.205 Need Not, and Should Not, Be Construed to Require A "Best Interests of The Embryo" Child Custody Approach.

A. Conflict with federal constitutional law

Section 1.205 is expressly subject to "the Constitution of the United States, and decisional interpretations thereof by the United States Supreme Court and specific provisions to the contrary in the statutes and constitution of this state." With respect to the first exception, it is common ground that the unborn are not "persons" within the meaning of the 14th Amendment to the U.S. Constitution, and thus have no rights of their own to the life, liberty, property, and equal protection of the laws guaranteed there. See *Roe v. Wade*, 410 U.S. 113, 158 (1973); TMLC Br. 15 ("the Supreme Court held that the unborn are not 'persons' under the Fourteenth Amendment and, thus, not [*sic*] are not entitled to its guarantee of the right to life").

Nonetheless, here, Appellant is asking the Court to enforce these exact rights—"continued life" chief among them—on behalf of constitutionally unrecognized entities, as against the asserted interests of those who do have constitutional status as "persons," including Mr. Gadberry in particular. Missouri courts have not had to confront that precise constitutional issue in the cases thus far, which have been limited to holding that the unborn are "persons" for purposes of criminal and tort liability for harm to those entities, by third parties, while their mothers carried them. See Appellant Br. at 15; TMLC Br. at 7–8. . . .

[N]ot one of the several reported cases around the country that have addressed embryo custody disputes over the last two decades or more has resolved custody by attempting to ascertain the best interests of the embryo as an entity with rights of its own. Rather, in various ways, each has sought to determine and balance the competing rights and interests of the adults who created the embryos. . . . ASRM believes that this focus on the wishes of the contributing adults, to the extent those wishes can be fairly determined and weighed, is the appropriate one, consistent with ASRM's consistent ethical guidance that embryos are unique entities worthy of special care and respect, but not people. . . .

THE AMERICAN SOCIETY FOR REPRODUCTIVE MEDICINE is an organization that advocates for the advancement and practice of reproductive medicine.

EXPLORING THE ISSUE

Should Embryos Produced During IVF Be Considered Children?

Critical Thinking and Reflection

1. The readings take contradictory positions on the question of whether there is a scientific or biological basis for determining whether an embryo is a person from the moment of conception. What biological reason does the ASRM give for thinking that very early stage embryos are not yet persons? Suppose that it became technological possible to cause twinning in a later-stage embryo; would that defeat the ASRM's argument, or would it mean that even later-stage embryos are not persons?

2. The first reason ASRM gives for rejecting the view that embryos are persons from the moment of conception is that the view would be profoundly harmful to couples who are seeking medical assistance in having children. What are the implications that the ASRM identifies? Should the decision whether am embryo is a person depend on the state of technologies for creating or using embryos?

3. The question of personhood in this case is a little different from the question of personhood when the embryo is already implanted in a woman's uterus and is developing into a fetus and progressing toward birth. Is this difference significant? Is it possible that the embryo could be considered a person in one context and not in another? Suppose, for example, that some other kind of cell—for example, a skin cell that has been bathed in a special mix of chemicals—could turn into a fetus if it were implanted in a woman's uterus. At what point, if any, should that entity be considered a person? How would these considerations support or undermine the position of Missouri Right to Life and the ASRM?

Is There Common Ground?

There are few debates less amenable to finding common ground than the debate over whether embryos are persons. In the reading above, the ASRM describes as common ground the rather controversial idea that unborn fetuses are not persons under the Constitution. Another gesture that the ASRM makes at common ground is its declaration that the "preembryo is due greater respect than other human tissue because of its potential to become a person and because of its symbolic meaning for many people," but while this idea goes some distance toward recognizing special moral significance for the unborn, it is hardly enough to satisfy those on the pro-life side of the debate.

Other attempts to find common ground are the ideas, often advanced by pro-choice advocates, that abortion should be rare and that it is more acceptable in the early stages than in the later stages of pregnancy. Abortion already occurs mostly in the early stages of pregnancy. According to the Centers for Disease Control, most abortions in the United States are performed during the first eight weeks of pregnancy, and the great majority are performed before the 12th week. Abortions performed later in pregnancy are requested usually because of fetal abnormalities, illness in the mother, or late diagnosis of pregnancy in a teenager. Abortions performed at this stage are the particularly controversial type known as intact dilation and extraction.

Additional Resources

In *Life Before Birth: The Moral and Legal Status of Embryos and Fetuses*, 2nd edition (Oxford, 2011), Bonnie Steinbock offers both an in-depth study of the abortion controversy and of some of the issues in reproductive medicine and stem cell research that turn on that controversy.

A much-discussed secular argument for a pro-life position is Don Marquis, "Why Abortion Is Immoral," *Journal of Philosophy*, April 1984.

A very widely read argument for a pro-choice position is Judith Jarvis Thompson, "A Defense of Abortion," *Philosophy and Public Affairs*, Winter 1971.

Internet References . . .

Abortion

http://www.thehastingscenter.org/briefingbook/
aborliton/

Arguments for and against Abortion

http://www.soc.ucsb.edu/sexinfo/article/
arguments-and-against-abortion

Should Abortion Be Legal?

http://abortion.procon.org

The Best Pro-Life Arguments for Secular Audiences

http://frc.org/arguments

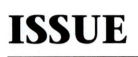

Selected, Edited, and with Issue Framing Material by:
Gregory E. Kaebnick, *The Hastings Center*

ISSUE

Should a Pregnant Woman Be Punished for Exposing Her Fetus to Risk?

YES: Liles Burke, from *Hope Elisabeth Ankrom v. State of Alabama*, Circuit Court of Coffee County (2011)

NO: Lynn M. Paltrow, from "Punishment and Prejudice: Judging Drug-Using Pregnant Women," Beacon Press (1999)

Learning Outcomes

After reading this issue, you will be able to:

- Discuss the implications of maternal responsibility during pregnancy.
- Discuss how environmental factors may affect a person's well-being and a person's responsibility for their behavior.
- Discuss how the debate about abortion is affecting public policy on other issues, including substance abuse and child welfare.

ISSUE SUMMARY

YES: Liles Burke sets out the majority opinion of the Alabama Court of Criminal Appeals in a case involving a pregnant woman who was found to have used cocaine while pregnant. Burke argues that Alabama law that forbids adults from exposing children to controlled substances applies in cases involving pregnant women and their fetuses.

NO: Attorney Lynn M. Paltrow argues that treating drug-using pregnant women as criminals targets poor, African American women while ignoring other drug usage and fails to provide the resources to assist them in recovery.

In 1989, fueled by the specter of an epidemic of drug use resulting in the birth of thousands of "crack babies," the Medical University of South Carolina established a program that required drug-using pregnant women to seek treatment and prenatal care or face criminal prosecution. This program applied only to patients attending the university's obstetric clinic, primarily poor black women, and not to private patients. Patients enrolled in the clinic saw a video and were given written information about the harmful effects of substance abuse during pregnancy. The information warned that the police, the court system, and child protective services in Charleston, South Carolina, might become involved if illegal drug use were detected.

Women who met certain criteria were required to undergo periodic urine screening for drugs. A patient who had a positive urine test or who failed to keep scheduled appointments for therapy or prenatal care could be arrested and placed in custody. If a woman delivered a baby who tested positive for drugs, she would be arrested immediately after her medical release and her newborn taken into protective custody. If the drug use was detected within the first 27 weeks of gestation, the patient was charged with possession of an illegal substance; after that date, the charge was possession and distribution of an illegal substance to a minor. If the drug use were detected during delivery, the woman would be charged with unlawful neglect of a child.

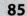

This stringent policy was developed as a result of clinicians' concern about the harmful effects of drug use on fetal development and prosecutors' desires to take a strong public stand condemning drug use. The Supreme Court of South Carolina upheld the law in a 1997 decision involving a woman, Cornelia Whitner, who admitted to using cocaine during pregnancy and whose baby was born with cocaine metabolites in his system. The court wrote that, "The abuse or neglect of a child at any time during childhood can exact a profound toll on the child herself as well as on society as a whole. However, the consequences of abuse or neglect that takes place after birth often pale in comparison to those resulting from abuse suffered by the viable fetus before birth."

Critics argued, however, that the law punished women without helping them correct their behavior. Although the law's stated goal was to get women into treatment, there were few places that women could receive treatment and the necessary support, such as transportation and child care. At the time, there was no women-only residential treatment center for substance-abusing pregnant women anywhere in the state.

The program was discontinued in September 1994 as the result of a settlement with the Civil Rights Division of the federal Department of Health and Human Services. By then, 42 pregnant women had been arrested. In recent years, however, similar cases have been tried in other states. In Alabama, prosecutors began filing charges against women under the state's 2006 chemical endangerment law, whose explicit goal was to prevent adults from bringing children to methamphetamine laboratories and other places where illegal substances are produced or distributed. Prosecutors argued that the law also applied to fetuses exposed to drugs while in the uterus. A long list of medical, legal, and public organizations filed legal briefs arguing against their interpretation of the law, but their prosecutors' position has been upheld by the Alabama Court of Criminal Appeals. Over 60 women have now been charged under the law.

In *Hope Elisabeth Ankrom v. State of Alabama*, Justice Liles Burke explains why a majority of the court's justices found that the state's chemical endangerment law includes a fetus within its definition of "child." Lynn Paltrow argues, however, that criminalization of drug use is a punitive response that rejects the humanity of the women who are denied treatment and support for recovering from their addiction.

YES ↩

Liles Burke

Hope Elisabeth Ankrom v. State of Alabama

Hope Elisabeth Ankrom pleaded guilty to chemical endangerment of a child, a violation of [Section 26-15-3.2 of the Code of Alabama]. . . . The trial court sentenced Ankrom to three years in prison, but the court suspended that sentence and placed her on one year of supervised probation. Ankrom appealed her conviction. We affirm.

Facts and Procedural History

At the guilty-plea hearing, the parties stipulated to the following facts:

"On January 31, 2009, the defendant, Hope Ankrom, gave birth to a son, [B.W.], at Medical Center Enterprise. Medical records showed that the defendant tested positive for cocaine prior to giving birth and that the child tested positive for cocaine after birth.

"Department of Human Resources worker Ashley Arnold became involved and developed a plan for the care of the child. During the investigation the defendant admitted to Ashley that she had used marijuana while she was pregnant but denied using cocaine.

"Medical records from her doctor show that he documented a substance abuse problem several times during her pregnancy and she had tested positive for cocaine and marijuana on more than one occasion during her pregnancy."

On February 18, 2009, Ankrom was arrested and charged with chemical endangerment of a child. On August 25, 2009, the grand jury indicted Ankrom. The indictment stated that Ankrom "did knowingly, recklessly, or intentionally cause or permit a child . . . to be exposed to, to ingest or inhale, or to have contact with a controlled substance, chemical substance, or drug paraphernalia as defined in Section 13A–12–260 of the Code of Alabama. . . .

Discussion

Ankrom alleges that based on the facts of this case, she cannot be convicted of violating § 26–15–3.2(a)(1), Ala. Code 1975. . . . [T]he issue before this Court is whether a mother who ingested a controlled substance during her pregnancy, may be prosecuted under § 26–15–3.2(a)(1), Ala.Code 1975, if at birth the infant tests positive for the controlled substance. We answer that legal question in the affirmative, and we conclude that based on the facts of this case, Ankrom's conviction was proper. . .

Turning to the merits of the present case, § 26–15–3.2(a)(1), Ala.Code 1975, provides:

> "(a) A responsible person commits the crime of chemical endangerment of exposing a child to an environment in which he or she does any of the following:
>> "(1) Knowingly, recklessly, or intentionally causes or permits a child to be exposed to, to ingest or inhale, or to have contact with a controlled substance, chemical substance, or drug paraphernalia as defined in Section 13A–12–260. A violation under this subdivision is a Class C felony."

Ankrom alleges that the term "child" in § 26–15–3.2, Ala.Code 1975, does not include a viable fetus. The State responds that the plain meaning of the term "child," as used in the statute, includes an unborn child.

. . . The legislature has stated that "[t]he public policy of the State of Alabama is to protect life, born, and unborn. This is particularly true concerning unborn life that is capable of living outside the womb." . . . Chapter 15 of Title 26, Ala.Code 1975, does not define the term "child." However, Chapters 14 and 16 of Title 26, Ala. Code 1975, define a "child" as a "person" under the age of 18 years. . . .

From Circuit Court of Coffee County, 2011.

Also, the Alabama Supreme Court has interpreted the term "minor child" in Alabama's wrongful-death-of-minor statute to include a viable fetus that received prenatal injuries causing death before a live birth. . . . Specifically, the Court held that "the parents of an eight and one-half month old stillborn fetus [are] entitled to maintain an action for the wrongful death of the child"; thus, the Court explicitly recognized the viable fetus as a "child." Eich, 293 Ala. at 100, 300 So. 2d at 358.

Furthermore, the dictionary definition of a word provides the meaning ordinary people would give the word. . . . According to Merriam–Webster's Collegiate Dictionary 214 (11th ed.2003), the word "child" is defined as "an unborn or recently born person." The word "child" is defined in Black's Law Dictionary 254 (8th ed.2004), as "[a] baby or fetus.". . .

. . . [W]e do not see any reason to hold that a viable fetus is not included in the term "child," as that term is used in § 26–15–3.2, Ala.Code 1975. Not only have the courts of this State interpreted the term "child" to include a viable fetus in other contexts, the dictionary definition of the term "child" explicitly includes an unborn person or a fetus. In everyday usage, there is nothing extraordinary about using the term "child" to include a viable fetus. For example, it is not uncommon for someone to state that a mother is pregnant with her first "child." Unless the legislature specifically states otherwise, the term "child" is simply a more general term that encompasses the more specific term "viable fetus." If the legislature desires to proscribe conduct against only a "viable fetus," it is necessary to use that specific term. However, if the legislature desires to proscribe conduct against a viable fetus and all other persons under a certain age, the term "child" is sufficient to convey that meaning. In fact, proscribing conduct against a "child" and a "viable fetus" would be redundant.

The term "child" in § 26–15–3.2, Ala.Code 1975, is unambiguous; thus, this Court must interpret the plain language of the statute to mean exactly what it says and not engage in judicial construction of the language in the statute. Also, because the statute is unambiguous, the rule of lenity does not apply. We do not see any rational basis for concluding that the plain and ordinary meaning of the term "child" does not include a viable fetus.

Ankrom advances three main arguments against interpreting the term "child" in § 26–15–3.2, Ala.Code 1975, to include a viable fetus: (1) The legislature has specifically included the term "fetus" or "unborn child" in other statutes when the legislature's intent was for the statute to apply to a fetus; (2) most courts from other jurisdictions have held that mothers could not be criminally prosecuted for prenatal substance abuse on the statutory theories of child abuse/endangerment or drug distribution;

and (3) the legislature has declined to amend § 26–15–3.2, Ala.Code 1975, to explicitly include an unborn child in the definition of the term "child." We will address each argument in turn.

Contrary to Ankrom's argument, the fact that the legislature has included the term "fetus" or "unborn child" in other statutes does not mean that the term "child" in § 26–15–3.2, Ala.Code 1975, does not include a viable fetus. Ankrom specifically points to § 26–23–3, Ala. Code 1975, as an example to support her argument. Section 26–23–3, Ala. Code 1975, provides: "Any physician who knowingly performs a partial-birth abortion within this state and thereby kills a human fetus shall be guilty of a Class C felony and upon conviction thereof shall be punished as prescribed by law." Ankrom states that "[t]here is no doubt in the plain meaning of that statute of which class it is designed to protect: human fetuses." . . . Ankrom then reasons that "[i]f the legislature had intended for § 26–15–3.2(a) to apply to a fetus, then the legislature would have specifically included that language as it has in other statutes." . . . However, the flaw in Ankrom's reasoning is that she misses the distinction between the use of the more specific term "human fetus" and the more general term "child." As stated earlier, the general term "child" encompasses the more specific term "fetus." Statutes such as § 26–23–3 can only apply to a fetus or unborn child because it is impossible to perform an abortion after a live birth has been completed, so using the more general term "child" in such a statute would be nonsensical. On the other hand, statutes such as § 26–15–3.2 may proscribe conduct against born and unborn children; thus, the more general term "child" is necessary. Therefore, Ankrom's first argument is without merit.

Next, we acknowledge the many decisions from appellate courts in other states holding that a mother cannot be criminally prosecuted for prenatal substance abuse under those states' child abuse/endangerment or drug-distribution statutes. . . . However, we find that those cases are either distinguishable from the present case or unpersuasive.

Some of the cases from other jurisdictions involved prosecutions under statutes forbidding delivery of a controlled substance and, unlike the present case, depended on statutory construction of the term "deliver." . . . In other cases, the courts noted that their states' homicide statutes did not apply to a fetus, unlike Alabama's homicide statute, which does apply to unborn children. . . .

In Collins, the Texas Court of Appeals held that, divergent from Alabama, "the [Texas] Penal Code does not proscribe any conduct with respect to a fetus, and the Legislature, by its definitions of 'child,' 'person,' and 'individual,' has specifically limited the application of our penal laws to conduct committed against a human being who has been born and is alive." . . . Similarly, in Dunn, the Washington Court of Appeals held that "[n]o Washington criminal case has ever included 'unborn child' or fetus in its definition of person." . . .

In Gray, unlike the present case, the mother was prosecuted under a statute that stated, in relevant part: "No person, who is the parent of a child under eighteen years of age shall create a substantial risk to the health of safety of the child, by violating a duty of care, protection, or support." . . . Noting that criminal statutes must be strictly construed, the Ohio Supreme Court interpreted that statute by defining the terms "parent" and "child" to apply only to the relationship between mothers and fathers and their born infants. . . .

Other courts have worried about the implications of holding a mother criminally liable under a child-endangerment statute for conduct harmful to her fetus. Specifically, other courts have worried that holding a mother liable under such statutes would open the proverbial floodgates to prosecution of pregnant women who ingest legal toxins, such as alcohol or nicotine, or engage in any behavior that could conceivably injure the fetus. . . . In Wade, the Missouri Court of Appeals stated that the logic of allowing prosecutions to protect the interest of the fetus "would be extended to cases involving smoking, alcohol ingestion, the failure to wear seatbelts, and any other conduct that might cause harm to a mother's unborn child. It is a difficult line to draw and, as such, our legislature has chosen to handle the problems of pregnant mothers through social service programs instead of the court system." . . . However, in the present case, we need not worry about such unlimited extensions because we are not dealing with a general endangerment statute. Section 26–15–3.2(a)(1), Ala.Code 1975, the only statute we are asked to construe, concerns only conduct involving controlled substances or drug paraphernalia. It does not concern conduct involving smoking, alcohol ingestion, failure to wear seatbelts, or any other potentially harmful conduct that does not involve controlled substances.

Other courts have examined policy issues, legislative history, or other extrinsic materials to reach their conclusions that a mother cannot be criminally prosecuted for prenatal substance abuse under those states' child-abuse/endangerment statutes. . . . However, we are not at liberty to engage in such a review because we hold that § 26–15–3.2(a)(1), Ala.Code 1975, is unambiguous on its face. See Pinigis v. Regions Bank, 977 So.2d 446, 451 (Ala.2007) (holding that "courts may examine extrinsic materials, including legislative history, to determine [legislative] intent" only "[i]f the statutory language is ambiguous").

Again, we find the cases from other states holding that a mother cannot be criminally prosecuted for prenatal substance abuse under those states' child-abuse/endangerment or drug-distribution statutes to be distinguishable from the present case. To the extent that they are not distinguishable, we find that their reasoning is unpersuasive.

Ankrom's final argument against interpreting the term "child" in § 26–15–3.2, Ala.Code 1975, to include a viable fetus alleges that we should not interpret the term "child" to include a viable fetus because the legislature recently attempted to amend § 26–15–3.2, Ala.Code 1975, to explicitly state that the term "child" includes a child in utero at any stage of development, but the amendment failed. However, " 'failed legislative proposals' are "a particularly dangerous ground on which to rest an interpretation of a prior statute." ' " ' Baney v. State, 42 So.3d 170, 174 (Ala.Crim.App.2009) . . . In the present case, we do not need to speculate as to why the proposed amendment failed. Again, we hold that § 26–15–3.2, Ala.Code 1975, is unambiguous on its face; thus, we must construe the statute to mean exactly what it says. . . .

Finally, Ankrom argues that § 26–15–3.2, Ala.Code 1975, as applied in the present case, is void for vagueness because, she says, the statute did not give her adequate notice that her conduct was proscribed. See Vaughn v. State, 880 So.2d 1178, 1195 (Ala.Crim.App.2003) (holding that "the void-for-vagueness doctrine requires that a penal statute define the criminal offense with sufficient definiteness that ordinary people can understand what conduct is prohibited and in a manner that does not encourage arbitrary and discriminatory enforcement," but "[t]his prohibition against excessive vagueness does not invalidate every statute which a reviewing court believes could have been drafted with greater precision" because "[m]any statutes will have some inherent vagueness, for [i]n most English words and phrases there lurk uncertainties"). Specifically, Ankrom alleges that "[t]he plain language of the statute does not give notice that its criminal sanctions apply to fetuses exposed to controlled substances, and for that reason, Ms. Ankrom is being deprived of her due process right to fair notice of what conduct is impermissible." . . . However, as we held above, the plain meaning of the term "child," as found in § 26–15–3.2, Ala.Code 1975, includes a viable fetus. Therefore, Ankrom had adequate notice that her conduct was proscribed; thus, her constitutional argument is without merit.

LILES BURKE is a justice on the Alabama Court of Criminal Appeals.

Lynn M. Paltrow

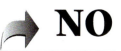 **NO**

Punishment and Prejudice: Judging Drug-Using Pregnant Women

The Villain Cocaine

In the late 1980s and into the 1990s newspapers, magazines, and television were full of stories documenting the devastating effects of cocaine and predicting a lost generation irredeemably damaged by the effects of their mothers' cocaine use. For example, in 1991 *Time* magazine ran a cover story on the subject.[1] Bold yellow letters read "Crack Kids" followed by the headline: "Their mothers used drugs, and now it's the children who suffer." The face of a tearful child filled the page beneath the words. . . .

The same year the *New York Times* ran a front page story entitled "Born on Crack and Coping with Kindergarten."[2] The story is accompanied by a photograph of a school teacher surrounded by young children. Underneath the caption reads: "I can't say for sure it's crack, said Ina R. Weisberg, a kindergarten teacher at P.S. 48 in the Bronx, but I can say that in all my years of teaching I've never seen so many functioning at low levels."

Throughout these years medical and popular journals, public school teachers and judges alike were willing to assume that if a child had a health or emotional problem and he or she had been exposed prenatally to cocaine, then cocaine and cocaine alone was the cause of the perceived medical or emotional problem. Rather than wait for careful research and evaluation of the drug's effect there was, as several researchers later criticized, a "rush to judgment" that blamed cocaine for a host of problems that the research simply has not borne out.[3]

Indeed, an article in the medical journal *Lancet* in 1989 found that scientific studies that concluded that exposure to cocaine prenatally had adverse effects on the fetus had a significantly higher chance of being published than more careful research finding no adverse effects.[4] The published articles, delineating the harmful effects on infants prenatally exposed to cocaine, reported brain damage, genitourinary malformations, and fetal demise as just a few of the dire results of a pregnant woman's cocaine use. Infants that survived the exposure were described as inconsolable, unable to make eye contact, emitting a strange high-pitched piercing wail, rigid and jittery. These early studies, however, had numerous methodologic flaws that made generalization from them completely inappropriate. For example, these studies were based on individual case reports or on very small samples of women who used more than one drug. Researchers often failed to control for the other drugs and problems the mother might have, and/or failed to follow up on the child's health.[5] The articles describing these studies were nevertheless relied upon to show that cocaine alone was the cause of an array of severe and costly health problems.

Like alcohol and cigarettes, using cocaine during pregnancy can pose risks to the woman and the fetus. More carefully controlled studies, however, are finding that cocaine is not uniquely or even inevitably harmful. For example, unlike the devastating and permanent effects of fetal alcohol syndrome, which causes permanent mental retardation, cocaine seems to act more like cigarettes and marijuana, increasing certain risks like low birth weight but only as one contributing factor and only in some pregnancies.[6] Epidemiological studies find that statistically speaking many more children are at risk of harm from prenatal exposure to cigarettes and alcohol. In fact, one recent publication on women and substance abuse has created the label "Fetal Tobacco Syndrome" to draw attention to the extraordinarily high miscarriage and morbidity rates associated with prenatal exposure to cigarette smoke.[7]

By the late 1980s it was already becoming clear to researchers in the field that the labels "crack babies" and "crack kids" were dangerous and counterproductive.[8] If one read far enough in the *Time* article—past the pictures of premature infants and deranged children—the story reported that

> [a]n increasing number of medical experts, however, vehemently challenge the notion that most crack kids are doomed. In fact, they detest the term crack kids, charging that it unfairly brands the children and puts them all into a single

dismal category. From this point of view, crack has become a convenient explanation for problems that are mainly caused by a bad environment. When a kindergartner from a broken home in the impoverished neighborhood misbehaves or seems slow, teachers may wrongly assume that crack is the chief reason, when other factors, like poor nutrition, are far more important.

Even the *New York Times* article about crack-exposed children in kindergarten eventually revealed that researchers "after extensive interviews [found] the problems in many cases were traced not to drug exposure but to some other traumatic event, death in the family, homelessness, or abuse, for example."[9] And despite the fact that school administrators "rarely know who the children are who have been exposed to crack . . . and the effects of crack are difficult to diagnose because they may mirror and be mixed up with symptoms of malnutrition, low birth-weight, lead poisoning, child abuse and many other ills that frequently afflict poor children," the article resorts to crack as the only reasonable explanation for an otherwise seemingly inexplicable phenomenon. . . .

The Public Responds

The public response to the media and medical journal reports was largely one of outrage. The harshest reaction was the call for the arrest of the pregnant women and new mothers who used drugs. Numerous states considered legislation to make it a crime for a woman to be pregnant and addicted.[10] Although not a single state legislature passed a new law creating the crime of fetal abuse, individual prosecutors in more than thirty states arrested women whose infants tested positive for cocaine, heroin, or alcohol. Many of these women were arrested for child abuse, newly interpreted as "fetal" abuse. Others, like Jennifer Johnson in Florida, were charged with delivery of drugs to a minor.[11] In that case, the prosecutor argued that the drug delivery occurred through the umbilical cord after the baby was born but before the umbilical cord was cut. Still other women were charged with assault with a deadly weapon (the weapon being cocaine), or feticide (if the woman suffered a miscarriage), or homicide (if the infant, once born, died). Some women were charged with contributing to the delinquency of a minor.

While arrests were almost always the result of the action of an individual prosecutor, in the state of South Carolina there was unprecedented coordination between health care providers, the prosecutor's office, and the police.

In 1989, the city of Charleston, South Carolina, established a collaborative effort among the police department,

the prosecutor's office, and a state hospital, the Medical University of South Carolina (MUSC), to punish pregnant women and new mothers who tested positive for cocaine. Under the policy, the hospital tested certain pregnant women for the presence of cocaine. Women were tested for the presence of cocaine to further criminal investigations, but the women never consented to these searches and search warrants were never obtained.

While the hospital refused to create a drug treatment program designed to meet the needs of pregnant addicts, or to put even a single trained drug counselor on its obstetrics staff, it did create a program for drug-testing certain patients, their in-hospital arrest, and removal to jail (where there was neither drug treatment nor prenatal care); the ongoing provision of medical information to the police and prosecutor's office; and tracking for purposes of ensuring their arrest. Some women were taken to jail while still bleeding from having given birth. They were handcuffed and shackled while hospital staff watched with approval. All but one of the women arrested were African American. The program itself had been designed by and entrusted to a white nurse who admitted that she believed that the "mixing of races was against God's will."[12] She noted in the medical records of the one white woman arrested that she lived "with her boyfriend who is a Negro."[13] . . .

Who Are These Mothers?

As a report from the Southern Regional Project on Infant Mortality observed:

> Newspaper reports in the 1980s sensationalized the use of crack cocaine and created a new picture of the "typical" female addict; young, poor, black, urban, on welfare, the mother of many children and addicted to crack. In interviewing nearly 200 women for this study, a very different picture of the "typical" chemically dependent woman emerges. She is most likely white, divorced or never married, age 31, a high school graduate, on public assistance, the mother of two or three children, and addicted to alcohol and one other drug. It is clear from the women we interviewed that substance abuse among women is not a problem confined to those who are poor, black, or urban, but crosses racial, class, economic and geographic boundaries.[14]

African American women have been disproportionately targeted for arrest and punishment, not because they use more drugs or are worse mothers, but because, as Dorothy Roberts explains, "[t]hey are the least likely to obtain adequate prenatal care, the most vulnerable to government monitoring, and the least able to conform to the white middle-class standard of motherhood. They are therefore the primary targets of government control."[15]

Beyond the stock images and prejudicial stereotypes, the media has given the public little opportunity to meet or get to know the pregnant women on drugs. If we never learn who they are it is inevitable that their drug use will seem inexplicably selfish and irresponsible. Yet, if we could meet them and learn their history, we might be able to begin to understand them and the problems that need to be addressed.

Let me give an example. In the popular television show *NYPD Blue* we get to know the irascible Detective Sipowicz. While he is neither handsome nor charming, we come to care for him. We learn that he is an alcoholic who is able to stop drinking and improve his life. When he has a massive relapse and behaves outrageously, effectively abandoning his new wife and their newborn son, committing crimes of violence and countless violations of his responsibilities as a police officer, we nevertheless want to forgive him and give him another chance.

We are able to sympathize, at least in part because we have been given the information about why he has relapsed. His first son, whom he has finally reconnected with, is murdered, and Sipowicz, who can't handle it emotionally, turns back to the numbing, relief-giving effects of alcohol.

Sipowicz, in the end, is supported by his police colleagues who cover up for him and give him yet another chance. By contrast, when the same program did an episode involving a heroin-addicted pregnant woman, whose drug habit leads her two older sons to a life of crime, we never get to know why she has turned to drugs. We do not know as we did with Sipowicz what could have driven her to this behavior. The viewer can only assume that her drug use is purely selfish, stemming from a thoughtless hedonism. Thus, she is not entitled to understanding, sympathy, or the many second chances Sipowicz's character routinely gets.

But like Sipowicz, pregnant women who use drugs also have histories and complex lives that affect their behavior and their chances of recovery. We know that substance abuse in pregnancy is highly correlated with a history of violent sexual abuse.[16] In one study 70 percent of the pregnant addicted women were found to be in violent battering relationships. A hugely disproportionate number, compared to a control group, were raped as children. Drugs appear to be used as a means to numb the pain of a violent childhood and adulthood. Like Vietnam veterans who self-medicated with drugs for their post-

traumatic stress disorders, at least some pregnant women also use drugs to numb the pain of violent and traumatic life experiences.[17]

Are their difficult childhoods or their experiences with violence an excuse for drug use? No. But the information begins to provide some idea of root causes that might need to be taken into consideration when trying to imagine the appropriate societal reaction. Will the threat of jail remove the trauma and pain that in many instances prompted the drug use and stands in the way of recovery? It is not that a woman who uses drugs is not responsible, but rather that we have to hold her responsible in a context that takes into account the obstacles, internal and external, that stand in the way of recovery. . . .

All pregnant women, not just poor ones, are routinely denied access to the limited drug treatment that exists in this country. In a landmark study in 1990, Dr. Wendy Chavkin surveyed drug treatment programs in New York City. She found that 54 percent flat out refused to take pregnant women.[18] Sixty-seven percent refused to take women who relied on Medicaid for payment, and 84 percent refused to take crack-addicted pregnant women.

One hospital in New York was sued for excluding women from drug treatment. The program argued that its exclusion of all women was justified and no different from its medical judgment to exclude all psychotics.[19] While New York State courts found that such exclusion violated state law, this did not automatically increase needed services. . . .

Other barriers also exist. [In the case of Jennifer Johnson, a pregnant Florida woman,] Judge Eaton ruled that "the defendant also made a choice to become pregnant and to allow those pregnancies to come to term." The prosecutor argued that "[w]hen she delivered that baby she broke the law." By saying this, the judge makes clear that it was having a child that was against the law. If Ms. Johnson had had an abortion she would not have been arrested—even for possessing drugs.[20] But this statement not only reveals a willingness to punish certain women for becoming mothers, it also reflects a host of widely held beliefs and assumptions about access to reproductive health services for women.

For example, implicit in this statement is the assumption that Ms. Johnson had sex and became pregnant voluntarily. Given the pervasiveness of rape in our society, assuming voluntary sexual relations may not be justified. Perhaps, though, the judge, like many others, simply thought that addicts have no business becoming pregnant in the first place. A South Carolina judge put it bluntly: "I'm sick and tired of these girls having these bastard babies on crack cocaine." Apparently concerned about his candor, he later explained: "They say you're not supposed to call them that but that's what they are . . . when I was a little boy, that's what they called them."[21]

On call-in radio talk shows someone inevitably asks why these mothers can't just be sterilized or injected with Depo Provera until they can overcome their drug problems and, while they are at it, their low socioeconomic status. The consistency of this view should not be surprising given our country's history of eugenics and sterilization abuse. Indeed, the U.S. Supreme Court has declared sterilization of men unconstitutional, but has never overturned its decision upholding the sterilization of women perceived to be a threat to society.[22]

The suggestion of sterilization, however, is particularly attractive if there is no explanation about why a pregnant woman with a drug problem would want to become pregnant or to have a child in the first place. But drug-using pregnant women become pregnant and carry to term for the same range of reasons all women do. Because contraception failed. Because they fell in love again and hoped this time they could make their family work. Because they are "prolife" and would never have an abortion. Because when they found out the beloved father of the baby was really already married, they thought it was too late to get a legal abortion. Because they do not know what their options might be. Because they have been abused and battered for so long they no longer believe they can really control any aspect of their lives including their reproductive lives. Because they wanted a child. Because their neighbors and friends, despite their drug use, had healthy babies and they believed theirs would be healthy too.

The threat of sterilization is just another punitive response that denies the humanity of the women themselves. Although Judge Eaton did not propose sterilization as part of the sentence he imposed on Ms. Johnson, as some judges in related cases have,[23] he undoubtedly assumed that Ms. Johnson could decide, once pregnant, whether or not to continue that pregnancy to term. Since 1976, however, the United States government has refused to pay for poor women's abortions and few states have picked up the costs.[24] In Florida, like most other states, the "choice" Judge Eaton spoke of does not exist for low-income women. . . .

Lack of access to abortion services is only one of the many barriers that exist for a drug-addicted pregnant woman who attempts to make responsible "choices." There are many other barriers that make it extremely difficult for pregnant women on drugs to get the kind of help and support they need. Access to services for drug-addicted women who are physically abused is also limited. For example, many battered women's shelters are set up to deal with women who have experienced violence, but are not equipped to support a woman who has become addicted to drugs as a way to numb the pain of the abuse.[25] Other barriers include lack of housing, employment, and access to prenatal care. As one of the few news stories to discuss these women's dilemmas explains:

> Soon after she learned she was pregnant, [Kimberly] Hardy [who was eventually prosecuted for delivery of drugs to a minor], convinced she had to get away from her crowd of crack users as well as her crumbling relationship with her [boyfriend] Ronald, took the kids home to Mississippi for the duration of her pregnancy. But by moving, she lost her welfare benefits, including Medicaid. Unable to pay for clinic visits, she had to go without prenatal care.[26]

And what about the men in their lives? Their contributions to the problem, physiologically and socially, are ignored or deliberately erased. Rarely in the media do we know what has happened to the potential fathers. Their drug use, abandonment, and battering somehow miraculously disappear from view.

Nevertheless, men often do play a significant role. For example, in California Pamela Rae Stewart was arrested after her newborn died. One of her alleged crimes contributing to the child's ultimate demise was having sex with her husband on the morning of the day of the delivery. Her husband, with whom she had had intercourse, was never arrested for fetal abuse. Indeed, the prosecutor's court papers argued that Ms. Stewart had "subjected herself to the rigors of intercourse," thereby totally nullifying the man's involvement or culpability.[27]

Prosecutors in South Carolina have also managed to ignore male culpability, even when it is the father who is supplying the pregnant woman with cocaine or other potentially harmful substances. Many women arrested in this state were not identified as substance addicted until after they had given birth, a point at which their drug use could not even arguably have a biological impact on the baby. Prosecutors argued that arrest was still justified because evidence of a woman's drug use during pregnancy is predictive of an inability to parent effectively. But fathers identified as drug users are not automatically presumed to be incapable of parenting. Indeed, when a man who happens to be a father is arrested for drunk driving, a crime that entails a serious lack of judgment and the use of a drug, he is not automatically presumed to be incapable of parenting and reported to the child welfare authorities. Prosecutors nevertheless rely on biological differences between mothers and fathers, arguing that a man's drug use could not have hurt the developing baby in the first place. However, studies indicate that male drug use can affect birth outcome: Studies on male alcohol use have demonstrated a relationship between male drinking and low birth weight in their children and a study of cocaine and men suggests that male drug use can also affect birth outcome.[28]

We continue to live in a society with double standards and extremely different expectations for men and women. Drug use by men is still glorified, while drug use by women is shameful, and by pregnant women a crime. This could not have been better demonstrated than by an advertising campaign by Absolut vodka. On Father's Day, as a promotional gimmick, Absolut sent 250,000 free ties to recipients of the *New York Times* Sunday edition. Scores of little sperm in the shape of Absolut vodka bottles swim happily on the tie's blue background. So while many call for arrest when a pregnant woman uses drugs or alcohol, fathers who drink are celebrated and, in effect, urged to "tie one on."

Of course, none of these arguments is made to suggest that women are not responsible for their actions or that they are unable to make choices that reflect free will. Rather, it is to say that popular expectations of what acting responsibly looks like and notions of "choice" have to be modified by an understanding of addiction as a chronic relapsing disease, of the degree to which our country has abandoned programs for poor women and children, and of the time, strength, and courage it takes for a drug-addicted woman to confront her history of drug use, violence, and abandonment. Compassion and significantly more access to coordinated and appropriate services will not guarantee that all of our mothers and children are healthy. But medical experts and both children's and women's rights advocates agree that such an approach is far more likely to improve health than are punishment and blame. . . .

The problem with treating the fetus as a person is that women will not simply continue to be less than equal, they will become nonpersons under the law. [To oppose the recognition of fetal personhood as a matter of law is not to deny the value and importance of potential life as a matter of religious belief, emotional conviction, or personal experience. Rather, by opposing such a new legal construct, we can avoid devastating consequences to women's health, prenatal health care, and women's hope for legal equality.—L.P.] No matter how much value we place on a fetus's potential life, it is still inside the woman's body. To pretend that the pregnant woman is separate is to reduce her to nothing more than, as one radio talk show host asserted, a "delivery system" for drugs to the fetus.

Notes

1. *Time Magazine* (13 May 1991).
2. Suzanne Dale, "Born on Crack and Coping with Kindergarten," *New York Times* (7 February 1991), A1.
3. Linda C. Mayes, R. H. Granger, M. H. Bornstein, and B. Zuckerman, "The Problem of Cocaine Exposure, A Rush to Judgment," *Journal of the American Medical Association* 267 (1992): 406.
4. Gideon Koren, Karen Graham, Heather Shear, and Tom Einarson, "Bias Against the Null Hypothesis: The Reproductive Hazards of Cocaine," *Lancet* (1989): 1, 1440–1442.
5. Mayes, "The Problem of Cocaine Exposure"; B. Lutiger, K. Graham, T. R. Einarson, and G. Koren, "Relationship Between Gestational Cocaine Use and Pregnancy Outcome: A Meta-Analysis," *Teratology* (1991): 44, 405–414.
6. Barry Zuckerman et al., "Effect of Maternal Marijuana and Cocaine Use on Fetal Growth," *New England Journal of Medicine* 320, no. 12 (23 March 1990): 762–768; Deborah A. Frank and Barry S. Zuckerman, "Children Exposed to Cocaine Prenatally: Pieces of the Puzzle," *Neurotoxicology and Teratology* 15 (1993): 298–300; Deborah A. Frank, Karen Breshahn, and Barry Zuckerman, "Maternal Cocaine Use: Impact on Child Health and Development," *Advances in Pediatrics* 40 (1993): 65–99.
7. Center on Addiction and Substance Abuse at Columbia University, *Substance Abuse and the American Woman* (1997); Joseph R. DiFranza and Robert A. Lew, "Effect of Maternal Cigarette Smoking on Pregnancy Complications and Sudden Death Syndrome," *Journal of Family Practice* 40 (1995): 385. Cigarette smoking has been linked to as many as 141,000 miscarriages and 4,800 deaths resulting from perinatal disorders, as well as 2,200 deaths from sudden infant death syndrome, nationwide.
8. American Academy of Pediatrics, Committee on Substance Abuse. Drug Exposed Infants, *Pediatrics* 86 (1990): 639.
9. Dale, "Born on Crack."
10. Allison Marshall, 1992, 1993, 1994 Legislative Update, in *National Association for Families and Addiction Research and Education Update* (Chicago, 1993, 1994, 1995).
11. *Johnson v. State,* 602 So.2d 1288 (Fla. 1992).
12. Brown Trial Transcript, *Ferguson et al. v. City of Charleston et al.,* U.S. District Court for the District of South Carolina, Charleston Division, C/A No. 2:93-2624-1 at 5:18–21 (Dec. 10, 1996).
13. Plaintiffs' Exhibit 119, *Ferguson et al. v. City of Charleston et al.,* U.S. District Court for the District

of South Carolina, Charleston Division, C/A No. 2:93-2624-1.

14. Shelley Geshan, "A Step Toward Recovery, Improving Access to Substance Abuse Treatment for Pregnant and Parenting Women," *Southern Regional Project on Infant Mortality* (1993): 1.

15. Dorothy Roberts, "Punishing Drug Addicts Who Have Babies: Women of Color, Equality, and the Right of Privacy," *Harvard Law Review* 104, no. 7 (1991): 1419, 1422.

16. Dianne O. Regan, Saundra M. Ehrlich, and Loretta P. Finnegan, "Infants of Drug Addicts: At Risk for Child Abuse, Neglect, and Placement in Foster Care," *Neurotoxicology and Teratology* 9 (1987): 315–319.

17. Sheigla Murphy and Marsha Rosenbaum, *Pregnant Women on Drugs: Combating Stereotypes and Stigma* (New Brunswick, N.J.: Rutgers University Press, 1999).

18. Wendy Chavkin, "Drug Addiction and Pregnancy: Policy Crossroads," *American Journal of Public Health* 80, no. 4 (April 1990): 483–487.

19. *Elaine W. v. Joint Diseases North General Hospital Inc.*, 613 N.E.2d 523 (N.Y. 1993).

20. Lynn M. Paltrow, "When Becoming Pregnant Is a Crime," *Criminal Justice Ethics* 9, no. 1 (Winter–Spring 1990): 41–47.

21. *State v. Crawley,* Transcript of Record (Ct. Gen. Sess. Anderson Cnty., S.C., Oct. 17, 1994).

22. *Skinner v. Oklahoma,* 316 U.S. 535 (1942); *Buck v. Bell,* 274 U.S. 200 (1927); Stephen J. Gould, "Carrie Buck's Daughter," *Natural History* (July 1984).

23. *People v. Johnson,* No. 29390 (Cal.Super.Ct. Jan. 2, 1991).

24. *Harris v. McRae,* 448 U.S. 297 (1980).

25. Amy Hill, "Applying Harm Reduction to Services for Substance Using Women in Violent Relationships," *Harm Reduction Coalition* 6 (Spring 1998): 7–8.

26. Jan Hoffman, "Pregnant, Addicted and Guilty?" *New York Times Magazine* (19 August 1990): 53.

27. Shelly Geshan, "A Step Toward Recovery, Improving Access to Substance Abuse Treatment for Pregnant and Parenting Women" Southern Regional Project on Infant Mortality (1993): 1.

28. Dorothy Roberts, "Punishing Drug Addicts who have Babies: Women of Color, Equality, and the Right of Privacy," Harvard Law Review 104, no. 7, (1991): 1419, 1422.

Lynn M. Paltrow is an attorney and executive director of National Advocates for Pregnant Women, New York.

EXPLORING THE ISSUE

Should a Pregnant Woman Be Punished for Exposing Her Fetus to Risk?

Critical Thinking and Reflection

1. The well-being of children is surely vitally important; how does the value attached to their well-being compare, as a matter of public policy, against the value of a woman's freedom and privacy?
2. Avoiding exposure to dangerous substances is about creating a good environment for the child; what is the responsibility of a person to make good decisions when environmental factors in their own life may not have helped them acquire good decision-making skills?
3. Does recognition that a child's well-being can be impaired by things that happen before the child is born lead one to conclude that a fetus is a person?
4. In your view, is protection of persons-to-be best achieved by criminalizing bad behavior or by fostering good behavior in mothers (and fathers)?

Is There Common Ground?

State policies similar to that developed by Alabama prosecutors remain highly contested. In New Mexico in May 2007, the Supreme Court struck down a law expanding the state's criminal child abuse law to drug-using pregnant women and fetuses. Courts in many other states have ruled similarly on this issue. However, according to the Guttmacher Institute, 15 states consider substance abuse during pregnancy to be child abuse under civil child-welfare statutes, and three consider it grounds for civil commitment. Some states also require health care professionals to report suspected prenatal drug abuse or to test for prenatal drug exposure if they suspect abuse. In 2012, *Ankrom v. State* and a similar case concerning a woman named Amanda Kimbrough were appealed from the Alabama Court of Criminal Appeals to the Supreme Court of Alabama. As of this writing, a ruling had not been issued.

Personhood laws have been introduced in a number of states. The measures have been struck down in Colorado, South Dakota, California, and Mississippi, but a bill signed into law in Oklahoma in February 2012 states that the laws of the state "shall be interpreted and construed to acknowledge on behalf of the unborn child at every stage of development all the rights, privileges, and immunities available to other persons, citizens, and residents of this state." Virginia lawmakers have suspended consideration of a similar law until at least 2013.

The approach tried in South Carolina to criminalize substance abuse in pregnancy has been limited by privacy concerns. In March 2001, the U.S. Supreme Court ruled in the case of *Ferguson v. City of Charleston* (121 S.C. 1281) that the Medical University of South Carolina's program to require drug-using pregnant women to seek treatment and prenatal care or face criminal prosecution was unconstitutional. The Court reversed the decision of the lower Fourth Circuit Court of Appeals and sent the case back to the circuit court for a factual determination of whether the women had actually consented to the search that led to their arrest and imprisonment. The circuit court had ruled that the searches were not "unreasonable searches" (prohibited under the Fourth Amendment to the Constitution) because of the "special need" to protect women and children from the consequences of cocaine use in pregnant women. The Supreme Court rejected this claim. But the Court's decision did not settle the public policy and ethical challenges that remain concerning drug use and pregnant women.

Additional Resources

An amicus brief filed in support of Hope Ankrom and Amanda Kimbrough on behalf of a list of organizations and individuals by the Drug Policy Alliance, National Advocates for Pregnant Women, and the Southern Poverty Law Center is available at http://advocatesforpregnantwomen.org/featured/in_the_alabama_supreme_court_1.php.

For information about the criminalization of substance abuse during pregnancy, see the Guttmacher Institute fact sheet, "Substance Abuse During Pregnancy," at www.guttmacher.org/statecenter/spibs /spib_SADP.pdf.

For more on the decision in Ferguson, see George Annas, "Testing Poor Pregnant Women for Cocaine: Physicians as Police Investigators," *The New England Journal of Medicine* (May 31, 2001) and Lawrence O. Gostin, "The Rights of Pregnant Women: The Supreme Court and Drug Use," *Hastings Center Report* (September–October, 2001).

For a book-length treatment of these issues, see Drew Humphries, *Crack Mothers: Pregnancy, Drugs, and the Media* (Ohio State University Press, 1999).

Internet References . . .

Guttmacher Institute Resources Page for Pregnancy

http://www.guttmacher.org/sections/pregnancy.php

MedlinePlus Page on Pregnancy and Substance Abuse

http://www.nlm.nih.gov/medlineplus /pregnancyandsubstanceabuse.html

National Advocates for Pregnant Women

www.advocatesforpregnantwomen.org/

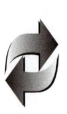

Unit 4

UNIT

Professional Integrity

*P*robably one of the reasons bioethics is recognized as a distinct area of inquiry within the broader field of ethics is that many of the core issues in it are about the distinct role in society held by physicians and other medical professionals, and the special social relationships they have with people in need of their expertise and assistance. The questions are not just about how individuals should treat each other, but also about how individuals who have taken on the role of physician, nurse, or pharmacist should use their special knowledge to serve society. Physicians are often said to be healers—to have committed themselves to promoting health and saving life; is it acceptable, then, for a physician to hurt or even kill someone? Physicians and other medical professionals take on their social roles not merely because society asks them to, but because they are moral beings themselves and they wanted those roles. May society ask them to do something that conflicts with their own moral judgments? Several issues in this volume involve such questions. This unit explores a couple of them in detail.

Selected, Edited, and with Issue Framing Material by:
Gregory E. Kaebnick, *The Hastings Center*

ISSUE

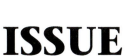

Should Physicians Be Allowed to Participate in Executions?

YES: David Waisel, from "Physician Participation in Capital Punishment," *Mayo Clinic Proceedings* (2007)

NO: Atul Gawande, from "When Law and Ethics Collide—Why Physicians Participate in Executions," *The New England Journal of Medicine* (2006)

Learning Outcomes

After reading this issue, you will be able to:

- Discuss the lethal injection method of execution in the United States, and explain the role of physicians in conducting them.
- Discuss whether the physician's medical role is consistent with participation in lethal injection executions.

ISSUE SUMMARY

YES: David Waisel, a professor of medicine, argues that if the state is to administer capital punishment, then physicians may honorably seek to help the condemned die as painlessly as possible.

NO: Physician and journalist Atul Gawande supports capital punishment but believes physicians, as healers, should play no role in it.

In France, during the reign of the Bourbon monarchs, the methods of execution included beheading with a sword or axe, hanging, burning at the stake, and being bludgeoned to death on the "breaking wheel." None of the methods were quick and painless; beheading often required multiple blows, and hanging takes several minutes when it works well. In 1791, during the French Revolution, Joseph-Ignace Guillotin, a physician who in 1789 had called for the reformation of capital punishment, devised a new beheading machine that allowed for quick and comparatively painless deaths. The machine proved, at least in one way, a great success: During the next few years, in the period known as the Reign of Terror, tens of thousands of people were publicly executed using guillotines.

Guillotin's involvement is often cited in a contemporary debate that has arisen over whether physicians should participate in executions. It shows there is a long history of physician involvement in them, and it illustrates one of the primary reasons for involving physicians: a humanitarian belief that if people are to be executed, then they should be executed with as little suffering as possible. (Before Guillotin, execution was often specifically designed to cause suffering.)

The most common method of execution employed in the United States today is lethal injection, and physicians' expertise is especially useful in carrying it out. Execution by lethal injection was proposed in 1977 by the Oklahoma medical examiner, who (like Guillotin) sought a more humane method of killing the condemned. The method he developed consists of three drugs administered in sequence: a fast-acting barbiturate to put the condemned person to sleep, a paralytic to completely immobilize him, and potassium chloride to kill him. As the YES and NO selections document, much can still go wrong in administering the drugs, and when things do go wrong, the results can be very painful for the person being executed and horrific to witness. Physicians' understanding of the drugs and how they interact, and their expertise in starting the intravenous saline drip through which the drugs are administered, can help ensure that lethal injection is administered well.

The question of whether physicians should be allowed to participate in executions is usually handled separately from the question of whether capital punishment itself is permissible. The American Medical Association's position, for example, is that the permissibility of capital punishment is a personal moral decision but that whether physicians may participate in it follows from a proper understanding of the physician's special role in society. "A physician, as a member of a profession dedicated to preserving life when there is hope of doing so," declares Current Opinion 2.06 of the AMA's Code of Medical Ethics, "should not be a participant in a legally authorized execution." Physician participation in execution, continues the opinion, would include not merely causing the condemned to die, but also assisting or supervising someone who does. The physician is permitted by AMA policy to give a condemned person medical treatment before execution and to certify the person's death afterward.

The YES and NO selections, both by esteemed physicians affiliated with Harvard Medical School, offer contrasting positions on the permissibility of physician participation in execution. In the YES selection, David Waisel, professor of anesthesia at Boston Children's Hospital, argues that concern for the welfare of the condemned makes physician participation permissible. If executions are to occur, they should be done humanely and physicians not only may participate in them, but in fact it is honorable for them to participate. In the NO selection, Atul Gawande, a surgeon at Brigham and Women's Hospital in Boston and professor of surgery at Harvard Medical School, argues that physicians' special healing role in society is incompatible with assisting in executions.

YES ↵

David Waisel

Physician Participation in Capital Punishment

If state administration of capital punishment is legal and ongoing, humane methods of execution should be sought and applied. In medieval times, the condemned and their families would bribe the executioner to make death quick and painless. In the 18th century, Dr Joseph-Ignace Guillotin proposed amending the French penal code to require executioners to use what is now known as the guillotine, believing that to be a more humane method of execution. In the United States, hanging was the predominant method of execution until electrocution was introduced as a more humane method in 1890.[1] One of the subtexts of electrocution was Thomas Edison's attempts to promote his direct current electricity by tainting the competing alternating current electricity through its association with the electric chair.[1] Cyanide gas was introduced in 1924.[2] Hanging, electrocution, and chemical asphyxiation were the primary methods of execution until the introduction of lethal injection in 1977.[2] Lethal injection has been the predominant form of execution in the 699 executions in the United States during the past 10 years.[3] Recent concerns about the technical issues surrounding legal execution, most specifically regarding drug delivery, have prompted some persons to suggest that physician participation in capital punishment would minimize these problems.

Opposing the involvement of physicians is the American Medical Association (AMA), which prohibits physician participation in legally authorized executions. According to the AMA's published position statements,[4] "An individual's opinion on capital punishment is the personal moral decision of the individual. A physician, as a member of a profession dedicated to preserving life when there is hope of doing so, should not be a participant in a legally authorized execution." The AMA further stated that physician participation in capital punishment "distorts the purpose and role of medicine and its professionals in the preservation of life. The use of physicians and medical technology in execution presents a conceptual contradiction for society and the public. The image of physician as executioner under circumstances mimicking medical care risks the general trust of the public."

The Code of Medical Ethics of the AMA prohibits physicians from "an action which would directly cause the death of the condemned [and] an action which would assist, supervise or contribute to the ability of another individual to directly cause the death of the condemned."[5] Prohibitions include nearly all aspects of lethal injection such as "selecting injection sites; starting intravenous lines as a port for a lethal injection device; prescribing, preparing, administering, or supervising injection drags or their doses or types; inspecting, testing, or maintaining lethal injection devices; and consulting with or supervising lethal injection personnel."[5]

In this commentary, I argue that poorly done executions needlessly hurt the condemned and that, in the case of lethal injections, the problems center not on the specific drugs chosen but on establishing and maintaining intravenous access and assessing for anesthetic depth. I argue that it is honorable for physicians to minimize the harm to these condemned individuals and that organized medicine has an obligation to *permit* physician participation in legal execution. By participation, I mean to the extent necessary to ensure a good death. This includes designing protocols both in general and for specific condemned persons and participating in the performance of these protocols, up to and including gaining intravenous access and giving drugs.

I will not address the policy of capital punishment. Although numerous issues surround capital punishment (appropriateness, fairness, and effectiveness as a crime deterrent, etc), they are beyond the scope of this article. The purpose of this commentary is to address physician participation in the ongoing practice of lethal injection.

From *Mayo Clinic Proceedings*, September 2007, pp. 1073–1080. Copyright © 2007 by Elsevier. Reprinted by permission via Rightslink.

The Need for Physician Participation

Lethal injection is the predominant form of execution in the United States, in part because it is considered more humane than hanging, electrocution, and chemical asphyxiation. In 1977, an anesthesiologist suggested a process that appeared to mimic a typical induction of anesthesia: sodium thiopental to cause unconsciousness, pancuronium bromide to paralyze the muscles, and (in the case of lethal injection) potassium chloride to stop the heart.[6]

In anesthetic practice, after a drug to induce anesthesia (like sodium thiopental) is given, anesthesiologists test for adequate depth of anesthesia, sometimes using a hands-on assessment like an eyelash reflex (touching the eyelashes to see if the eyelids flutter). A normal induction dose of 3 to 5 mg/kg of thiopental would be expected to produce unconsciousness in approximately 30 seconds and peak respiratory depression in 1 to 1.5 minutes.[7] It is not uncommon for respiratory attempts to return shortly thereafter. Pancuronium bromide, a paralytic with no anesthetic properties, is given in a dose of 1 mg/kg and within 4 minutes [and] produces muscle relaxation to facilitate tracheal intubation.[8]

San Quentin Operational Procedure No. 770 describes how a typical lethal execution is to be done;[9] 2 intravenous lines are inserted, and saline flows through 1 of the lines. Individuals other than the condemned person leave the room. The door is sealed. Through injection ports located outside the room, 5 g of sodium thiopental (ie, 10 times the 500-mg induction of anesthesia dose for a man weighing 100 kg) is given in "[A] steady even flow . . . maintained with only a minimum amount of force applied to the syringe plunger." The intravenous line is then flushed with 20 cm³ of normal saline. Two syringes of 50 mg of pancuronium bromide in 50 cm³ of diluent (ie, a total of 100 mg, 10 times the 10-mg dose given for a man weighing 100 kg) are then "injected with slow, even pressure on the syringe plunger," and the intravenous line is flushed with 20 cm³ of normal saline. Two syringes of 50 mEq of potassium chloride in 50 cm³ of diluent (a total of 100 mEq of potassium chloride) are then injected.[9]

If this process is performed correctly, the inmate will be unconscious before receiving pancuronium bromide and potassium chloride.[7,10] These massive doses of sodium thiopental should both stop breathing and cause unconsciousness in 1 minute.[11] In the absence of a hands-on assessment of anesthetic depth, sustained apnea becomes a reasonable surrogate for adequate delivery of the massive doses of sodium thiopental. Sustained apnea guarantees a sufficient depth of anesthesia.

In contrast, spontaneous ventilation after sodium thiopental indicates that the desired dose of sodium thiopental was *not* delivered. Spontaneous ventilation does not indicate awareness, but it also does not confirm anesthesia.

The presence of apnea after administration of pancuronium bromide is not a guarantee that the sodium thiopental was delivered. A dose that is 3 times a normal intubating dose of pancuronium (ie, 30 mg instead of 10 mg in a man weighing 100 kg) will cause muscle relaxation within 1 minute.[8] Thus, only a fraction of the pancuronium bromide needs to be successfully administered to cause apnea. Apnea after pancuronium bromide, instead of after sodium thiopental, does not indicate that the inmate was anesthetized before the pancuronium bromide. If the inmate was not anesthetized before the administration of pancuronium bromide and potassium chloride, the inmate may have the sensation of paralysis without anesthesia (known as awareness) and may feel the burning of the highly concentrated potassium chloride.

One problem with lethal injection is obtaining venous access, leading to extensive and painful attempts, including placement of central venous access.[12] A more concerning problem is inadequate medication delivery during the execution. This can occur from technical errors and procedural errors (Table 1). For example, in 6 executions since 1999 in California, the condemned had reactions such as respirations and tachycardia, which may have been consistent with awareness or pain.[11] The possible patterns of successful and botched lethal injection are listed in Table 2 and Table 3.

Other problems exist with drug delivery. In 1994 in Illinois, with use of a machine to inject the sodium thiopental and pancuronium bromide, the intravenous catheter clogged, leaving the inmate snorting and his belly "heaving up and down with the breathing."[14] After the botched execution, the spokesman for the corrections department stated, "It looks like the two drugs just don't mix . . . they get tacky and don't flow when they come together."[18] The same problem had happened the only previous time the machine was used 4 years earlier.

In 1995 in Missouri, the arm restraint functioned as a tourniquet, prolonging the process and bringing into question the sensations of the condemned person.[21] The county coroner said that the heartbeat stopped several minutes after the strap was loosened, suggesting that the sodium thiopental, pancuronium bromide, and potassium chloride entered the bloodstream at the same time, not giving the sodium thiopental time to work, and increasing the likelihood that the condemned person was aware while paralyzed or felt the burning from the

Table 1

Sources of Error in Lethal Execution

Steps of execution	Sources of potential error
1. Prepare medications, including mixing sodium thiopental from powder	Improper and improvisational mixing of sodium thiopental[10,13]
2. Obtain intravenous access	Difficulty[14,15]
	Not placed intravascularly[16]
	Protocols do not address what should happen if obtaining peripheral venous access is not possible[9,15]
3. Inject sodium thiopental	Burning and blistering if injected into subcutaneous tissues[16,17]
	Human error[10,13]
4. Assess anesthetic depth	Not assessed, improperly assessed, false proxies of anesthesia[15]
	Individual not physically present to assess depth of anesthesia[10,13,15]
	Inadequate human skill[10,15]
5. Inject pancuronium bromide	Muscle relaxation may hide signs of inmate distress[10,13,15]
	Precipitation with sodium thiopental[15,18,19]
6. Repeat doses of pancuronium bromide and potassium chloride if necessary	Poorly designed protocols, no repeated doses of sodium thiopental[10,15]
7. Other problems	Deviation from protocols[15]
	Absence of written protocol[13]
	Inadequate records; no assessment of the quality of executions[10, 15]
	No meaningful training, supervision, and oversight of the execution team[10,13,15,20]
	Inadequate lighting, overcrowded conditions and poorly designed facilities in which the execution team must work[10,13,15]
	Lack of respect for "solemn" task of executions[9]

Table 2

Proper and Improper Drug Administration Procedures for Lethal Injection*

Procedure	Consequence
Proper: STP→Apnea→P→KCL	Time is given for inmate to be anesthetized by sodium thiopental, as confirmed by apnea, then paralyzed, then given potassium chloride
Improper: STP→P→Apnea→KCL	Inmate is administered paralytic medication before becoming apneic, raising the possibility that insufficient sodium thiopental was delivered to the venous circulation. Inmate may be aware of being paralyzed and may feel the burning of potassium chloride. With 100 mg of pancuronium bromide being administered, even one-third of the intended dose would cause paralysis within 1 min
Improper: STP, P, KCL (at the same time)	No time is given for the sodium thiopental to work and no time is taken to assess whether the sodium thiopental has caused apnea
Improper: STP→P→KCL→→→P, KCL	In some protocols, the pancuronium bromide and potassium chloride are repeated at 10 min if the inmate is not dead. This indicates that the drugs were not delivered adequately (ie, insufficient doses) to the venous system (because if they had been, the inmate would be dead). Repeating pancuronium bromide and potassium chloride without the sodium thiopental increases the likelihood of awareness

*KCL = potassium chloride; P = pancuronium bromide; STP = sodium thiopental.

potassium chloride. The inmate was "gasping, slightly convulsing" 7 minutes after initiation of the lethal injection.[21] The coroner declared that it was "a little error. It's not like the guy suffered."[21]

In 2006 in Ohio, after a difficult insertion of an intravenous line, the execution team chose not to insert a second intravenous line (as apparently called for by prison procedures)[22] and injected the drugs. The inmate appeared

Table 3

Five Specific Cases of Lethal Injection in California*[11]

Inmate, year	Minutes										
	0	1	2	3	4	5	6	7	8	9	10
Siripongs, 1999	STP				P	Apnea					
Babbitt, 1999	STP			P		Apnea					
Rich, 2000	STP		P/apnea								
Anderson, 2002	STP		P			Apnea					
Allen, 2006	STP									P	Apnea

*All cases follow the example of STP→P→Apnea→KCL. One case, Williams, 2005, is not included because inadequate recordkeeping makes it unclear whether apnea occurred concurrent with the pancuronium bromide (6 min after sodium thiopental) or concurrent with the potassium chloride (12 min after sodium thiopental and 6 min after pancuronium bromide). KCL = potassium chloride; P = pancuronium bromide; STP = sodium thiopental.

to have fallen asleep, with shallow breathing. But shortly thereafter, he "raised his head and, frustrated, shook it back and forth, repeatedly declaring, 'it don't work.'"[22] The execution team obtained additional intravenous access, mistakenly connected the intravenous line to the failed intravenous catheter, administered the drugs, noticed a reaction by the inmate, subsequently reconnected the intravenous line to the correct catheter, and administered the drugs. The inmate "raised his head about a dozen times and appeared to try to speak"[22] before dying.

In 2006 in Florida, 2 intravenous catheters were placed in the condemned person, and it appears that both catheters infiltrated into the surrounding tissues, so that the drugs were injected into the tissues and not into the veins.[16] "More than 20 minutes after the first injection, [the inmate] appeared to be mouthing words, clenching his jaw, and grimacing."[23] The inmate received a second dose of drugs.[23] Likely as a result of the drugs entering the tissues instead of the vein, the inmate had footlong "chemical blisters on both of his arms."[16] An anesthesiologist familiar with the case testified that the accounts of the inmate breathing "like a fish out of water" were consistent with a "person who is partially paralyzed and struggling for breath."[16] This event led the Governor of Florida to declare a moratorium on state executions pending a report from a concurrently designated commission.

Attempts to tweak operating procedures for lethal injection are insufficient. The Morales Memorandum of Intended Decision reported that in February 2006, officials in California decided that "a continuous infusion of sodium thiopental during the administration of pancuronium bromide and potassium chloride would be added."[10] As in the 1994 case in Illinois, such an approach would lead to a precipitate being formed and subsequent clogging of the intravenous catheter.

If the problem is the delivery of the drugs and the assessment of anesthetic depth before injection of a paralytic and potassium chloride, then a person who is wholly competent at managing intravenous infusions and assessing for anesthetic depth is needed for humane lethal injection. Although nonphysicians *could* perform this procedure (as the AMA has argued), they would need to be trained by physicians to develop these skills. In the absence of extensive teaming and refresher courses for nonphysicians (which would seemingly fly in the face of the AMA statement), the most skilled individuals would be those who intravenously inject medications routinely to obtain an end result.

Arguments Regarding Roles of Physicians and the Government

Physicians have an obligation to be altruistic. Some interpret this obligation to prohibit physician participation in the execution of an unwilling individual (reports of condemned persons choosing to die rather than prolong their stay on death row notwithstanding[24]), even if the condemned person desires the aid of a physician to make death more humane. The AMA addresses this point directly: "While physician participation may potentially add some degree of humaneness to the execution of an individual, it does not outweigh the greater harm of causing death to the individual."[4]

Death, however, is not the sole issue. Physicians are permitted to let people die, such as in the withdrawal or withholding of care. Physicians are even permitted to be a proximate cause of death, in the sense that sometimes the medications needed to treat pain and discomfort unintentionally hasten death. Public policy has shifted in some countries and states to allow physicians to assist in the death of a patient. For example, from 1998 to 2002 in Oregon, 129 people self-administered legally prescribed lethal medications.[25] It is even becoming accepted that physicians may directly cause death. In the Netherlands, termination of life on request and assistance with suicide are not treated as criminal offenses if certain requirements are met.[26] The primary distinction is that in the aforementioned examples, death is considered in the best interest of the patient by the patient or concerned surrogate decisionmakers. In capital punishment, death is involuntary and is not in the best interest of the individual.

If one accepts the premise that physician participation will lead to more humane executions, does the fact that death is not in the inmate's best interest obviate a request for relief from suffering? Does physician participation mean that physicians are acting as tools of the government, helping the state carry out judicial punishment? More to the point, does acting in a manner concordant with the goals of the government make a physician a tool of the government?

Some argue that physician participation constitutes inappropriate use of physicians as a tool of the government.[27] Historically, when the government has used physicians to implement policies that did not benefit the individuals affected, the health of the society benefited. For example, physician participation in quarantine of individuals with infectious diseases, while limiting the freedom of movement of some individuals, resulted in an overall health benefit of minimizing the spread of disease. This societal health benefit legitimizes physician participation in quarantine, but physician participation in capital punishment provides no societal health benefit. According to Truog (Robert D. Truog, MD, Professor of Medical Ethics, Anesthesia, & Pediatrics, Harvard Medical School),[27] "A physician's participation in capital punishment does nothing to promote the moral community of medicine. Indeed, such participation offends the sense of community by prostituting medical knowledge and skills to serve the purposes of the state and its criminal justice system."[27] If the physician's primary role is to ensure a successful execution, such that a physician would be willing to do it in an inhumane way, then the physician is being used as a tool of the government to further state goals. But a legitimate question is whether the physician is acting as a tool of the individual to

minimize suffering and further the individual's goals or whether the physician is acting as a tool of the government to ensure a successful execution. Although the outcome may be death, the act of the physician may be solely to provide comfort. In this case, a physician is not acting as a tool of the government; he is acting as a physician whose goals temporarily align with the goals of the government. Clearly, there are potential harms in permitting physicians to act in this way. But these harms need to be weighed against the benefits to the condemned. Physicians are responding to the immediate goals of the condemned. To prohibit this aid because the use of the physician as a tool for the individual (good reason) happens to occur in conjunction with the use of the physician as a tool for the government (bad reason) requires a compelling reason to forego our responsibilities to the individual. Indeed, a principled stance of prohibition regressively harms society's most vulnerable individuals. Consider this: a prison warden "testified that he believes a 'successful execution' is simply one where 'the inmate ends up dead at the end of the process.' When asked whether he considered a successful execution to mean anything else, he responded, 'I'm thinking not.'"[10] If you were to be executed, would you prefer to have a competent and caring individual obtain venous access quickly and minimize any chance of pain or awareness?

This argument, of course, is susceptible to comparison with the Nazi concentration camp physicians' argument that they were "morally neutral bystanders" who followed the law and who compassionately spared concentration camp "subhumans" from a slower and more painful death.[28] But I argue that this is too free an analogy. The process by which the laws are developed and the underlying intent of the laws (as well as can be surmised) [is] relevant in determining whether government authorization makes physician participation in capital punishment legitimate and permissible. We live in a society open to free speech and public protest, one in which citizens have a remarkable ability to participate in the development of laws and policies. Furthermore, capital punishment is public and avidly discussed, not hidden. Of importance, Nazi physicians thought "they were acting for the good of the whole nation and society."[28] Such notions of prioritizing the state (or even certain communities) over individuals often lead to harm. In Nazi Germany, the purpose of the government intervention (concentration camps, genocide, etc) was the actualization of political goals. In contrast, capital punishment does not advance a comprehensive political goal.

Slippery Slope Arguments Regarding Other Harms of Participation

Some worry that permitting physician participation in capital punishment will erode a physician's ability to be compassionate and independent, will make it easier to permit physicians to participate in government-sanctioned killing, and will harm public trust.[5,12,27,29] These arguments are rooted in the psychological slippery slope by claiming that one event will lead to another. The usefulness of the slippery slope argument is suspect.

We should always be concerned about permitting actions that would lead us down the psychological slippery slope to causing harm. However, the problem with many slippery slope arguments is that they do not precisely clarify how permitting the debated action will lead to another, often unspecified, action. In a different context, Burgess (John Burgess, BA, MA, DPhil, Faculty of Arts, University of Wollongong, New South Wales, Australia)[30] labeled this the One Great Slippery Slope Argument: "[I]f we adopt . . . a particular change in our practices it just might start a slide into a moral deterioration that ends with our committing Nazi-style atrocities." The argument that a slope exists is often used as a poor substitute for an argument about how the debated action will cause the slide down the slope. Furthermore, while uncritically accepting as legitimate the sketchy possibility that society could slide down the slope, slippery slope supporters often demand a detailed argument about how it could not occur.[30]

A good psychological slippery slope argument is detailed and modest.[30] The arguments connecting disaster with physician participation in capital punishment do not provide a clear and detailed account of how participation leads to calamity. Consider the most extreme and visceral argument, that permitting physician participation would be the first step down the slope to Nazi-like atrocities.[29,31] Such a descent would require a series of extraordinary events that culminate in a self-serving totalitarian regime and a dominant social group, whose primary concern is the health of the social organism and the exploitation of an identified other.[30] Perhaps most importantly, the Nazi premise of society as a biological organism led to the concept of medicalized killing as "killing as therapeutic imperative."[32] This medicalized view of society legitimized removing the disease (ie, killing) of those "unfit to live," just like antibiotics kill bacteria or a surgeon removes an appendix. This thinking provided a rationale for society (and thus physicians) to kill. There is no reason to believe that physician participation in capital punishment would lead to such a radical restructuring of society and society's views.

With that preamble, we will examine the claims. We do not know the effects of self-chosen participation in executions on a physician's ability to act with compassion and independence. We do have information on the effects on members of execution teams who carry out executions (eg, secure inmate, obtain intravenous access, inject medications) in 3 Southern states.[33] Individuals on execution teams use selective moral disengagement, moral justification, economic and security justification, dehumanization, and nonresponsibility to be able to perform executions. Executioners compartmentalize work and home life, construe participation in executions as a positive activity with "high moral and societal purposes," and become more desensitized as they participate in more executions. Lifton (Robert Jay Lifton, MD, is a psychiatrist who has studied and written extensively on mental adaptations to war, atrocities, and war crimes)[32] described compartmentalization in the context of Nazi physicians as the experience of the "doubling" of the self, in which the 2 selves are partitioned from each other. This mechanism of "doubling" enabled Nazi physicians to be evil at one moment and caring in the next moment and is what Lifton thought permitted specific individuals with what appeared to be relatively appropriate moral values to slide, incrementally, into performing atrocities. The concern is that compartmentalization by physicians participating in capital punishment could similarly harm physicians.

However, the application of this study of prison workers to physicians is unclear. Physicians participating in capital punishment have the ability to view their actions as helping the condemned. Indeed, to me, participation in a horrible detail to benefit another person is true altruism. Additionally, that article did not consider what sort of interventions may help those who participate in capital punishment (eg, caps on number of cases in which an individual participates, mandatory counseling). Even if a few willing physicians were harmed, it is hard to construct a detailed slippery slope argument that connects a few physicians undergoing compartmentalization with widespread societal harms. Furthermore, of importance, physicians will not be required to participate because most states have conscience clauses that permit caregivers to opt out of care they deem morally objectionable.[34]

Beyond the effect on specific physicians, there is concern that permitting physicians to appear to be tools of the government by participating in capital punishment will make it psychologically easier for physicians to be used in inappropriate ways.[27,29] Although this may be true, the possibility of an event is not the step-by-step connection between an event and a specified harm that constitutes evidence in a slippery slope argument. In addition, I argue that our society is more than capable of withstanding the psychological slippery slope.

One argument that supports the slippery slope claim is that physicians were prime leaders in Nazi Germany and if the physicians of that time had held the line and had not acquiesced in devaluing human life (as physicians in the United States would by aiding the process of capital punishment), it is unlikely that Nazi Germany would have happened.

The idea that protesting physicians could have been a bulwark against harm in Nazi Germany is speculative counterfactual history. Proponents of this argument highlight that physician participation in the Nazi party eclipsed other professions; 45% of doctors joined the party, a full 20% more than lawyers and teachers and greater than 35% more than the general population.[35] However, the many physicians who joined the party around 1937 tended to be unemployed. Their desire for participation most likely had to do with navigating the central bureaucracy of medicine and a craving for "enduring professional and socioeconomic security and desired recognition."[35] Thus, rather than lead change, most party physicians were "petty opportunists" who joined in response to the societal changes.[31]

Finally, it has been argued that physician involvement, even if or especially because of government imprimatur, will lead to a loss of public trust, perhaps leading patients to wonder about what these physicians and what medicine will do to them. Patients may wonder, for example, that if physicians are "used to killing" people, then what would hold physicians back from making recommendations not in the patient's best interests.

The concerns about how physician participation in capital punishment would lead to a loss of public trust would have to be explicated. To me, this can be no more harmful to the public trust than the 40-year Tuskegee Syphilis Study, in which the US Public Health Service withheld treatment from African American men to determine the effects of syphilis; the government radiation experiments, in which many were experimented on without their knowledge or consent; the Sunbeam fiasco, in which the AMA agreed to and then renounced a deal to endorse Sunbeam medical products that the AMA had no plans to test; and the inability of journal editors to police themselves for conflicts of interests and the withholding or fabrication of information such as with cloning.[36-40] These examples are not presented to say that one wrong

should permit another. They are presented to say that, to me, these are likely more harmful to the public trust. The effects of these were more widespread. Yet organized medicine has weathered these events. If permitting physician participation in capital punishment is a matter of weighing the risks and benefits of participation, then using the argument of loss of public trust to prohibit participation would require that harm from the loss of public trust be substantial. No evidence suggests that physician participation in capital punishment would be more damaging to the public trust than these events. Indeed, organized medicine has already weathered physician participation in capital punishment "at every stage, whether preparing for, participating in, or monitoring executions."[41]

The Misapplied Argument of Palatability

A misplaced argument is that physician involvement will make executions smoother and thus more palatable, decreasing the likelihood of abolishing the death penalty.[41] Therefore, physicians, dedicated to improving the quality of life as the patient defines it, should not participate in any action that increases acceptance of capital punishment.[42] The implicit assumption is that physicians, by definition, should oppose capital punishment.[42] This connection, however, has no place in this discussion. It is organized medicine's obligation to lead, and organized medicine is free to make statements regarding the appropriateness of capital punishment. But to use participation as a stalking horse for abolition of capital punishment is disingenuous. This discussion is not about the appropriateness of capital punishment; this discussion is about physician participation in capital punishment.

The Value and Strength of Society

I have used the idea that our free and open society is a powerful bulwark against the potential harms of physician participation in capital punishment. I am fully aware that many enlightened and open societies have sunk into totalitarianism. It would be arrogant to suggest that our society is incapable of such a fall. But that does not mean it is likely that physician participation in capital punishment would be the tipping point or would even be contributory. I contend that, like the Nazi society, such a fall would be a function of widespread socioeconomic factors and that egregious medical abuse would follow, not precede, societal changes. I may be naive, but I believe our society has successfully weathered challenges, and I have faith in the strengths of our society and the sturdiness of its processes. In support of this argument, consider the experiences with physician aid-in-dying in Oregon and with euthanasia in the Netherlands, both of which some considered potential pathways to disaster.[43] In Oregon, the 5-year experience indicated no improprieties in physician aid-in-dying. In the Netherlands, the rate of uncommon improprieties, such as nonvoluntary euthanasia, has remained stable, with no indication of impending disaster.[44] In contrast, in an interview study, leaders in the Netherlands appeared disturbingly complacent about reports of euthanasia without explicit patient request.[45] Whether such unsettling attitudes will lead to future harms is unknown. Nonetheless, these 2 examples indicate that the presence of a slippery slope does not necessarily lead to descent down the slope. I argue that this stability is in large part due to society. In regard to analogies with Nazi Germany, we must be capable of and willing to make distinctions. To argue that the wanton torturing and killing of at least 11 million individuals is equivalent to the extensive processes of capital punishment is fallacious both by numbers and by process. Indeed, to me, comparisons to Nazi Germany are absurd, and if I had my way, this discussion would proceed without those analyses.

Is This Discussion Necessary?

Capital punishment could easily be performed without the use of venous access. The use of medications associated with treatment of humans for capital punishment is an accident, the result of a decision to ask a physician rather than a veterinarian for help. One can imagine, for example, that a veterinarian could provide an acceptable alternative, such as subcutaneous administration of etorphine hydrochloride (a synthetic opioid) and acepromazine maleate (a phenothiazine) to effectively cause cardiopulmonary arrest. Indeed, with subcutaneous injection, concerns about intravenous lethal injection would be nonexistent, and most of the problems discussed in this article would be moot. Although the literature is sparse, I imagine a number of combinations could be delivered subcutaneously or intramuscularly that would anesthetize an inmate before causing death.

Recommendations

The current AMA policy increases the chances of a botched execution. It seems cruel to permit capital punishment but not to permit participation of those who are capable of performing it humanely. If capital punishment is a reality in the United States, then for the sake of the condemned organized medicine should address how it should be performed. The AMA statement should be revised to address complex issues, some of which I briefly discuss.

Astute readers will note that I have avoided the use of the term *patients* when referring to inmates. I now advocate for the use of the word *patient* in this context. I conceptualize physician participation in capital punishment as an altruistic practice of medicine. The future *patient* should request physician participation, and the physician should be licensed to practice medicine in that state. To emphasize the altruistic nature of the service, physicians should refuse payment for this service. Although the fact that physicians are performing capital punishment should be public knowledge, specific physicians who perform capital punishment should be permitted to remain anonymous. I do realize that this connotes shame, but anonymity is necessary to protect a physician and his or her family from retaliation. Physicians who serve this *patient* community should receive counseling, and studies should be implemented to determine whether there should be limitations, such as the number of executions that a physician may perform. Physicians should be permitted to be involved in other ways to improve the humaneness of capital punishment, such as publicly suggesting and debating protocols or initiating and managing databases. Indeed, permitting physician participation in developing protocols is likely the best way to achieve humane executions while enabling physicians not to directly participate in the act of lethal injection.[10]

One issue that has come to the forefront is whether the government should be able to mandate physician participation.[13] It would be hard to argue that the government's interest is altruistic, that is, focused on removing harm from the patient. The government's interest is better understood as being able to achieve capital punishment as easily as possible. Permitting the government to mandate physician participation is wrongheaded because it verges on making the physician a tool of the government, not of the patient.

Some have suggested that the appropriate physician to perform capital punishment is the anesthesiologist.[10,13] To be sure, there are superficial similarities in appearance between capital punishment and induction of anesthesia. But such similarities are an accident of history. Many physicians, including intensivists and emergency department physicians, have the ability to manage intravenous infusions and assess for anesthetic depth or suggest alternative drugs. Indeed, although this article is focused on physician participation, many of these arguments are equally valid for others who develop caregiver-patient relationships and have the requisite skills. Space does not allow a detailed analysis for different professions.

Physician participation in capital punishment does have associated harms. But the question is whether the harms outweigh the benefits. Because the potential benefits are sufficiently clear and the potential harms are poorly explicated, we should permit physician participation in capital punishment.

References

1. Jones GR. Judicial electrocution and the prison doctor. *Lancet.* 1990;335(8691):713–714.
2. Bohm RM. *Deathquests: An Introduction to the Theory and Practice of Capital Punishment in the United States.* Cincinnati, OH: Anderson Publishing; 1999.
3. Death Penalty Information Center. Execution database: years selected 1997–2006. Available at: www.deathpenaltyinfo.org/executions.php. Accessed July 3, 2007.
4. Council on Ethical and Judicial Affairs, American Medical Association. Physician participation in capital punishment. *JAMA.* 1993;270(3):365–368.
5. Council on Ethical and Judicial Affairs, American Medical Association. Capital punishment. In: *Code of Medical Ethics: Current Opinions with Annotations 2006–2007.* Chicago, IL: American Medical Association; 2006:E-2.06.
6. Denno DW. When legislatures delegate death: the troubling paradox behind state use of electrocution and lethal injection and what it says about us. *Ohio State Law* J. 2002;63:63–260.
7. Reves JG, Glass PSA, Lubarsky DA, McEvoy MD. Intravenous nonopioid anesthetics. In: Miller RD, ed. *Miller's Anesthesia.* 6th ed. Philadelphia, PA: Elsevier Churchill Livingstone; 2005:317–378.
8. Naguib M, Lien CA. Pharmacology of muscle relaxants and their antagonists. In: Miller RD, ed. *Miller's Anesthesia.* Vol 1.6th ed. Philadelphia, PA: Elsevier Churchill Livingstone; 2005:481–572.
9. California State Prison, San Quentin. San Quentin Operational Procedure No. 770. Revised date: 6/13/03. Available at: www.law.berkeley.edu/clinics/dpclinic /Lethal%20Injection%20Documents/California/Morales /Morales%20Dist%20Ct.Cp/Ex%20A%20to%20TRO%20 motion%20(Procedure%20No.%20770).pdf. Accessed July 3, 2007.
10. *Morales v Tilton* 465 F Supp 2d 972 (ND Cal), December 15, 2006.
11. *Morales v Hickman* 415 F Supp 2d 1037 (ND Cal), February 14, 2006.
12. Gawande A. When law and ethics collide—why physicians participate in executions. *N Engl J Med.* 2006;354(12):1221–1229.
13. *Taylor v Crawford* 445 F3d 1095 (8th Cir 2006).
14. Chapman R. Witnesses describe killer's 'macabre' final few minutes. *Chicago Sun-Times.* May 11 , 1994:5.
15. Brief for Amicus Curiae, Darick Demorris Walker, Supporting Petitioner re *Hill v McDonough,* US 2006 WL 558286. Available at: www.law.berkeley.edu/clinics /dpclinic/Lethal%20Injection%20Documents/Florida /Hill2006.03.06%20amicus%20walker.pdf. Accessed July 5, 2007.
16. Tisch C. Doctor: execution flawed at start. *St. Petersburg Times.* February 13, 2007:1B.
17. Reich DL, Kaplan JA. Complications of cardiovascular access. In: Benumof JL, Saidman LJ, eds. *Anesthesia and Perioperative Complications.* St. Louis, MO: Mosby-Year Book Inc; 1992:16–37.
18. Fornek S. Bad drug mix delayed execution. *Chicago Sun-Times.* May 12, 1994:12.
19. Morton WD, Lerman J. The effect of pancuronium on the solubility of aqueous thiopentone. *Can J Anaesth.* 1987;34(l):87–89.
20. Executioner needs precise training in carrying out lethal injections. *Tampa Tribune.* February 13, 2007:10.
21. O'neil T. Too-tight strap hampered execution; coroner: chemical flow was impeded. *St. Louis Post-Dispatch.* May 5, 1995:1B.
22. Provance J, Hall C. Problems bog down execution of Clark. *Toledo Blade.* May 3, 2006:Al.
23. Whoriskey P, Geis S. Lethal injection is on hold in 2 states. *The Washington Post.* December 16, 2006:A1.
24. Overall M, Smith M. 22-year-old killer gets early execution; sped-up law adds witnesses. *The Tulsa World.* May 8, 1997:A1.
25. Hedberg K, Hopkins D, Kohn M. Five years of legal physician-assisted suicide in Oregon [letter]. *N Engl J Med.* 2003;348(10):961–964.
26. van der Maas PJ, van der Wal G, Haverkate I, et al. Euthanasia, physician-assisted suicide, and other medical practices involving the end of life in the Netherlands, 1990–1995. *N Engl J Med.* 1996;335(22):1699–1705.
27. Truog RD, Brennan TA. Participation of physicians in capital punishment. *N Engl J Med.* 1993;329(18):1346–1350.
28. Pellegrino ED, Thomasma DC. Dubious premises—evil conclusions: moral reasoning at the Nuremberg trials. *Comb Q Healthc Ethics.* Spring 2000; 9(2):261–274.
29. Freedman AM, Halpern AL. The erosion of ethics and morality in medicine: physician participation

in legal executions in the United States. NY *Law Sch Law Rev.* 1996;41(1):169–188.

30. Burgess JA. The great slippery-slope argument. *J Med Ethics.* 1993;19 (3): 169–174.

31. Lerner BH, Rothman DJ. Medicine and the Holocaust: learning more of the lessons [editorial]. *Ann Intern Med.* 1995;122(10):793–794.

32. Lifton RJ. *The Nazi Doctors: Medical Killing and the Psychology of Genocide.* New York, NY: Basic Books; 1986:15–16.

33. Osofsky MJ, Bandura A, Zimbardo PG. The role of moral disengagement in the execution process. *Law Hum Behav.* 2005;29(4):371–393.

34. Charo RA. The celestial fire of conscience—refusing to deliver medical care. *N Engl J Med.* 2005;352(24):2471–2473.

35. Kater MH. Criminal physicians in the third reich: towards a group portrait. In: Nicosia FR, Huener J, eds. *Medicine and Medical Ethics in Nazi Germany.* New York, NY: Bergbahn Books; 2002:77–92.

36. Jones JH. *Bad Blood: The Tuskegee Syphilis Experiments.* New York, NY: The Free Press; 1993.

37. United States Advisory Committee on Human Radiation Experiments. *The Human Radiation Experiments.* New York, NY: Oxford University Press; 1996.

38. Broken deal costs A.M.A. $9.9 million. *New York Times.* August 3, 1998:A12.

39. Our conflicted medical journals [editorial]. *New York Times.* July 23, 2006;4:11.

40. Bosman J. Reporters find science journals harder to trust, but not easy to verify. *New York Times.* February 13, 2006:C1.

41. Emanuel LL, Bienen LB. Physician participation in executions: time to eliminate anonymity provisions and protest the practice [editorial]. *Ann Intern Med.* 2001;135(10):922–924.

42. Stop killing people who kill people [editorial]. *Lancet.* 2007;369:343.

43. Snyder L, Sulmasy DP, Ethics and Human Rights Committee, American College of Physicians-American Society of Internal Medicine. Physician-assisted suicide. *Ann Intern Med.* 2001;135(3):209–216.

44. Onwuteaka-Philipsen BD, van der Heide A, Koper D, et al. Euthanasia and other end-of-life decisions in the Netherlands in 1990, 1995, and 2001. *Lancet.* 2003;362(9381):395–399.

45. Cohen-Almagor R. Non-voluntary and involuntary euthanasia in The Netherlands: Dutch perspectives. *Issues Law Med.* Spring 2003;18(3):239–257.

DAVID WAISEL is an associate professor of anesthesia at Children's Hospital Boston.

Atul Gawande

→ NO

When Law and Ethics Collide—Why Physicians Participate in Executions

On February 14, 2006, a U.S. District Court issued an unprecedented ruling concerning the California execution by lethal injection of murderer Michael Morales. The ruling ordered that the state have a physician, specifically an anesthesiologist, personally supervise the execution, or else drastically change the standard protocol for lethal injections.[1] Under the protocol, the anesthetic sodium thiopental is given at massive doses that are expected to stop breathing and extinguish consciousness within one minute after administration; then the paralytic agent pancuronium is given, followed by a fatal dose of potassium chloride.

The judge found, however, that evidence from execution logs showed that six of the last eight prisoners executed in California had not stopped breathing before technicians gave the paralytic agent, raising a serious possibility that prisoners experienced suffocation from the paralytic, a feeling much like being buried alive, and felt intense pain from the potassium bolus. This experience would be unacceptable under the Constitution's Eighth Amendment protections against cruel and unusual punishment. So the judge ordered the state to have an anesthesiologist present in the death chamber to determine when the prisoner was unconscious enough for the second and third injections to be given—or to perform the execution with sodium thiopental alone.

The California Medical Association, the American Medical Association (AMA), and the American Society of Anesthesiologists (ASA) immediately and loudly opposed such physician participation as a clear violation of medical ethics codes. "Physicians are healers, not executioners," the ASA's president told reporters. Nonetheless, in just two days, prison officials announced that they had found two willing anesthesiologists. The court agreed to maintain their anonymity and to allow them to shield their identities from witnesses. Both withdrew the day before the execution, however, after the Court of Appeals for the Ninth Circuit added a further stipulation requiring them

personally to administer additional medication if the prisoner remained conscious or was in pain.[2] This they would not accept. The execution was then postponed until at least May, but the court has continued to require that medical professionals assist with the administration of any lethal injection given to Morales.

This turn of events is the culmination of a steady evolution in methods of execution in the United States. On July 2, 1976, in deciding the case of *Gregg v. Georgia*, the Supreme Court legalized capital punishment after a decade-long moratorium on executions. Executions resumed six months later, on January 17, 1977, in Utah, with the death by firing squad of Gary Gilmore for the killing of Ben Bushnell, a Provo motel manager.

Death by firing squad, however, came to be regarded as too bloody and uncontrolled. (Gilmore's heart, for example, did not stop until two minutes afterward, and shooters have sometimes weakened at the trigger, as famously happened in 1951 in Utah when the five riflemen fired away from the target over Elisio Mares's heart, only to hit his right chest and cause him to bleed slowly to death.)[3]

Hanging came to be regarded as still more inhumane. Under the best of circumstances, the cervical spine is broken at C2, the diaphragm is paralyzed, and the prisoner suffocates to death, a minutes-long process.

Gas chambers proved no better: asphyxiation from cyanide gas, which prevents cells from using oxygen by inactivating cytochrome oxidase, took even longer than death by hanging, and the public revolted at the vision of suffocating prisoners fighting for air and then seizing as the hypoxia worsened. In Arizona, in 1992, for example, the asphyxiation of triple murderer Donald Harding took 11 minutes, and the sight was so horrifying that reporters began crying, the attorney general vomited, and the prison warden announced he would resign if forced to conduct another such execution.[4] Since 1976, only 2 prisoners have been executed by firing squad, 3 by hanging, and 12 by gas chamber.[5]

Electrocution, thought to cause a swifter, more acceptable death, was used in 74 of the first 100 executions after *Gregg*. But officials found that the electrical flow frequently arced, cooking flesh and sometimes igniting prisoners—postmortem examinations frequently had to be delayed for the bodies to cool—and yet some prisoners still required repeated jolts before they died. In Alabama, in 1979, for example, John Louis Evans III was still alive after two cycles of 2600 V; the warden called Governor George Wallace, who told him to keep going, and only after a third cycle, with witnesses screaming in the gallery, and almost 20 minutes of suffering did Evans finally die.[3] Only Florida, Virginia, and Alabama persisted with electrocutions with any frequency, and under threat of Supreme Court review, they too abandoned the method.

Lethal injection now appears to be the sole method of execution accepted by courts as humane enough to satisfy Eighth Amendment requirements—largely because it medicalizes the process. The prisoner is laid supine on a hospital gurney. A white bedsheet is drawn to his chest. An intravenous line flows into his or her arm. Under the protocol devised in 1977 by Dr. Stanley Deutsch, the chairman of anesthesiology at the University of Oklahoma, prisoners are first given 2500 to 5000 mg of sodium thiopental (5 to 10 times the recommended maximum), which can produce death all by itself by causing complete cessation of the brain's electrical activity followed by respiratory arrest and circulatory collapse. Death, however, can take up to 15 minutes or longer with thiopental alone, and the prisoner may appear to gasp, struggle, or convulse. So 60 to 100 mg of the paralytic agent pancuronium (10 times the usual dose) is injected one minute or so after the thiopental. Finally, 120 to 240 meq of potassium is given to produce rapid cardiac arrest.

Officials liked this method. Because it borrowed from established anesthesia techniques, it made execution like familiar medical procedures rather than the grisly, backlash-inducing spectacle it had become. (In Missouri, executions were even moved to a prison-hospital procedure room.) It was less disturbing to witness. The drugs were cheap and routinely available. And officials could turn to doctors and nurses to help with technical difficulties, attest to the painlessness and trustworthiness of the technique, and lend a more professional air to the proceedings.

But medicine balked. In 1980, when the first execution was planned using Dr. Deutsch's technique, the AMA passed a resolution against physician participation as a violation of core medical ethics. It affirmed that ban in detail in its 1992 Code of Medical Ethics. Article 2.06 states, "A physician, as a member of a profession dedicated to preserving life when there is hope of doing so, should not be a participant in a legally authorized execution," although an individual physician's opinion about capital punishment remains "the personal moral decision of the individual." It states that unacceptable participation includes prescribing or administering medications as part of the execution procedure, monitoring vital signs, rendering technical advice, selecting injection sites, starting or supervising placement of intravenous lines, or simply being present as a physician. Pronouncing death is also considered unacceptable, because the physician is not permitted to revive the prisoner if he or she is found to be alive. Only two actions were acceptable: provision at the prisoner's request of a sedative to calm anxiety beforehand and certification of death after another person had pronounced it.

The code of ethics of the Society of Correctional Physicians establishes an even stricter ban: "The correctional health professional shall . . . not be involved in any aspect of execution of the death penalty." The American Nurses Association (ANA) has adopted a similar prohibition. Only the national pharmacists' society, the American Pharmaceutical Association, permits involvement, accepting the voluntary provision of execution medications by pharmacists as ethical conduct.

States, however, wanted a medical presence. In 1982, in Texas, Dr. Ralph Gray, the state prison medical director, and Dr. Bascom Bentley agreed to attend the country's first execution by lethal injection, though only to pronounce death. But once on the scene, Gray was persuaded to examine the prisoner to show the team the best injection site.[6] Still, the doctors refused to give advice about the injection itself and simply watched as the warden prepared the chemicals. When he tried to push the syringe, however, it did not work. He had mixed all the drugs together, and they had precipitated into a clot of white sludge. "I could have told you that," one of the doctors reportedly said, shaking his head.[3] Afterward, Gray went to pronounce the prisoner dead but found him still alive. Though the doctors were part of the team now, they did nothing but suggest allowing time for more drugs to run in.

Today, all 38 death-penalty states rely on lethal injection. Of 1012 murderers executed since 1976, 844 were executed by injection.[5] Against vigorous opposition from the AMA and state medical societies, 35 of the 38 states explicitly allow physician participation in executions. Indeed, 17 require it: Colorado, Florida, Georgia, Idaho, Louisiana, Mississippi, Nevada, North Carolina, New Hampshire, New Jersey, New Mexico, Oklahoma, Oregon, South Dakota, Virginia, Washington, and Wyoming. To protect participating physicians from license challenges for violating ethics codes, states commonly provide legal immunity and promise anonymity. Nonetheless, several physicians have faced such challenges, though none have lost their licenses as yet.[7] And despite the promised anonymity, several states have produced the physicians in court to vouch publicly for the legitimacy and painlessness of the procedure.

States have affirmed that physicians and nurses—including those who are prison employees—have a right to refuse to participate in any way in executions. Yet they have found physicians and nurses who are willing to participate. Who are these people? And why do they do it?

It is not easy to find answers to these questions. The medical personnel are difficult to identify and reluctant to discuss their roles, even when offered anonymity. Among the 15 medical professionals I located who have helped with executions, however, I found 4 physicians and 1 nurse who agreed to speak with me; collectively, they have helped with at least 45 executions. None were zealots for the death penalty, and none had a simple explanation for why they did this work. The role, most said, had crept up on them.

Dr. A has helped with about eight executions in his state. He was extremely uncomfortable talking about the subject. Nonetheless, he sat down with me in a hotel lobby in a city not far from where he lives and told me his story.

Almost 60 years old, he is board certified in internal medicine and critical care, and he and his family have lived in their small town for 30 years. He is well respected. Almost everyone of local standing comes to see him as their primary care physician—the bankers, his fellow doctors, the mayor. Among his patients is the warden of the maximum-security prison that happens to be in his town. One day several years ago, they got talking during an appointment. The warden complained of difficulties staffing the prison clinic and asked Dr. A if he would be willing to see prisoners there occasionally. Dr. A said he would. He'd have made more money in his own clinic—the prison paid $65 an hour—but the prison was important to the community, he liked the warden, and it was just a few hours of work a month. He was happy to help.

Then, a year or two later, the warden asked him for help with a different problem. The state had a death penalty, and the legislature had voted to use lethal injection exclusively. The executions were to be carried out in the warden's prison. He needed doctors, he said. Would Dr. A help? He would not have to deliver the lethal injection. He would just help with cardiac monitoring. The warden gave the doctor time to consider it.

"My wife didn't like it," Dr. A told me. "She said, 'Why do you want to go there?'" But he felt torn. "I knew something about the past of these killers." One of them had killed a mother of three during a convenience-store robbery and then, while getting away, shot a man who was standing at his car pumping gas. Another convict had kidnapped, raped, and strangled to death an 11-year-old girl. "I do not have a very strong conviction about the death penalty, but I don't feel anything negative about it for such people either. The execution order was given legally by the court. And morally, if you think about the animal behavior of some of these people. . . . " Ultimately, he decided to participate, he said, because he was only helping with monitoring, because he was needed by the warden and his community, because the sentence was society's order, and because the punishment did not seem wrong.

At the first execution, he was instructed to stand behind a curtain watching the inmate's heart rhythm on a cardiac monitor. Neither the witnesses on the other side of the glass nor the prisoner could see him. A technician placed two IV lines. Someone he could not see pushed the three drugs, one right after another. Watching the monitor, he saw the sinus rhythm slow, then widen. He recognized the peaked T waves of hyperkalemia followed by the fine spikes of ventricular fibrillation and finally the flat, unwavering line of an asystolic arrest. He waited half a minute, then signaled to another physician who went out before the witnesses to place his stethoscope on the prisoner's unmoving chest. The doctor listened for 30 seconds and then told the warden the inmate was dead. Half an hour later, Dr. A was released. He made his way through a side door, past the crowd gathered outside, and headed home.

In three subsequent executions there were difficulties, though, all with finding a vein for an IV. The prisoners were either obese or past intravenous drug users, or both. The technicians would stick and stick and, after half an hour, give up. This was a possibility the warden had not prepared for. Dr. A had placed numerous lines. Could he give a try?

OK, Dr. A decided. Let me take a look.

This was a turning point, though he didn't recognize it at the time. He was there to help, they had a problem, and so he would help. It did not occur to him to do otherwise.

In two of the prisoners, he told me, he found a good vein and placed the IV. In one, however, he could not find a vein. All eyes were on him. He felt responsible for the situation. The prisoner was calm. Dr. A remembered the prisoner saying to him, almost to comfort him, "No, they can never get the vein." The doctor decided to place a central line. People scrambled to find a kit.

I asked him how he placed the line. It was like placing one "for any other patient," he said. He decided to place it in the subclavian vein, because that is what he most commonly did. He opened the kit for the triple-lumen catheter and explained to the prisoner everything he was going to do. I asked him if he was afraid of the prisoner. "No," he said. The man was perfectly cooperative. Dr. A put on sterile gloves, gown, and mask. He swabbed the man's skin with antiseptic.

"Why?" I asked.

"Habit," he said. He injected local anesthetic. He punctured the vein with one stick. He checked to make sure he had good, nonpulsatile flow. He threaded the guidewire, the dilator, and finally the catheter. All went smoothly. He flushed the lines, secured the catheter to the skin with a stitch, and put a clean dressing on, just as he always does. Then he went back behind the curtain to monitor the lethal injection.

Only one case seemed to really bother him. The convict, who had killed a policeman, weighed about 350 pounds. The team placed his intravenous lines without trouble. But after they had given him all three injections, the prisoner's heart rhythm continued. "It was an agonal rhythm," Dr. A said. "He was dead," he insisted. Nonetheless, the rhythm continued. The team looked to Dr. A. His explanation of what happened next diverges from what I learned from another source. I was told that he instructed that another bolus of potassium be given. When I asked him if he did, he said, "No, I didn't. As far as I remember, I didn't say anything. I think it may have been another physician." Certainly, however, all boundary lines had been crossed. He had agreed to take part in the executions simply to pronounce death, but just by being present, by having expertise, he had opened himself to being called on to do steadily more, to take responsibility for the execution itself. Perhaps he was not the executioner. But he was darn close to it.

I asked him whether he had known that his actions—everything from his monitoring the executions to helping officials with the process of delivering the drugs—violated the AMA's ethics code. "I never had any inkling," he said. And indeed, the only survey done on this issue, in 1999, found that just 3 percent of doctors knew of any guidelines governing their participation in executions.[8] The humaneness of the lethal injections was challenged in court, however. The state summoned Dr. A for a public deposition on the process, including the particulars of the execution in which the prisoner required a central line. His local newspaper printed the story. Word spread through his town. Not long after, he arrived at work to find a sign pasted to his clinic door reading, "THE KILLER DOCTOR." A challenge to his medical license was filed with the state. If he wasn't aware of the AMA's stance on the issue earlier, he was now.

Ninety percent of his patients supported him, he said, and the state medical board upheld his license under a law that defined participation in executions as acceptable activity for a physician. But he decided that he wanted no part of the controversy anymore and quit. He still defends what he did. Had he known of the AMA's position, though, "I never would have gotten involved," he said.

Dr. B spoke to me between clinic appointments. He is a family physician, and he has participated in some 30 executions. He became involved long ago, when electrocution was the primary method, and then continued through the transition to lethal injections. He remains a participant to this day. But it was apparent that he had been more cautious and reflective about his involvement than Dr. A had. He also seemed more troubled by it.

Dr. B, too, had first been approached by a patient. "One of my patients was a prison investigator," he said. "I never quite understood his role, but he was an intermediary between the state and the inmates. He was hired to monitor that the state was taking care of them. They had the first two executions after the death penalty was reinstated, and there was a problem with the second one, where the physicians were going in a minute or so after the event and still hearing heartbeats. The two physicians were doing this out of courtesy, because the facility was in their area. But the case unnerved them to the point that they quit. The officials had a lot of trouble finding another doctor after that. So that was when my patient talked to me."

Dr. B did not really want to get involved. He was in his 40s then. He'd gone to a top-tier medical school. He'd protested the Vietnam War in the 1960s. "I've gone from a radical hippie to a middle-class American over the years," he said. "I wasn't on any bandwagons anymore." But his patient said the team needed a physician only to pronounce death. Dr. B had no personal objection to capital punishment. So in the moment—"it was a quick judgment"—he said OK, "but only to do the pronouncement."

The execution was a few days later by electric chair. It was an awful sight, he said. "They say an electrocution is not an issue. But when someone comes up out of that chair six inches, it's not for nothing." He waited a long while before going out to the prisoner. When he did, he performed a systematic examination. He checked for a carotid pulse. He listened to the man's heart three times with a stethoscope. He looked for a pupil response with his pen light. Only then did he pronounce the man dead.

He thought harder about whether to stay involved after that first time. "I went to the library and researched it," and that was when he discovered the AMA guidelines. As he understood the code, if he did nothing except make a pronouncement of death, he would be acting properly and ethically. (This was not a misreading. The AMA only later distinguished between pronouncing death, which it now considers unethical, and certifying death after someone has made the initial pronouncement, which it considers ethical.)

Knowing the guidelines reassured him about his involvement and made him willing to continue. They also emboldened him to draw thicker boundaries around his participation. During the first lethal injections, he and another physician "were in the room when they were administering the drugs," he said. "We could see the telemetry. We could see a lot of things. But I had them remove us from that area. I said I do not want any access to the monitor or the EKGs. . . . A couple times they asked me about recommendations in cases in which there were venous access problems. I said, 'No. I'm not going to assist in any way.' They would ask about amounts of medicines. They had problems getting the medicines. But I said I had no interest in getting involved in any of that."

Dr. B kept himself at some remove from the execution process, but he would be the first to admit that his is not an ethically pristine position. When he refused to provide additional assistance, the execution team simply found others who would. He was glad to have those people there. "If the doctors and nurses are removed, I don't think [lethal injections] could be competently or predictably done. I can tell you I wouldn't be involved unless those people were involved."

"I agonize over the ethics of this every time they call me to go down there," he said. His wife knew about his involvement from early on, but he could not bring himself to tell his children until they were grown. He has let almost no one else know. Even his medical staff is unaware.

The trouble is not that the lethal injections seem cruel to him. "Mostly, they are very peaceful," he said. The agonizing comes instead from his doubts about whether anything is accomplished. "The whole system doesn't seem right," he told me toward the end of our conversation. "I guess I see more and more [executions], and I really wonder. . . . It just seems like the justice system is going down a dead-end street. I can't say that [lethal injection] lessens the incidence of anything. The real depressing thing is that if you don't get to these people before

the age of three or four or five, it's not going to make any difference in what they do. They've struck out before they even started kindergarten. I don't see [executions] as saying anything about that."

The medical people most wary of speaking to me were those who worked as full-time employees in state prison systems. Nonetheless, two did agree to speak, one a physician in a Southern state prison and the other a nurse who had worked in a prison out West. Both were less uncertain about being involved in executions than Dr. A or Dr. B.

The physician, Dr. C, was younger than the others and relatively junior among his prison's doctors. He did not trust me to keep his identity confidential, and I think he worried for his job if anyone found out about our conversation. As a result, although I had independent information that he had participated in at least two executions, he would speak only in general terms about the involvement of doctors. But he was clear about what he believed.

"I think that if you're going to work in the correctional setting, [participating in executions] is potentially a component of what you need to do," he said. "It is only a tiny part of anything that you're doing as part of your public health service. A lot of society thinks these people should not get any care at all." But in his job he must follow the law, and it obligates him to provide proper care, he said. It also has set the prisoners' punishment. "Thirteen jurors, citizens of the state, have made a decision. And if I live in that state and that's the law, then I would see it as being an obligation to be available."

He explained further. "I think that if I had to face someone I loved being put to death, I would want that done by lethal injection, and I would want to know that it is done competently."

The nurse saw his participation in fairly similar terms. He had fought as a Marine in Vietnam and later became a nurse. As an Army reservist, he served with a surgical unit in Bosnia and in Iraq. He worked for many years on critical care units and, for almost a decade, as nurse manager for a busy emergency department. He then took a job as the nurse-in-charge for his state penitentiary, where he helped with one execution by lethal injection.

It was the state's first execution by this method, and "at the time, there was great naiveté about lethal injection," he said. "No one in that state had any idea what was involved." The warden had the Texas protocol and thought it looked pretty simple. What did he need medical personnel for? The warden told the nurse that he would start the IVs himself, though he had never started one before.

"Are you, as a doctor, going to let this person stab the inmate for half an hour because of his inexperience?" the nurse asked me. "I wasn't." He said, "I had no qualms. If this is to be done correctly, if it is to be done at all, then I am the person to do it."

This is not to say that he felt easy about it, however. "As a Marine and as a nurse . . . , I hope I will never become someone who has no problem taking another person's life." But society had decided the punishment and had done so carefully with multiple judicial reviews, he said. The convict had killed four people even while in prison. He had arranged for an accomplice to blow up the home of a county attorney he was angry with while the attorney, his wife, and their child were inside. When the accomplice turned state's evidence, the inmate arranged for him to be tortured and killed at a roadside rest stop. The nurse did not disagree with the final judgment that this man should be put to death.

The nurse took his involvement seriously. "As the leader of the health care team," he said, "it was my responsibility to make sure that everything be done in a way that was professional and respectful to the inmate as a human being." He spoke to an official with the state nursing board about the process, and although involvement is against the ANA's ethics code, the board said he could do everything except push the drugs.

So he issued the purchase request to the pharmacist supplying the drugs. He did a dry run with the public citizen chosen to push the injections and with the guards to make sure they knew how to bring the prisoner out and strap him down. On the day of the execution, the nurse dressed as if for an operation, in scrubs, mask, hat, and sterile gown and gloves. He explained to the prisoner exactly what was going to happen. He placed two IVs and taped them down. The warden read the final order to the prisoner and allowed him his last words. "He didn't say anything about his guilt or his innocence," the nurse said. "He just said that the execution made all of us involved killers just like him."

The warden gave the signal to start the injection. The nurse hooked the syringe to the IV port and told the citizen to push the sodium thiopental. "The inmate started to say, 'Yeah, I can feel . . . ' and then he passed out." They completed the injections and, three minutes later, he flatlined on the cardiac monitor. The two physicians on the scene had been left nothing to do except pronounce the inmate dead.

I have personally been in favor of the death penalty. I was a senior official in the 1992 Clinton presidential campaign and in the administration, and in that role I defended the President's stance in support of capital punishment. I have no illusions that the death penalty deters anyone from murder. I also have great concern about the ability of our justice system to avoid putting someone innocent to death. However, I believe there are some human beings who do such evil as to deserve to die. I am not troubled that Timothy McVeigh was executed for the 168 people he had killed in the Oklahoma City bombing, or that John Wayne Gacy was for committing 33 murders. The European Union refuses to participate in any way in the trial of Saddam Hussein because of the court's insistence on allowing the death penalty as a possible punishment, but given Hussein's role in the massacre of more than 100,000 people, the European position only puzzles me.

Still, I have always regarded involvement in executions by physicians and nurses as wrong. The public has granted us extraordinary and exclusive dispensation to administer drugs to people, even to the point of unconsciousness, to put needles and tubes into their bodies, to do what would otherwise be considered assault, because we do so on their behalf—to save their lives and provide them comfort. To have the state take control of these skills for its purposes against a human being—for punishment—seems a dangerous perversion. Society has trusted us with powerful abilities, and the more willing we are to use these abilities against individual people, the more we risk that trust. The public may like executions, but no one likes executioners.

My conversations with the physicians and the nurse I had tracked down, however, rattled both of these views—and no conversation more so than one I had with the final doctor I spoke to. Dr. D is a 45-year-old emergency physician. He is also a volunteer medical director for a shelter for abused children. He works to reduce homelessness. He opposes the death penalty because he regards it as inhumane, immoral, and pointless. And he has participated in six executions so far.

About eight years ago, a new jail was built down the street from the hospital where he worked, and it had an infirmary "the size of our whole emergency room." The jail needed a doctor. So, out of curiosity as much as anything, Dr. D began working there. "I found that I loved it," he said. "Jails are an underserved niche of health care." Jails, he pointed out, are different from prisons in that they house people who are arrested and awaiting trial. Most are housed only a few hours to days and then released. "The substance abuse and noncompliance is high. The people have a wide variety of medical needs. It is a fascinating population. The setting is very similar to the ER. You can make a tremendous impact on people and on public health." Over time, he shifted more and more of his work to the jail system. He built a medical group for the jails in his area and soon became an advocate for correctional medicine.

Three years ago, the doctors who had been involved in executions in his state pulled out. Officials asked Dr. D if his group would take the contract. Before answering, he went to witness an execution. "It was a very emotional experience for me," he said. "I was shocked to witness something like this." He had opposed the death penalty since college, and nothing he saw made him feel any differently. But, at the same time, he felt there were needs that he as a correctional physician could serve.

He read about the ethics of participating. He knew about the AMA's stance against it. Yet he also felt an obligation not to abandon inmates in their dying moments. "We, as doctors, are not the ones deciding the fate of this individual," he said. "The way I saw it, this is an end-of-life issue, just as with any other terminal disease. It just happens that it involves a legal process instead of a medical process. When we have a patient who can no longer survive his illness, we as physicians must ensure he has comfort. [A death-penalty] patient is no different from a patient dying of cancer—except his cancer is a court order." Dr. D said he has "the cure for this cancer"—abolition of the death penalty—but "if the people and the government won't let you provide it, and a patient then dies, are you not going to comfort him?"

His group took the contract, and he has been part of the medical team for each execution since. The doctors are available to help if there are difficulties with IV access, and Dr. D considers it their task to ensure that the prisoner is without pain or suffering through the process. He himself provides the cardiac monitoring and the final determination of death. Watching the changes on the two-line electrocardiogram tracing, "I keep having that reflex as an ER doctor, wanting to treat that rhythm," he said. Aside from that, his main reaction is to be sad for everyone involved—the prisoner whose life has led to this, the victims, the prison officials, the doctors. The team's payment is substantial—$18,000—but he donates his portion to the children's shelter where he volunteers.

Three weeks after speaking to me, he told me to go ahead and use his name. It is Dr. Carlo Musso. He helps with executions in Georgia. He didn't want to seem as if he was hiding anything, he said. He didn't want to invite trouble, either. But activists have already challenged his license and his membership in the AMA, and he is resigned to the fight. "It just seems wrong for us to walk away, to abdicate our responsibility to the patients," he said.

There is little doubt that lethal injection can be painless and peaceful, but as courts have recognized, this requires significant medical assistance and judgment—for placement of intravenous lines, monitoring of consciousness, and adjustments in medication timing and dosage. In recent years, medical societies have persuaded two states, Kentucky and Illinois, to pass laws forbidding physician participation in executions. Nonetheless, officials in each of these states intend to continue to rely on medical supervision, employing nurses and nurse-anesthetists instead. How, then, to reconcile the conflict between government efforts to ensure a medical presence and our ethical principles forbidding it? Are our ethics what should change?

The doctors' and nurse's arguments for competence and comfort in the execution process do have some force. But however much they may wish to be there for an inmate, it seems clear that the inmate is not really their patient. Unlike genuine patients, an inmate has no ability to refuse the physicians' "care"—indeed, the inmate and his family are not even permitted to know the physician's identity. And the medical assistance provided primarily serves the government's purposes—not the inmate's needs as a patient. Medicine is being made an instrument of punishment. The hand of comfort that more gently places the IV, more carefully times the bolus of potassium, is also the hand of death. We cannot escape this truth. The ethics codes seem right.

It is this truth that persuades me that we should seek a legal ban on the participation of physicians and nurses in executions. And if it turns out that executions cannot then be performed without, as the courts put it, "unconstitutional pain and cruelty," the death penalty should be abolished.

It is far from clear that a society that punishes its most evil murderers with life imprisonment is worse off than one that punishes them with death. But a society in which the government actively subverts core ethical principles of medical practice is patently worse off for it. The government has shown willingness to use medical skills against individuals for its own purposes—having medical personnel assist in the interrogation of prisoners, for example, place feeding tubes for force-feeding them, and help with executing them. As medical abilities advance, government interest in our skills will only increase. Preserving the integrity of our ethics could not be more important.

The four physicians and the nurse I spoke to all acted against long-standing principles of their professions. Their actions have made our ethics codes effectively irrelevant in society. Yet, it must be said, most took their moral duties seriously. It is worth reflecting on this truth as well.

The easy thing for any doctor or nurse is simply to follow the written rules. But each of us has a duty not to follow rules and laws blindly. In medicine, we face conflicts about what the right and best actions are in all kinds of areas: relief of suffering for the terminally ill, provision of narcotics for patients with chronic pain, withdrawal of care for the critically ill, abortion, and executions, to name just a few. All have been the subject of professional rules and government regulation, and at times those rules and regulations will be wrong. We will then be called on to make a choice. We must do our best to choose intelligently and wisely.

Sometimes, however, we will be wrong—as I think the doctors and nurses are who have used their privileged skills to make possible 844 deaths by lethal injection thus far. We each should then be prepared to accept the consequences. Unlike Dr. Musso, however, nearly all these doctors and nurses have sought to keep their actions hidden in order not to face the consequences. In the final analysis, I think this is what makes their actions seem particularly troubling. We cannot blame them for their impulse to hide. But we cannot admire them either.

References

1. Michael Angelo Morales v. Roderick Q. Hickman, No. C 06 219 JF, (Dist. Ct. Northern Dist. of Cal. February 14, 2006).
2. Michael Angelo Morales v. Roderick Q. Hickman, No. CV 06 00926 JF (9th Cir. February 20, 2006).
3. Trombley S. The execution protocol: inside America's capital punishment industry. New York: Crown, 1992.
4. Solotaroff I. The last face you'll ever see: the private life of the American death penalty. New York: HarperCollins, 2001:7.
5. Death Penalty Information Center execution database. Accessed March 1, 2006, at http://www.deathpenaltyinfo.org/executions.php.
6. Breach of trust: physician participation in executions in the United States. Philadelphia: American College of Physicians, 1994.
7. Norbut M. Complaint cites Georgia doctors who took part in executions. American Medical News. July 4, 2005:1.
8. Farber NJ, Aboff BM, Weiner J, Davis EB, Boyer EG, Ubel PA. Physicians' willingness to participate in the process of lethal injections for capital punishment. Ann Intern Med 2001;135:884–8.

ATUL GAWANDE practices general and endocrine surgery at Brigham and Women's Hospital in Boston. He is also a professor of surgery at Harvard Medical School and a professor in the Department of Health Policy and Management at the Harvard School of Public Health.

EXPLORING THE ISSUE

Should Physicians Be Allowed to Participate in Executions?

Critical Thinking and Reflection

1. How do you understand the physician's social role, and do you think it would be undermined by allowing physicians to participate in executions? Why or why not?
2. How morally important is it to conduct executions in such a way that the condemned do not suffer, and if that goal is important, what is the best way to accomplish it? Is physician participation necessary or helpful? Are there ways physicians might participate that would be more appropriate to their social role?

Is There Common Ground?

It is natural to think that moral debates should be solved by moral arguments. But what if the moral arguments have all been marshaled and articulated in the best way possible, and still there is disagreement? The hope that good moral argument should always eventually lead to moral agreement is what the philosopher Norman Daniels once called the philosopher's dream. In place of that dream, Daniels proposes that we must fall back on a political solution: We must organize our public institutions in such a way that personal differences can be allowed to continue. We should compromise. For Daniels, permitting such individual differences of opinion is part of the task of a liberal state.

Of course, whether a political compromise is possible or desirable on the issue of physician participation in lethal injection executions is itself controversial. In February 2010, the American Board of Anesthesiology declared that it would no longer provide board certification to anesthesiologists who participate in capital punishment. Losing board certification undermines a physician's ability to practice medicine, since board certification is an important professional credential.

In a recent, controversial paper, Lawrence Nelson and Brandon Ashby argue against the ABA's stance and for political compromise on this issue. They argue that there are "principled and morally serious arguments" behind both the pro and the con positions on permitting physicians to participate in execution by lethal injection, and that individual physicians should therefore be allowed to make their own decisions about participation. Nelson and Ashby believe that professional medical organizations "should not impose organizational sanctions that significantly impede or destroy physicians' ability to practice medicine."

Additional Resources

The paper by Lawrence Nelson and Brandon Ashby is "Rethinking the Ethics of Physician Participation in Lethal Injection Execution," *Hastings Center Report* (May–June 2011). The position of the American Board of Anesthesiology is found in "Anesthesiologists and Capital Punishment," at www.theaba.orgpdfCapitalPunishmentCommentary.pdf.

The position of the American Medical Association is found in, "Code of Medical Ethics Opinion 2.211—Physician-Assisted Suicide," at http://www.ama-assn.org/ama/pub/physician-resources/medical-ethics/code-medical-ethics/opinion2211.page?

The New England Journal of Medicine featured a round-table discussion on physician participation in execution. Atul Gawande, Deborah W. Denno, Robert D. Truog, and David Waisel, "Physicians and Execution— Highlights from a Discussion of Lethal Injection," *The New England Journal of Medicine* (vol. 358, January 31, 2008). Video of the roundtable discussion is available at www.nejm.org/doi/full/10.1056/NEJMp0800378.

For a forceful argument against permitting physician participation, see L.L. Emanuel and L.B. Bienen, "Physician Participation in Executions: Time to Eliminate Anonymity and Protest the Practice," *Annals of Internal Medicine* (vol. 135, no. 10, 2001).

Ty Alper offers insight into physicians' views about lethal injection executions and their willingness to participate them in "The Truth about Physician Participation in Lethal Injection Executions," *North Carolina Law Review* (vol. 88, 2010).

Deborah Deno provides a study of lethal injection protocols around the United States. Deno argues that states have produced "grossly inadequate protocols that severely restrict sufficient understanding of how executions are performed and heighten the likelihood of unconstitutionality." Deborah Deno, "The Lethal Injection Quandary: How Medicine Has Dismantled the Death Penalty," *Fordham Law Review* (vol. 76, 2007).

Internet References . . .

Death Penalty Information Center

> http://www.deathpenaltyinfo.org/

National Coalition to Abolish the Death Penalty

> http://www.ncadp.org/

ProCon.org

> http://deathpenalty.procon.org/

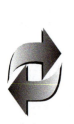

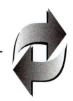

Selected, Edited, and with Issue Framing Material by:
Gregory E. Kaebnick, *The Hastings Center*

ISSUE

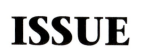

Should Pharmacists Be Allowed to Deny Prescriptions on Grounds of Conscience?

YES: Donald W. Herbe, from "The Right to Refuse: A Call for Adequate Protection of a Pharmacist's Right to Refuse Facilitation of Abortion and Emergency Contraception," *Journal of Law and Health* (2002/2003)

NO: Julie Cantor and Ken Baum, from "The Limits of Conscientious Objection—May Pharmacists Refuse to Fill Prescriptions for Emergency Contraception?" *The New England Journal of Medicine* (2004)

Learning Outcomes

After reading this issue, you will be able to:

- Discuss the considerations in favor and against granting pharmacists a right to refuse to fill a prescription if they believe the drug will be used in a way they find deeply objectionable on moral or religious grounds.
- Explain the use of mifepristone (RU-486) to produce a very early abortion.
- Explain the concepts of "conscience clause" and a "right of conscience."

ISSUE SUMMARY

YES: Law student Donald W. Herbe asserts that pharmacists' moral beliefs concerning abortion and emergency contraception are genuinely fundamental and deserve respect. He proposes that professional pharmaceutical organizations lead the way to recognizing a true right of conscience, which would eventually result in universal legislation protecting against all potential ramifications of choosing conscience.

NO: Julie Cantor, a lawyer, and Ken Baum, a physician and lawyer, reject an absolute right to object, as well as no right to object, to these prescriptions but assert that pharmacists who cannot or will not dispense a drug have a professional obligation to meet the needs of their customers by referring them elsewhere.

Under U.S. law and practice, a person who objects on grounds of conscience or religious belief to performing certain acts has considerable protections. To force someone to perform an act totally forbidden by his or her religion would be a profound violation of ethical and human rights. But there are limits to exercising this right. Right now there is no military draft in the United States; however, all young men must register with the Selective Service Agency on their 18th birthday. If there were to be

a military draft, a conscientious objector would have to demonstrate that he has a strongly held religious or moral belief, not just a political one, against participation in the military. Conscientious objectors could request alternative community service, such as caring for the elderly, or serving in the military as a noncombatant, for example, as a medic. In the Vietnam War, some conscientious objectors were jailed for their refusal to serve.

Conscientious objection has ethical implications for medical personnel as well. Physicians, for example, may refrain from performing procedures that are legal but repugnant to them on moral grounds. Just as in the military example, there are limits. Physicians cannot ethically refuse to provide life-saving or emergency treatment to a person on the grounds that the individual is a murderer or has committed an act that violates the physician's religion. They can refuse to perform abortions on grounds of conscience, but ethical codes require them to refer patients to another provider. Nurses have less discretion than physicians because they are employees of hospitals and are subject to disciplinary action. Nevertheless, they too can establish grounds for refusing to assist in an abortion procedure, sterilization, or the withdrawal of life-sustaining treatment.

The issue is murkier, however, when it comes to pharmacists, who are generally self-employed, or pharmacy employees. They do not directly participate in the acts they find objectionable, but they make those acts possible by dispensing medications. What are their options and obligations?

Birth control pills and emergency contraception medications, which are basically high doses of regular birth control pills taken to prevent pregnancy after unprotected sexual intercourse, have been on the market for years. Some pharmacists object to dispensing these medications. The issue became much more controversial when in September 2000 the Food and Drug Administration (FDA) approved the drug mifepristone as safe and effective. This drug, formerly known as RU-486 after Russel Uclaf, its initial French manufacturer, had been marketed in Europe for several years. Mifepristone is a synthetic steroid that blocks progesterone, preventing an implanted fertilized egg from developing. It must be taken within 49 days of conception and followed within 48 hours by a second drug, misoprostol, related to the hormone prostaglandin. Taken together, the two drugs act as a chemical form of early abortion. Emergency contraception, on the other hand, is not a form of abortion, since no conception has taken place.

And it is here that some pharmacists have drawn the line. Believing strongly that abortion is immoral, they want the legal right to exercise their religious beliefs and ethical right by refusing to dispense the drugs for this purpose and to be protected from losing their jobs, or other repercussions. Should they be allowed to do so and without referring women to another, more willing pharmacist?

The YES and NO selections present different points of view. Donald Herbe sees the exercise of conscientious objection as fundamental to pharmacists' human rights and calls for legislation to protect them from any kind of repercussions or discrimination. While recognizing that pharmacists have a legitimate interest in avoiding conflicts of conscience, Julie Cantor and Ken Baum believe that because pharmacists are licensed and have a professional obligation to serve the public, they must make alternative options available to customers who seek legal prescription drugs they find objectionable.

YES ⤶

Donald W. Herbe

The Right to Refuse: A Call for Adequate Protection of a Pharmacist's Right to Refuse Facilitation of Abortion and Emergency Contraception

Introduction

The ability to convince an individual, through the art of honest persuasion, of the righteousness of a belief is celebrated; however, in failure of such persuasion, compelling that person to act contradictory to their retained ideal is detestable. The free will to reject a movement or disagree with a practice is the sort of liberty this Nation was founded upon, yet today the potential exists that many in the pharmaceutical profession will be forced into behaviors repugnant to their basic standards of goodness and morality. The proliferation of abortive and contraceptive drug therapies has thrust many pharmacists into roles as facilitators of practices they oppose on fundamental levels without a corresponding ability to opt out of such action.

When a patient desires drug therapies that, in the eyes of the pharmacist, are likely to destroy an unborn human life, the pro-life pharmacist is left in an unsettling position: accommodate the patient and breach basic moral principles *or* adhere to conscience and risk liability and disciplinary action.

Section I: Anti-Reproduction Pills and the Pharmacist's Role

The Pills

On September 28, 2000, the Food and Drug Administration (FDA) approved the drug mifepristone, formerly known as RU-486, for use in the United States as an abortifacient. Mifepristone had previously been approved and is currently used in some European countries, including France, England, and Sweden. Although mifepristone has other potential uses, such as postcoital contraception and daily-use birth control, its FDA approved use is as an early pregnancy abortifacient.

Mifepristone acts as an anti-hormone and precludes a woman's uterus from retaining an *implanted* fertilized egg. The drug blocks progesterone, an essential hormone in the acceptance and retention of an implanted egg within a woman's uterus; and, when taken in concurrence with misoprostol, induces a spontaneous abortion. The fact that the mifepristone abortion regimen acts to destroy an implanted egg as opposed to a fertilized yet not implanted egg, is what distinguishes it from emergency contraception.

Drugs used post-coitally with the intent to prevent the development of a pregnancy are referred to as emergency contraception. This labeling as emergency contraception is a bit conclusory, as the definition of whether use of such drugs is contraception or abortion lies at the heart of the controversy over them. However, for purposes of convenience and clarity, this Note will refer to drug regimens consumed post-intercourse for the purpose of preventing the onset or continuance of pregnancy as emergency contraception (EC), as that is the term that has been attached to them in modern medical, social, and political arenas.

Notwithstanding this controversy, the physical and biological effects of orally administered EC, often referred to as the morning-after pill, are not in dispute. EC may prevent the development of a pregnancy by inhibiting any of four successive biological events, either pre or post fertilization, necessary to establish and maintain a pregnancy. EC works before fertilization by either suppressing ovulation, like regular birth-control pills, or preventing fertilization of an egg by inhibiting the movement of the sperm or the egg. If an egg becomes fertilized, then EC may disrupt transport of the fertilized egg to the uterus or, if the transport through the fallopian tube is complete, prevent the implantation of the fertilized egg in the woman's uterus. EC is most effective when used up to seventy-two hours after unprotected intercourse and becomes completely ineffective after implantation occurs, usually six or seven days after intercourse.

The Pharmacist's Role

During the past twenty years emergency contraception pills (ECPs) have been available to and used by American women. During this time frame non-emergency oral contraceptives (those taken as a daily pre-intercourse regimen) were used off-label as emergency contraception and were distributed as such "primarily in hospital emergency rooms, reproductive health clinics, and university health centers." These medical facilities would repackage oral contraceptives for use as emergency contraception; pharmacies associated with certain clinics would repackage oral contraceptives into EC regimens and label them as such; and private physicians would instruct patients to take a larger dosage of their regular birth control pills as EC.

In 1998 the FDA approved the Preven Emergency Contraceptive Kit, an EC based on the Yuzpe regimen. In 1999, the FDA also approved Plan B, another EC regimen. While different regimens of oral contraceptives had been distributed and used before 1998 as emergency contraceptives, Preven and Plan B are the first regimens specifically approved by the FDA as safe and effective emergency contraceptives, to be packaged and marketed as such. Additionally, modified doses of oral contraceptives, not specifically packaged for use as an EC, can still be prescribed in doses that would effect emergency contraception if doctor and patient desire such a method.

Emergency contraception pills are classified as prescription drugs, and "states are delegated the power and responsibility of determining which health care professionals . . . have prescriptive authority." Currently, many states have authorized collaborative practices that have expanded the role of pharmacists. These collaborative practices generally authorize greater independence of the pharmacist to initiate drug therapies not specifically prescribed by a patient's physician or other authorized health care professional. In other words, some patients may not require a prescription from their doctor before being distributed certain medications or drugs from a pharmacist. However, with the exception of Washington, California, and Alaska, states do not authorize this expanded pharmacist role in the distribution of ECPs. Pharmacists are generally limited to dispensing ECPs specifically prescribed by some other authorized health care professional. Other general duties of a pharmacist in the distribution of ECPs may include counseling and educating women on EC use at the time the prescription is filled.

In Washington, California, and Alaska, pharmacists have the dual authority to prescribe *and* dispense ECPs under each state's respective collaborative practices. Generally speaking, the pharmacist may dispense ECPs in accordance with "standardized procedures or protocols developed by the pharmacist and an authorized prescriber[.]" Thus, a woman need not receive authorization from her doctor prior to buying ECPs; the pharmacist acts not as a third party or indirect provider of ECPs, but as a direct provider in accordance with a general collaborative protocol.

If pro-choice groups and the American Medical Association have their way, pharmacists will have no future role in ECPs. This is because these groups support an FDA reclassification of ECPs as over-the-counter (OTC) drugs, rather than prescription. Many pro-choice groups claim as a top goal the persuasion of the FDA to reclassify ECPs as OTC. If OTC status were granted, then "women would be able to get ECPs without encountering any type of health care provider."

OTC status for ECPs is not generally supported by pharmacists however, and is not likely in today's political climate. Advocates on both sides of the issue believe the Bush administration, with its influence on the FDA, will delay or negate a switch in classification from prescription to OTC. The behavioral and social policy concerns raised by ECPs "may make switching ECPs to OTC status a politically unpopular move." In any event, ECPs are currently available only by prescription.

Many restrictions have been imposed by the FDA in the use and distribution of mifepristone. First, the drug can only be used during the first forty-nine days after a woman's last menstrual cycle. Also, the drug is distributed to women directly from doctors and certain health clinics. Mifepristone "is not and will not be available in pharmacies[.]" Thus, under the current FDA restrictions, pharmacists have no role in mifepristone-induced abortions.

While current mifepristone use is much lower than expected since its FDA approval and subsequent availability to the public, some signals suggest that future use or access may become more widespread. A survey of doctors by the Kaiser Family Foundation discovered that twenty-three percent of doctors said they were "likely" to offer mifepristone in 2002; up from the seven percent that actually provided the drug since its approval. Also, health centers offering mifepristone have reported a ninety-nine percent rate of abortion in women who have taken the drug. An expected increase in availability, a near perfect rate of achieving the desired ends of abortion, together with continued efforts by pro-choice groups, such as Planned Parenthood, to increase accessibility to abortion, could be the impetus to pharmaceutical distribution of mifepristone in the future.

FDA approval of mifepristone and ECPs, such as Preven and Plan B, has made drug related reproductive therapy a real and potentially widespread option for women. Marketing campaigns by women's and abortion-rights groups and the drug manufacturers themselves will further introduce these drug options to women. This drug therapy revolution of sorts has expanded the pharmacist's role in the provision of emergency contraception, and perhaps, in the future, the provision of mifepristone.

The more women that are aware of and desire EC, the more involved and important pharmacists will become in the contraception process. One can imagine that if more and more states adopt the liberal EC distribution procedures of Washington and California, then pharmacists would become the primary providers of ECPs. And if mifepristone distribution restrictions are relaxed, pharmacists could feasibly become key players in the furnishing of abortion drugs as well. Whether they like it or not, pharmacists are being thrust into the role of common, everyday providers of controversial reproductive medications, and this position may put some pharmacists in the predicament of having to choose between their moral convictions regarding EC and abortion and the patient's wishes. . . .

The Pharmacist's Professional Ethical Obligations

Pharmacy is a profession, and much like the professions of medicine and law, entails a duty to assure and promote the patient's best interests. As professionals, pharmacists are expected to give priority to the patient's interests over their own immediate interests. As key players in the implementation of drug therapies, pharmacists are expected to withhold drugs "from those who have no authority to use them" and not to withhold "medications from those who do have authority to use them."

The patient's best interests are the pharmacist's primary commitment and concern. Among other things, pharmacists are expected to "help individuals achieve optimum benefit from their medications, to be committed to their welfare, and to maintain their trust"; to place "concern for the well-being of the patient at the center of professional practice" taking into consideration the "needs stated by the patient"; and to hold "the patient's welfare paramount." Further, patient autonomy and "personal and cultural differences among patients" must be respected by the pharmacist. These professional duties, and others, encompass the "collective conscience" of the

pharmaceutical profession, and their implementation by each pharmacist is considered a moral obligation.

When presented with a validly authorized prescription for a legal medication, by a patient aware of the risks involved in taking the medication, and for whom the medication would be reasonably safe, the aforementioned principles and expectations leave the pharmacist with an ethical duty to fill and dispense the prescription. The duty to dispense in these circumstances may give rise to a serious conflict between the pharmacist's personal conviction concerning abortion and her professional duty to the patient.

In 1998, the American Pharmaceutical Association (APhA), and subsequently various other pharmaceutical organizations, eased the conflict between personal and professional morals by adopting policies recognizing a pharmacist's right to refuse dispensing medications based on the pharmacist's personal beliefs. However, if the pharmacist exercises her right of conscience and refuses to fill the prescription, the duty to the patient is not extinguished, and could be fulfilled by referring the patient to another pharmacist or distributor. In any event, "the patient should not be required to abide by the pharmacist's personal, moral decision." For many pharmacists, a referral would be no more than passive participation in the activity they initially refused to actively assist. Thus the dilemma, while transformed into whether to refer or not, is equally troublesome to the pharmacist.

Section II: The Potential Ramifications of Choosing Conscience

The pharmacist who ultimately decides that her moral convictions regarding abortion outweigh her professional obligation to the patient may refuse to fill the prescription and refer the patient to another pharmacist; or, the pharmacist with conscientious objection may refuse to dispense and refuse to refer. While the former decision will, in practical terms, shield the pharmacist from most negative consequences, the latter decision could have serious implications for the pharmacist, including employment termination or demotion, civil tort liability, or disciplinary action from the state pharmacy board. . . .

❧❀❧

Legal protection must serve two purposes in order to appropriately ensure a pharmacist's right of conscientious refusal: 1) prevent and deter detrimental recriminatory action against the pharmacist; and 2) provide adequate remedies in the case that the pharmacist is sued or disciplined. The most efficient and effective means to these ends is the enactment of state and federal legislation.

The first step to successful enactment of pharmacist conscience legislation in each state and the United States is the cooperation of local, regional, and national pharmaceutical associations. The American Pharmaceutical Association took a large positive step when it adopted its pharmacist conscience clause. However, in the same pronouncement it rejected adoption of a policy encouraging enactment of state and national legal protection of the right of conscience. If pharmacists themselves, as represented by their professional associations and organizations, do not call for state and national legislative action, the road to adequate protection will be more difficult.

In any event, an effective conscience statute should take into consideration many complex issues including broad protection against recriminatory action, efficient administration of pharmacies, and accommodation of patients. First and foremost the conscience clause should serve its purpose stating clearly that no pharmacist shall be required to dispense abortion or EC drugs, nor shall any pharmacist be required to refer to another pharmacist who will dispense abortion or EC drugs. Although pharmacists currently have no role in the distribution of mifepristone, the abortion language should nonetheless be included as the potential for future pharmaceutical access exists. Next, the conscience statute should prohibit discrimination, civil liability, and professional disciplinary action that result from exercising the aforementioned rights of refusal. The statute should also encompass provisions prohibiting discrimination in the hiring process so as to preclude pharmacy-employers from screening applicants to avoid hiring pro-life pharmacists in the first place. Finally, the statute should provide adequate methods of deterrence. Employment discrimination could be deterred through its criminalization or by providing an express cause of action in tort as a remedy to the discriminatory hiring, firing, demotion, or promotion of pharmacists.

Employer and patient considerations should also exist in a pharmacist conscience clause. Prior notification of a pharmacist's beliefs regarding abortion and EC should be disclosed to the employer so as to enable efficient administration of the pharmacy. Further, patients should be put on notice in advance regarding when pharmacists with moral objections to abortion and EC will be on duty. For example, schedules could be posted conspicuously within a pharmacy as to when abortion and EC drugs will and will not be available to customer-patients. This will enable patients to avoid the hassle of going to a pharmacy and having their prescription refused. In any event, matters such as the aforementioned should be considered when drafting a pharmacist conscience clause.

Conclusion

Pharmacists, like other professionals such as physicians and attorneys, have a general duty to ensure their client's best interests, and thus must put the health of patients above all other considerations. Thus, it would seem to follow, when a pharmacist is presented with a valid prescription of what is safe for the patient to consume, the drugs should be distributed without dispute. However, to require that a pharmacist, or any professional, participate in what she would equate to the taking of a human life should never be a principle of professional ethics.

Certain issues, because of their inherent complexity and ambiguity, must be resolved, with guidance from religion, philosophy, and science, in the heart and mind of each individual. The commencement of human life and the relative sanctity of unborn life are issues that fall within this category of subjective individual determination. The thoughtful decision should be respected and free from vilifying recrimination. If a pharmacist, in her heart of hearts, concludes that accommodating prescriptions for abortive and EC medications is akin to directly facilitating the destruction of a precious human life, a refusal to accommodate such prescriptions should be protected under the law and within the profession. A safeguard of the right to refuse is imminently necessary as abortive drugs and EC become more widespread and risk of liability and loss of employment may compel many pharmacists to disregard their sacred beliefs or reap the consequences of their objections. Proactive acceptance of a pharmacist's conscientious objection to abortion and EC within the pharmaceutical community would pave the way to legislative protection already afforded doctors and nurses.

DONALD W. HERBE is an attorney in Cleveland, Ohio.

Julie Cantor and Ken Baum   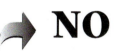 **NO**

The Limits of Conscientious Objection— May Pharmacists Refuse to Fill Prescriptions for Emergency Contraception?

Health policy decisions are often controversial, and the recent determination by the Food and Drug Administration (FDA) not to grant over-the-counter status to the emergency contraceptive Plan B was no exception. Some physicians decried the decision as a troubling clash of science, politics, and morality.[1] Other practitioners, citing safety, heralded the agency's prudence.[2] Public sentiment mirrored both views. Regardless, the decision preserved a major barrier to the acquisition of emergency contraception—the need to obtain and fill a prescription within a narrow window of efficacy. Six states have lowered that hurdle by allowing pharmacists to dispense emergency contraception without a prescription.[3–8] In those states, patients can simply bypass physicians. But the FDA's decision means that patients cannot avoid pharmacists. Because emergency contraception remains behind the counter, pharmacists can block access to it. And some have done just that.

Across the country, some pharmacists have refused to honor valid prescriptions for emergency contraception. In Texas, a pharmacist, citing personal moral grounds, rejected a rape survivor's prescription for emergency contraception.[9] A pharmacist in rural Missouri also refused to sell such a drug,[10] and in Ohio, Kmart fired a pharmacist for obstructing access to emergency and other birth control.[11] This fall, a New Hampshire pharmacist refused to fill a prescription for emergency contraception or to direct the patron elsewhere for help. Instead, he berated the 21-year-old single mother, who then, in her words, "pulled the car over in the parking lot and just cried."[12] Although the total number of incidents is unknown, reports of pharmacists who refused to dispense emergency contraception date back to 1991[13] and show no sign of abating.

Though nearly all states offer some level of legal protection for health care professionals who refuse to provide certain reproductive services, only Arkansas, Mississippi, and South Dakota explicitly protect pharmacists who refuse to dispense emergency and other contraception.[14] But that list may grow. In past years, legislators from nearly two dozen states have taken "conscientious objection"—an idea that grew out of wartime tension between religious freedom and national obligation[15] and was co-opted into the reproductive-rights debate of the 1970s[16]—and applied it to pharmacists. One proposed law offers pharmacists immunity from civil lawsuits, criminal liability, professional sanctions, and employment repercussions.[17] Another bill, which was not passed, would have protected pharmacists who refused to transfer prescriptions.[18]

This issue raises important questions about individual rights and public health. Who prevails when the needs of patients and the morals of providers collide? Should pharmacists have a right to reject prescriptions for emergency contraception? The contours of conscientious objection remain unclear. This article elucidates those boundaries and offers a balanced solution to a complex problem. Because the future of over-the-counter emergency contraception is in flux, this issue remains salient for physicians and their patients.

Arguments in Favor of a Pharmacist's Right to Object

Pharmacists Can and Should Exercise Independent Judgment

Pharmacists, like physicians, are professionals. They complete a graduate program to gain expertise, obtain a state license to practice, and join a professional organization with its own code of ethics. Society relies on pharmacists to instruct patients on the appropriate use of medications and to ensure the safety of drugs prescribed in combination.

Courts have held that pharmacists, like other professionals, owe their customers a duty of care.[19] In short, pharmacists are not automatons completing tasks; they are integral members of the health care team. Thus, it seems inappropriate and condescending to question a pharmacist's right to exercise personal judgment in refusing to fill certain prescriptions.

Professionals Should Not Forsake Their Morals as a Condition of Employment

Society does not require professionals to abandon their morals. Lawyers, for example, choose clients and issues to represent. Choice is also the norm in the health care setting. Except in emergency departments, physicians may select their patients and procedures. Ethics and law allow physicians, nurses, and physician assistants to refuse to participate in abortions and other reproductive services.[14,20] Although some observers argue that active participation in an abortion is distinct from passively dispensing emergency contraception, others believe that making such a distinction between active and passive participation is meaningless, because both forms link the provider to the final outcome in the chain of causation.

Conscientious Objection Is Integral to Democracy

More generally, the right to refuse to participate in acts that conflict with personal ethical, moral, or religious convictions is accepted as an essential element of a democratic society. Indeed, Oregon acknowledged this freedom in its Death with Dignity Act,[21] which allows health care providers, including pharmacists, who are disquieted by physician-assisted suicide to refuse involvement without fear of retribution. Also, like the draftee who conscientiously objects to perpetrating acts of death and violence, a pharmacist should have the right not to be complicit in what they believe to be a morally ambiguous endeavor, whether others agree with that position or not. The reproductive-rights movement was built on the ideal of personal choice; denying choice for pharmacists in matters of reproductive rights and abortion seems ironic.

Arguments Against a Pharmacist's Right to Object

Pharmacists Choose to Enter a Profession Bound by Fiduciary Duties

Although pharmacists are professionals, professional autonomy has its limits. As experts on the profession of pharmacy explain, "Professionals are expected to exercise special skill and care to place the interests of their clients above their own immediate interests."[22] When a pharmacist's objection directly and detrimentally affects a patient's health, it follows that the patient should come first. Similarly, principles in the pharmacists' code of ethics weigh against conscientious objection. Given the effect on the patient if a pharmacist refuses to fill a prescription, the code undermines the right to object with such broadly stated objectives as "a pharmacist promotes the good of every patient in a caring, compassionate, and confidential manner," "a pharmacist respects the autonomy and dignity of each patient," and "a pharmacist serves individual, community, and societal needs."[23] Finally, pharmacists understand these fiduciary obligations when they choose their profession. Unlike conscientious objectors to a military draft, for whom choice is limited by definition, pharmacists willingly enter their field and adopt its corresponding obligations.

Emergency Contraception Is Not an Abortifacient

Although the subject of emergency contraception is controversial, medical associations,[24] government agencies,[25] and many religious groups agree that it is not akin to abortion. Plan B and similar hormones have no effect on an established pregnancy, and they may operate by more than one physiological mechanism, such as by inhibiting ovulation or creating an unfavorable environment for implantation of a blastocyst.[26] This duality allowed the Catholic Health Association to reconcile its religious beliefs with a mandate adopted by Washington State that emergency contraception must be provided to rape survivors.[27] According to the association, a patient and a provider who aim only to prevent conception follow Catholic teachings and state law. Also, whether one believes that pregnancy begins with fertilization or implantation, emergency contraception cannot fit squarely within the concept of abortion because one cannot be sure that conception has occurred.

Pharmacists' Objections Significantly Affect Patients' Health

Although religious and moral freedom is considered sacrosanct, that right should yield when it hinders a patient's ability to obtain timely medical treatment. Courts have held that religious freedom does not give health care providers an unfettered right to object to anything involving birth control, an embryo, or a fetus.[28,29] Even though the Constitution protects people's beliefs, their actions may be regulated.[30] An objection must be balanced with the burden it imposes on others. In some cases, a pharmacist's objection imposes his or her religious beliefs on a patient. Pharmacists may decline to fill prescriptions for emergency contraception because they believe that the drug ends a life. Although the patient may disapprove of abortion, she may not share the pharmacist's beliefs about contraception. If she becomes pregnant, she may then face the question of abortion—a dilemma she might have avoided with the morning-after pill.

Furthermore, the refusal of a pharmacist to fill a prescription may place a disproportionately heavy burden on those with few options, such as a poor teenager living in a rural area that has a lone pharmacy. Whereas the savvy urbanite can drive to another pharmacy, a refusal to fill a prescription for a less advantaged patient may completely bar her access to medication. Finally, although Oregon does have an opt-out provision in its statute regulating assisted suicide, timing is much more important in emergency contraception than in assisted suicide. Plan B is most effective when used within 12 to 24 hours after unprotected intercourse.[31] An unconditional right to refuse is less compelling when the patient requests an intervention that is urgent.

Refusal Has Great Potential for Abuse and Discrimination

The limits to conscientious objection remain unclear. Pharmacists are privy to personal information through prescriptions. For instance, a customer who fills prescriptions for zidovudine, didanosine, and indinavir is logically assumed to be infected with the human immunodeficiency virus (HIV). If pharmacists can reject prescriptions that conflict with their morals, someone who believes that HIV-positive people must have engaged in immoral behavior could refuse to fill those prescriptions. Similarly, a pharmacist who does not condone extramarital sex might refuse to fill a sildenafil prescription for an unmarried man. Such objections go beyond "conscientious" to become invasive. Furthermore, because a pharmacist does not know a patient's history on the basis of a given prescription, judgments regarding the acceptability of a prescription may be medically inappropriate. To a woman with Eisenmenger's syndrome, for example, pregnancy may mean death. The potential for abuse by pharmacists underscores the need for policies ensuring that patients receive unbiased care.

Toward Balance

Compelling arguments can be made both for and against a pharmacist's right to refuse to fill prescriptions for emergency contraception. But even cogent ideas falter when confronted by a dissident moral code. Such is the nature of belief. Even so, most people can agree that we must find a workable and respectful balance between the needs of patients and the morals of pharmacists.

Three possible solutions exist: an absolute right to object, no right to object, or a limited right to object. On balance, the first two options are untenable. An absolute right to conscientious objection respects the autonomy of pharmacists but diminishes their professional obligation to serve patients. It may also greatly affect the health of patients, especially vulnerable ones, and inappropriately brings politics into the pharmacy. Even pharmacists who believe that emergency contraception represents murder and feel compelled to obstruct patients' access to it must recognize that contraception and abortion before fetal viability remain legal nationwide. In our view, state efforts to provide blanket immunity to objecting pharmacists are misguided. Pharmacies should follow the prevailing employment-law standard to make reasonable attempts to accommodate their employees' personal beliefs.[32] Although neutral policies to dispense medications to all customers may conflict with pharmacists' morals, such policies are not necessarily discriminatory, and pharmacies need not shoulder a heightened obligation of absolute accommodation.

Complete restriction of a right to conscientious objection is also problematic. Though pharmacists voluntarily enter their profession and have an obligation to serve patients without judgment, forcing them to abandon their morals imposes a heavy toll. Ethics and law demand that a professional's morality not interfere with the provision of care in life-or-death situations, such as a ruptured ectopic pregnancy.[29] Whereas the hours that elapse between intercourse and the intervention of emergency contraception are crucial, they do not meet that strict test. Also, patients who face an objecting pharmacist do have options, even if they are less preferable than having the prescription immediately filled. Because of these caveats, it is difficult to demand by law that pharmacists relinquish individual morality to stock and fill prescriptions for emergency contraception.

We are left, then, with the vast middle ground. Although we believe that the most ethical course is to treat patients compassionately—that is, to stock emergency contraception and fill prescriptions for it—the totality of the arguments makes us stop short of advocating a legal duty to do so as a first resort. We stop short for three reasons: because emergency contraception is not an absolute emergency, because other options exist, and because, when possible, the moral beliefs of those delivering care should be considered. However, in a profession that is bound by fiduciary obligations and strives to respect and care for patients, it is unacceptable to leave patients to fend for themselves. As a general rule, pharmacists who cannot or will not dispense a drug have an obligation to meet the needs of their customers by referring them elsewhere. This idea is uncontroversial when it is applied to common medications such as antibiotics and statins; it becomes contentious, but is equally valid, when it is applied to emergency contraception. Therefore, pharmacists who object should, as a matter of ethics and law, provide alternatives for patients.

Pharmacists who object to filling prescriptions for emergency contraception should arrange for another pharmacist to provide this service to customers promptly. Pharmacies that stock emergency contraception should ensure, to the extent possible, that at least one nonobjecting pharmacist is on duty at all times. Pharmacies that do not stock emergency contraception should give clear notice and refer patients elsewhere. At the very least, there should be a prominently displayed sign that says, "We do not provide emergency contraception. Please call Planned Parenthood at 800-230-PLAN (7526) . . . for assistance." However, a direct referral to a local pharmacy or pharmacist who is willing to fill the prescription is preferable. Objecting pharmacists should also redirect prescriptions for emergency contraception that are received by telephone to another pharmacy known to fill such prescriptions. In rural areas, objecting pharmacists should provide referrals within a reasonable radius.

Notably, the American Pharmacists Association has endorsed referrals, explaining that "providing alternative mechanisms for patients . . . ensures patient access to drug products, without requiring the pharmacist or the patient to abide by personal decisions other than their own."[33] A referral may also represent a break in causation between the pharmacist and distributing emergency contraception, a separation that the objecting pharmacist presumably seeks. And, in deference to the law's normative value, the rule of referral also conveys the importance of professional responsibility to patients. In areas of the country where referrals are logistically impractical, professional obligation may dictate providing emergency contraception, and a legal mandate may be appropriate if ethical obligations are unpersuasive.

Inevitably, some pharmacists will disregard our guidelines, and physicians—all physicians—should be prepared to fill gaps in care. They should identify pharmacies that will fill patients' prescriptions and encourage patients to keep emergency contraception at home. They should be prepared to dispense emergency contraception or instruct patients to mimic it with other birth-control pills. In Wisconsin, family-planning clinics recently began dispensing emergency contraception, and the state set up a toll-free hotline to help patients find physicians who will prescribe it.[34] Emergency departments should stock emergency contraception and make it available to rape survivors, if not all patients.

In the final analysis, education remains critical. Pharmacists may have misconceptions about emergency contraception. In one survey, a majority of pharmacists mistakenly agreed with the statement that repeated use of emergency contraception is medically risky.[35] Medical misunderstandings that lead pharmacists to refuse to fill prescriptions for emergency contraception are unacceptable. Patients, too, may misunderstand or be unaware of emergency contraception.[36] Physicians should teach patients about this option before the need arises, since patients may understand their choices better when they are not under stress. Physicians should discuss emergency contraception during office visits, offer prescriptions in advance of need, and provide education through pamphlets or the Internet. Web sites . . . allow users to search for physicians who prescribe emergency contraception by ZIP Code, area code, or address, and Planned Parenthood offers extensive educational information . . . , including details about off-label use of many birth-control pills for emergency contraception.

Our principle of a compassionate duty of care should apply to all health care professionals. In a secular society, they must be prepared to limit the reach of their personal objection. Objecting pharmacists may choose to find employment opportunities that comport with their morals—in a religious community, for example—but when they pledge to serve the public, it is unreasonable to expect those in need of health care to acquiesce to their personal convictions. Similarly, physicians who refuse to write prescriptions for emergency contraception should follow the rules of notice and referral for the reason previously articulated: the beliefs of health care providers should not trump patient care. It is difficult enough to be faced with the consequences of rape or of an unplanned pregnancy; health care providers should not make the situation measurably worse.

Former Supreme Court Chief Justice Charles Evans Hughes called the quintessentially American custom of respect for conscience a "happy tradition"[37]—happier, perhaps, when left in the setting of a draft objection than when pitting one person's beliefs against another's reproductive health. Ideally, conflicts about emergency contraception will be rare, but they will occur. In July, 11 nurses in Alabama resigned rather than provide emergency contraception in state clinics.[38] As patients understand their birth-control options, conflicts at the pharmacy counter and in the clinic may become more common. When professionals' definitions of liberty infringe on those they choose to serve, a respectful balance must be struck. We offer one solution. Even those who challenge this division of burdens and benefits should agree with our touchstone—although health professionals may have a right to object, they should not have a right to obstruct.

References

1. Drazen JM, Greene MF, Wood AJJ. The FDA, politics, and Plan B. N Engl J Med 2004;350:1561–2.
2. Stanford JB, Hager WD, Crockett SA. The FDA, politics, and Plan B. N Engl J Med 2004;350:2413–4.
3. Alaska Admin. Code tit. 12, § 52.240 (2004).
4. Cal. Bus. & Prof. Code § 4052 (8) (2004).
5. Hawaii Rev. Stat. § 461-1 (2003).
6. N.M. Admin. Code § 16.19.26.9 (2003).
7. Wash. Rev. Code § 246-863-100 (2004).
8. Me. Rev. Stat. Ann. tit.32, §§ 13821-13825 (2004).
9. Pharmacist refuses pill for victim. Chicago Tribune. February 11, 2004:C7.
10. Simon S. Pharmacists new players in abortion debate. Los Angeles Times. March 20, 2004:A18.
11. Sweeney JF. May a pharmacist refuse to fill a prescription? Plain Dealer. May 5, 2004:E1.
12. Associated Press. Pharmacist refuses to fill morning after prescription.
13. Sauer M. Pharmacist to be fired in abortion controversy. St. Petersburg Times. December 19, 1991:1B.
14. State policies in brief: refusing to provide health services. New York: Alan Guttmacher Institute, September 1, 2004.
15. Seeley RA. Advice for conscientious objectors in the armed forces. 5th ed. Philadelphia: Central Committee for Conscientious Objectors, 1998:1–2.
16. 42 U.S.C. § 300a-7 (2004).
17. Mich. House Bill No. 5006 (As amended April 21, 2004).
18. Oregon House Bill No. 2010 (As amended May 11, 1999).
19. Hooks Super X, Inc. v. McLaughlin, 642 N.E. 2d 514 (Ind. 1994).
20. Section 2.01. In: Council on Ethical and Judicial Affairs. Code of medical ethics: current opinions with annotations. 2002–2003 ed. Chicago: American Medical Association, 2002.
21. Oregon Revised Statute § 127.885 § 4.01 (4) (2003).
22. Fassett WE, Wicks AC. Is pharmacy a profession? In: Weinstein BD, ed. Ethical issues in pharmacy. Vancouver, Wash.: Applied Therapeutics, 1996:1–28.
23. American Pharmacists Association. Code of ethics for pharmacists: preamble.
24. Hughes EC, ed. Obstetric-gynecologic terminology, with section on neonatology and glossary of congenital anomalies. Philadelphia: F.A. Davis, 1972.
25. Commodity Supplemental Food Program, 7 C.F.R. § 247.2 (2004).
26. Glasier A. Emergency postcoital contraception. N Engl J Med 1997;337:1058–64.
27. Daily reproductive health report: state politics & policy: Washington governor signs law requiring hospitals to offer emergency contraception to rape survivors. Menlo Park, Calif.: Kaisernetwork, April 2, 2002.
28. Brownfield v. Daniel Freeman Marina Hospital, 208 Cal. App. 3d 405 (Cal. Ct. App. 1989).
29. Shelton v. Univ. of Medicine & Dentistry, 223 F.3d 220 (3d Cir. 2000).
30. Tribe LH. American constitutional law. 2nd ed. Mineola, N.Y.: Foundation Press, 1988:1183.
31. Brody JE. The politics of emergency contraception. New York Times. August 24, 2004:F7.
32. Trans World Airlines v. Hardison, 432 U.S. 63 (1977).
33. 1997–98 APhA Policy Committee report: pharmacist conscience clause. Washington, D.C.: American Pharmacists Association, 1997.
34. Politics wins over science. Capital Times. May 13, 2004:16A.
35. Alford S, Davis L, Brown L. Pharmacists' attitudes and awareness of emergency contraception for adolescents. Transitions 2001;12(4):1–17.
36. Foster DG, Harper CC, Bley JJ, et al. Knowledge of emergency contraception among women aged 18 to 44 in California. Am J Obstet Gynecol 2004; 191:150–6.
37. United States v. Macintosh, 283 U.S. 605, 634 (1931) (Hughes, C.J., dissenting).
38. Elliott D. Alabama nurses quit over morning-after pill. Presented on All Things Considered. Washington, D.C.: National Public Radio, July 28, 2004 (transcript). *Copyright © 2004 Massachusetts Medical Society.*

Julie Cantor is an attorney at Yale University School of Medicine.

Ken Baum is a physician and attorney at the firm of Wiggin and Dana, New Haven, Connecticut.

EXPLORING THE ISSUE

Should Pharmacists Be Allowed to Deny Prescriptions on Grounds of Conscience?

Critical Thinking and Reflection

1. How do you believe individual rights should be balanced against the social good? Individual freedom of speech and freedom to refuse vaccinations are typically thought to be limited in certain cases in which exercising those freedoms may lead to social harms; how does this balancing principle translate to the case of pharmacists filling prescriptions?
2. Does filling a prescription make a pharmacist complicit in the woman's use of the drug? Explain your reasoning.
3. If a pharmacist refuses to fill a prescription but helps a woman find someone else who will fill it, is the pharmacist as complicit in the woman's act as if he had filled the prescription himself? Explain your reasoning.

Is There Common Ground?

In November 2004, the FDA announced a labeling change for mifepristone. Because the FDA and the manufacturer Danco Laboratories had received reports of serious side effects, the warning label was changed to reflect this new information.

Both the U.S. federal government and the great majority of states have laws protecting conscientious objectors in health care. The Illinois Health Care Right of Conscience Act is particularly detailed and protects physicians, health care personnel, health care facilities, and health care payers who refuse to participate in services that are contrary to their conscience. In April 2005, however, Gov. Rod Blagojevich issued an emergency rule requiring pharmacies to fill prescriptions for birth control and mifepristone "without delay." Bills have been introduced that specifically include pharmacists in the Health Care Right of Conscience Act.

As of 2012, six states (Arizona, Arkansas, Georgia, Idaho, Mississippi, and South Dakota) have laws specifically recognizing a pharmacist's right of conscientious objection. A California law requires pharmacists to dispense these drugs unless the employer approves the refusal and the woman has another way of filling the prescription. A New Jersey law prohibits pharmacists from refusing to fill prescriptions on moral, religious, or ethical grounds.

Additional Resources

The National Conference of State Legislatures monitors state legislative activity on conscience clause laws. See www.ncsl.org/programs/health/conscienceclauses.htm.

A national survey of physicians found that physicians who were male, religious, and had moral objections to controversial but legal procedures like administering terminal sedation in dying patients or prescribing birth control to teenagers without parental approval were less likely to report that doctors must disclose information or refer patients for these medical procedures (Farr A. Curlin et al., "Religion, Conscience, and Controversial Clinical Practices," *The New England Journal of Medicine* [February 8, 2007]).

In "Pharmacies, Pharmacists, and Conscientious Objection," Mark R. Wicclair argues that the health needs of patients and the professional obligations of pharmacists limit the extent to which they may refuse to assist patients who have lawful prescriptions for medically indicated drugs (*Kennedy Institute of Ethics Journal* [vol. 16, no. 3, 2006]). On the other hand, Brian P. Knestout asserts that "conscience clauses" protect medical professionals who do not wish to perform or assist in procedures related to abortion, sterilization, or euthanasia ("An Essential Prescription: Why Pharmacist-Inclusive Clauses Are

Necessary," *Journal of Contemporary Health Lawand Policy*, [Spring 2006]).

Adrienne Asch compares conscientious objections to health care practices to similar behavior in times of war and offers limited support for these exceptions to professional responsibility ("Two Cheers for Conscience Exceptions," *Hastings Center Report* [November–December 2006]).

Internet References . . .

Guttmacher Institute, Resources, Services and Financing

http://www.guttmacher.org/sections/services.php

The Hastings Center

http://www.thehastingscenter.org/

The National Conference of State Legislatures

www.ncsl.org/

Unit 5

UNIT

The Development and Use of Biotechnology

*N*ew medical and biological science and technologies have created enormous possibilities for understanding heredity and its influence on disease, for identifying and perhaps treating people who are at risk for genetic diseases, and for changing human bodies in ways that have nothing to do with the treatment of disease. A deeper understanding of the mysteries of life and mastery of techniques for synthesizing or editing genomes put humans in the place, perhaps, of creating new forms of life. Such organisms could be specially designed to serve various human needs or wants, or they might be specially designed to serve environmental purposes. All scientific and technical breakthroughs bring unresolved questions, however. And the track record is not always great: The abuse of genetic information (much of it misinformation) in the past haunt efforts today to use this information wisely and compassionately, and the human capacity to alter the environment has brought mixed results. We have made agriculture possible through breeding and hybridization technologies, but we have also done significant environmental harm through our efforts to use and control species. What impact will medical and biological knowledge and technology have on our lives and futures, and on the lives and futures of our children? These are some of the challenging issues raised in this unit.

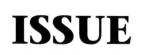

Selected, Edited, and with Issue Framing Material by:
Gregory E. Kaebnick, *The Hastings Center*

ISSUE

Is the Use of Medical Tools to Enhance Human Beings Morally Troubling?

YES: President's Council on Bioethics, from *Beyond Therapy: Biotechnology and the Pursuit of Happiness,* U.S. Government Printing Office (2003)

NO: Ronald Bailey, from "The Case for Enhancing People" *The New Atlantis* (2011)

Learning Outcomes
After reading this issue, you will be able to:
• Discuss a range of arguments for and against using medical technologies to enhance human bodies and behavior.
• Identify some claims commonly made about human nature in the debate about enhancement.

ISSUE SUMMARY

YES: The President's Council on Bioethics, a presidential body formed by President Bush, argues that biotechnological interventions for making people better than normal raise profound concerns about the relationship between humans and nature, human identity, and human happiness.

NO: The libertarian science writer Ronald Bailey maintains that enhancements will only help people live better lives.

Perhaps more than any other people, Americans seem to be obsessed with self-improvement. Each year there is a flood of new books and television commercials promoting ways to be richer, thinner, smarter, happier, healthier, more successful, attractive, or all of the above. Whatever one's presumed character or bodily flaw, there is a remedy. And for parents, there is an additional opportunity (sometimes presented as an obligation) to make one's children richer, thinner, smarter, happier, or all of the above.

Traditionally, most of these strategies for improving ourselves or our children are activities or experiences—education, exercise, summer camps, yoga, and so on. But what if we could change that? What if the self-improvement could be achieved with much less work, or without real work at all—in effect dropping the kinds of activities that the term "self-improvement" brings to mind and more directly *enhancing* ourselves or our children?

The most obvious targets for enhancement include physical form and functioning, cognitive functioning, and mood or temperament, but conceivably we could even go beyond the traditional targets of self-improvement and enhance such seeming givens of human life as lifespan, so that we lived hundreds of years or more.

Increasingly, if incrementally, biotechnologies seem to offer this promise. A biotechnological enhancement strategy that is by now relatively familiar is the use of pharmaceuticals, such as performance-enhancing drugs in sports (discussed in issue 13) or cognitive enhancers, such as Ritalin, in the classroom. Certain antidepressants are thought to have the ability to enhance mood. Surgery sometimes offers another familiar though limited route to enhancement, at least of bodily form.

Foreseeable sometime in the future is enhancement through genetic manipulation. This could happen by identifying genes that confer improved capabilities (which is much more difficult than news stories usually suggest, but may for at least some traits prove feasible) and transferring them into a person's somatic cells—into muscles to produce superior physical performance, for example—or into germline cells—that is, the cells that produce gametes—so that the changes would be passed from generation to generation. The first method would allow individuals to seek genetic enhancements for themselves or for their children, if the genes were transferred into their children's bodies, and the second would be a way of enhancing both one's children and subsequent generations.

The basic idea of genetic enhancement is arguably not new. Germline genetic enhancement has been practiced for centuries in animal husbandry and agriculture. By breeding for certain characteristics, animals and plants have been created to better meet human purposes. The largest Great Dane and the smallest Pekinese, and all the dog breeds in between, are descended from a handful of wolves tamed by humans in Asia nearly 15,000 years ago. Over the last 500 years, humans have practiced breeding techniques that account for vastly different appearances and characteristics of modern dogs.

Applying these techniques to humans—the theory of eugenics or "better genes"—also has a long but disastrous history. Its advocates, many of them in the United States in the twentieth century, advocated the elimination of "undesirable" people by preventing them from reproducing through involuntary sterilization. In the most malevolent form of eugenics, of course, the Nazi regime in Germany in the 1930s wanted to create a "master race" by encouraging reproduction among blonde, blue-eyed, tall Aryan types and eliminating from the gene pool—through murder—those other population groups, such as Jews and gypsies.

While these eugenics methods are not only barbarous and morally corrupt, the idea of enhancing one's capacities and those of future generations has been given new life by scientific advances in genetics. Being able to manipulate genes—the very core of human inheritance—opens up a new world of possibilities. Already animals like sheep and cows have been cloned, that is, their genomes were transferred into eggs to create animals that are genetically identical (although the animals are never entirely identical because of uterine and environmental differences). In principle, if the genetic contributions to traits can be identified, it might eventually be possible to use genetic enhancement to conduct a new eugenics—a "liberal eugenics"—in which the birth of people with desirable traits is promoted although people with undesirable traits are not targeted or suppressed.

Enhancement raises an assortment of ethical questions. Even if it is possible to enhance an individual's height, beauty, intelligence, or capacity for happiness, is it desirable? If these techniques proved to be safe and effective, would they be distributed fairly throughout society?

These questions are at the core of the following selections. The President's Council on Bioethics, a presidential commission during the administration of George W. Bush that was chaired by the physician and philosopher Leon Kass, argues that there are a number of moral problems with enhancement, whether it is undertaken for one's own benefit or to benefit one's children. Ronald Bailey, a libertarian science writer, is dismissive of the PCB's concerns.

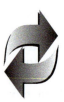

YES ↵

President's Council on Bioethics

Beyond Therapy: Biotechnology and the Pursuit of Happiness

Before proceeding, we wish to reiterate our intention in this inquiry, so as to avoid misunderstanding. In offering our synopsis of concerns, we are not making predictions; we are merely pointing to possible hazards, hazards that become visible only when one looks at "the big picture." More important, we are not condemning either biotechnological power or the pursuit of happiness, excellence, or self-perfection. Far from it. We eagerly embrace biotechnologies as aids for preventing or correcting bodily or mental ills and for restoring health and fitness. We even more eagerly embrace the pursuits of happiness, excellence, and self-improvement, for ourselves, our children, and our society. Desires for these goals are the source of much that is good in human life. Yet, as has long been known, these desires can be excessive. Worse, they can be badly educated regarding the nature of their object, sometimes with tragic result: we get what we ask for only to discover that it is very far from what we really wanted. Finally, they can be pursued in harmful ways and with improper means, often at the price of deforming the very goals being sought. To guard against such outcomes, we need to be alert in advance to the more likely risks and the more serious concerns. We begin with those that are more obvious and familiar.

Familiar Sources of Concern

The first concerns commonly expressed regarding any uses of biotechnology beyond therapy reflect, not surprisingly, the dominant values of modern America: health and safety, fairness and equality, and freedom. The following thumbnail sketches of the issues should suffice to open the questions—though of course not to settle them.

A. Health: Issues of Safety and Bodily Harm

In our health-conscious culture, the first reason people worry about any biotechnical intervention, whatever its intended purpose, is safety. This will surely be true regarding "elective" uses of biotechnology that aim beyond therapy. Athletes who take steroids to boost their strength may later suffer premature heart disease. College students who snort Ritalin to increase their concentration may become addicted. Melancholics taking mood-brighteners to change their outlook may experience impotence or apathy. To generalize: no biological agent used for purposes of self-perfection or self-satisfaction is likely to be entirely safe. This is good medical common sense: anything powerful enough to enhance system A is likely to be powerful enough to harm system B (or even system A itself), the body being a highly complex yet integrated whole in which one intervenes partially only at one's peril. And it surely makes sense, ethically speaking, that one should not risk basic health pursuing a condition of "better than well."

Yet some of the interventions that might aim beyond therapy—for example, genetic enhancement of muscle strength, retardation of aging, or pharmacologic blunting of horrible memories or increasing self-esteem—may, indirectly, lead also to improvements in general health. More important, many good things in life are filled with risks, and free people—even if properly informed about the magnitude of those risks—may choose to run them if they care enough about what they might gain thereby. . . .

B. Unfairness

An obvious objection to the use of enhancement technologies, especially by participants in competitive activities, is that they give those who use them an unfair advantage: blood doping or steroids in athletes, stimulants in students taking the SATs, and so on. This issue . . . has been well aired by the International Olympic Committee and the many other athletic organizations who continue to try to formulate rules that can be enforced, even as the athletes and their pharmacists continue to devise ways to violate those rules and escape detection. Yet as we saw, the fairness question can be turned on its head, and some people see in biotechnical intervention a way to compensate for the

From the President's Council on Bioethics, October 2003.

"unfairness" of natural inequalities—say, in size, strength, drive, or native talent. Still, even if everyone had equal access to genetic improvement of muscle strength or mind-enhancing drugs, or even if these gifts of technology would be used only to rectify the inequalities produced by the unequal gifts of nature, an additional disquiet would still perhaps remain: The disquiet of using such new powers in the first place or at all, even were they fairly distributed. . . .

C. Equality of Access

A related question concerns inequality of access to the benefits of biotechnology, a matter of great interest to many Members of this Council. . . . The issue of distributive justice is more important than the issue of unfairness in competitive activities, especially if there are systemic disparities between those who will and those who won't have access to the powers of biotechnical "improvement." Should these capabilities arrive, we may face severe aggravations of existing "unfairnesses" in the "game of life," especially if people who need certain agents to treat serious illness cannot get them while other people can enjoy them for less urgent or even dubious purposes. If, as is now often the case with expensive medical care, only the wealthy and privileged will be able to gain easy access to costly enhancing technologies, we might expect to see an ever-widening gap between "the best and the brightest" and the rest. The emergence of a biotechnologically improved "aristocracy"—augmenting the already cognitively stratified structure of American society—is indeed a worrisome possibility, and there is nothing in our current way of doing business that works against it. Indeed, unless something new intervenes, it would seem to be a natural outcome of mixing these elements of American society: our existing inequalities in wealth and status, the continued use of free markets to develop and obtain the new technologies, and our libertarian attitudes favoring unrestricted personal freedom for all choices in private life.

Yet the situation regarding rich and poor is more complex, especially if one considers actual benefits rather than equality or relative well-being. The advent of new technologies often brings great benefits to the less well off, if not at first, then after they come to be mass-produced and massmarketed and the prices come down. (Consider, over the past half-century, the spread in the United States of refrigerators and radios, automobiles and washing machines, televisions and VCRs, cell phones and personal computers, and, in the domain of medicine, antibiotics, vaccines, and many expensive diagnostic and therapeutic procedures.) To be sure, the gap between the richest and the poorest may increase, but in absolute terms the poor

may benefit more, when compared not to the rich but to where they were before. . . .

D. Liberty: Issues of Freedom and Coercion, Overt and Subtle

A concern for threats to freedom comes to the fore whenever biotechnical powers are exercised by some people upon other people. We encountered it in our discussion of "better children" (the choice of a child's sex or the drugmediated alteration of his or her behavior . . .), as well as in the coerced use of anabolic steroids by the East German Olympic swimmers. . . . This problem will of course be worse in tyrannical regimes. But there are always dangers of despotism within families, as many parents already work their wills on their children with insufficient regard to a child's independence or long-term needs, jeopardizing even the "freedom to be a child." To the extent that even partial control over genotype—say, to take a relatively innocent example, musician parents selecting a child with genes for perfect pitch—would add to existing social instruments of parental control and its risks of despotic rule, this matter will need to be attended to. Leaving aside the special case of children, the risk of overt coercion does not loom large in a free society. On the contrary, many enthusiasts for using technology for personal enhancement are libertarian in outlook; they see here mainly the enlargement of human powers and possibilities and the multiplication of options for private choice, both of which they see as steps to greater human freedom. They look forward to growing opportunities for more people to earn more, learn more, see more, and do more, and to choose—perhaps several times in one lifetime—interesting new careers or avocations. And they look with suspicion at critics who they fear might want to limit their private freedom to develop and use new technologies for personal advancement or, indeed, for any purpose whatsoever. The coercion they fear comes not from advances in technology but from the state, acting to deny them their right to pursue happiness or self-improvement by the means they privately choose.

Yet no one can deny that people living in free societies, and even their most empowered citizens, already experience more subtle impingements on freedom and choice, operating, for example, through peer pressure. What is freely permitted and widely used may, under certain circumstances, become practically mandatory. If most children are receiving memory enhancement or stimulant drugs, failure to provide them for your child might be seen as a form of child neglect. If all the defensive linemen are on steroids, you risk mayhem if you go against them chemically pure. And, a point subtler still, some critics complain that, as with cosmetic surgery, Botox, and breast implants, many of the enhancement technologies of the future will very likely be used in slavish adherence to certain socially defined and merely fashionable notions of "excellence" or improvement, very likely shallow and conformist. If these fears are realized, such exercises of individual freedom, suitably multiplied, might compromise the freedom to be an individual.

This special kind of reduction of freedom—let's call it the problem of conformity or homogenization—is of more than individual concern. In an era of mass culture, itself the byproduct of previous advances in communication, manufacture, and marketing techniques, the exercise of uncoerced private choices may produce untoward consequences for society as a whole. Trends in popular culture lead some critics to worry that the self-selected nontherapeutic uses of the new biotechnical powers, should they become widespread, will be put in the service of the most common human desires, moving us toward still greater homogenization of human society—perhaps raising the floor but also lowering the ceiling of human possibility, and reducing the likelihood of genuine freedom, individuality, and greatness. . . .

Essential Sources of Concern

Our familiar worries about issues of safety, equality, and freedom, albeit very important, do not exhaust the sources of reasonable concern. When richly considered, they invite us to think about the deeper purposes for the sake of which we want to live safely, justly, and freely. And they enable us to recognize that even the safe, equally available, noncoerced and non-faddish uses of biomedical technologies to pursue happiness or self-improvement raise ethical and social questions, questions more directly connected with the essence of the activity itself: the use of technological means to intervene into the human body and mind, not to ameliorate their diseases but to change and improve their normal workings. Why, if at all, are we bothered by the voluntary self-administration of agents that would change our bodies or alter our minds? What is disquieting about our attempts to improve upon human nature, or even our own particular instance of it?

The subject being relatively novel, it is difficult to put this worry into words. We are in an area where initial revulsions are hard to translate into sound moral arguments. Many people are probably repelled by the idea of drugs that erase memories or that change personalities, or of interventions that enable seventy-year-olds to bear children or play professional sports, or, to engage in some wilder imaginings, of mechanical implants that

would enable men to nurse infants or computer-brain hookups that would enable us to download the Oxford English Dictionary. But can our disquiet at such prospects withstand rational, anthropological, or ethical scrutiny? Taken one person at a time, with a properly prepared set of conditions and qualifications, it will be hard to say what is wrong with any biotechnical intervention that could improve our performances, give us (more) ageless bodies, or make it possible for us to have happier souls. Indeed, in many cases, we ought to be thankful for or pleased with the improvements our biotechnical ingenuity is making possible. . . .

A. Hubris or Humility: Respect for "the Given"

A common, man-on-the-street reaction to the prospects of biotechnological engineering beyond therapy is the complaint of "man playing God." If properly unpacked, this worry is in fact shared by people holding various theological beliefs and by people holding none at all. Sometimes the charge means the sheer prideful presumption of trying to alter what God has ordained or nature has produced, or what should, for whatever reason, not be fiddled with. Sometimes the charge means not so much usurping Godlike powers, but doing so in the absence of God-like knowledge: the mere playing at being God, the hubris of acting with insufficient wisdom. . . .

One revealing way to formulate the problem of hubris is what one of our Council Members has called the temptation to "hyper-agency," a Promethean aspiration to remake nature, including human nature, to serve our purposes and to satisfy our desires. This attitude is to be faulted not only because it can lead to bad, unintended consequences; more fundamentally, it also represents a false understanding of, and an improper disposition toward, the naturally given world. The root of the difficulty seems to be both cognitive and moral: the failure properly to appreciate and respect the "giftedness" of the world. Acknowledging the giftedness of life means recognizing that our talents and powers are not wholly our own doing, nor even fully ours, despite the efforts we expend to develop and to exercise them. It also means recognizing that not everything in the world is open to any use we may desire or devise. Such an appreciation of the giftedness of life would constrain the Promethean project and conduce to a much-needed humility. Although it is in part a religious sensibility, its resonance reaches beyond religion.

Human beings have long manifested both wondering appreciation for nature's beauty and grandeur and reverent awe before nature's sublime and mysterious power. . . . [A]ppreciating that the given world—including our natural powers to alter it—is not of our own making could induce a welcome attitude of modesty, restraint, and humility. Such a posture is surely recommended for anyone inclined to modify human beings or human nature for purposes beyond therapy.

Yet the respectful attitude toward the "given," while both necessary and desirable as a restraint, is not by itself sufficient as a guide. The "giftedness of nature" also includes smallpox and malaria, cancer and Alzheimer disease, decline and decay. Moreover, nature is not equally generous with her gifts, even to man, the most gifted of her creatures. Modesty born of gratitude for the world's "givenness" may enable us to recognize that not everything in the world is open to any use we may desire or devise, but it will not by itself teach us which things can be tinkered with and which should be left inviolate. Respect for the "giftedness" of things cannot tell us which gifts are to be accepted as is, which are to be improved through use or training, which are to be housebroken through self-command or medication, and which opposed like the plague. . . .

B. "Unnatural" Means: The Dignity of Human Activity

Until only yesterday, teaching and learning or practice and training exhausted the alternatives for acquiring human excellence, perfecting our natural gifts through our own efforts. But perhaps no longer: biotechnology may be able to do nature one better, even to the point of requiring less teaching, training, or practice to permit an improved nature to shine forth. As we noted earlier, the insertion of the growth-factor gene into the muscles of rats and mice bulks them up and keeps them strong and sound without the need for nearly as much exertion. Drugs to improve alertness (today) or memory and amiability (tomorrow) could greatly relieve the need for exertion to acquire these powers, leaving time and effort for better things. What, if anything, is disquieting about such means of gaining improvement?

The problem cannot be that they are "artificial," in the sense of having man-made origins. Beginning with the needle and the fig leaf, man has from the start been the animal that uses art to improve his lot by altering or adding to what nature alone provides. Ordinary medicine makes extensive use of similar artificial means, from drugs to surgery to mechanical implants, in order to treat disease. If the use of artificial means is absolutely welcome in the activity of healing, it cannot be their unnaturalness alone that disquiets us when they are used to make people "better than well."

Still, in those areas of human life in which excellence has until now been achieved only by discipline and effort, the attainment of similar results by means of drugs, genetic engineering, or implanted devices looks to many people (including some Members of this Council) to be "cheating" or "cheap." Many people believe that each person should work hard for his achievements. Even if we prefer the grace of the natural athlete or the quickness of the natural mathematician—people whose performances deceptively appear to be effortless—we admire also those who overcome obstacles and struggle to try to achieve the excellence of the former. This matter of character—the merit of disciplined and dedicated striving—is surely pertinent. For character is not only the source of our deeds, but also their product. As we have already noted, healthy people whose disruptive behavior is "remedied" by pacifying drugs rather than by their own efforts are not learning self-control; if anything, they may be learning to think it unnecessary. People who take pills to block out from memory the painful or hateful aspects of a new experience will not learn how to deal with suffering or sorrow. A drug that induces fearlessness does not produce courage.

Yet things are not so simple. Some biotechnical interventions may assist in the pursuit of excellence without in the least cheapening its attainment. And many of life's excellences have nothing to do with competition or overcoming adversity. Drugs to decrease drowsiness, increase alertness, sharpen memory, or reduce distraction may actually help people interested in their natural pursuits of learning or painting or performing their civic duty. Drugs to steady the hand of a neurosurgeon or to prevent sweaty palms in a concert pianist cannot be regarded as "cheating," for they are in no sense the source of the excellent activity or achievement. And, for people dealt a meager hand in the dispensing of nature's gifts, it should not be called cheating or cheap if biotechnology could assist them in becoming better equipped—whether in body or in mind.

Nevertheless, . . . there remains a sense that the "naturalness" of means matters. It lies not in the fact that the assisting drugs and devices are artifacts, but in the danger of violating or deforming the nature of human agency and the dignity of the naturally human way of activity. In most of our ordinary efforts at self-improvement, whether by practice, training, or study, we sense the relation between our doings and the resulting improvement, between the means used and the end sought. . . . In contrast, biotechnical interventions act directly on the human body and mind to bring about their effects on a passive subject, who plays little or no role at all.

C. Identity and Individuality

With biotechnical interventions that skip the realm of intelligible meaning, we cannot really own the transformations nor can we experience them as genuinely ours. And we will be at a loss to attest whether the resulting conditions and activities of our bodies and our minds are, in the fullest sense, our own as human. But our interest in identity is also more personal. For we do not live in a generic human way; we desire, act, flourish, and decline as ourselves, as individuals. To be human is to be someone, not anyone—with a given nature (male or female), given natural abilities (superior wit or musical talent), and—most important—a real history of attachments, memories, and experiences, acquired largely by living with others.

In myriad ways, new biotechnical powers promise (or threaten) to transform what it means to be an individual: giving increased control over our identity to others, as in the case of genetic screening or sex selection of offspring by parents; inducing psychic states divorced from real life and lived experience; blunting or numbing the memories we wish to escape; and achieving the results we could never achieve unaided, by acting as ourselves alone.

To be sure, in many cases, biomedical technology can restore or preserve a real identity that is slipping away: keeping our memory intact by holding off the scourge of Alzheimer disease; restoring our capacity to love and work by holding at bay the demons of self-destroying depression. In other cases, the effect of biotechnology on identity is much more ambiguous. By taking psychotropic drugs to reduce anxiety or overcome melancholy, we may become the person we always wished to be—more cheerful, ambitious, relaxed, content. But we also become a different person in the eyes of others, and in many cases we become dependent on the continued use of psychotropic drugs to remain the new person we now are. . . .

D. Partial Ends, Full Flourishing

Beyond the perils of achieving our desired goals in a "less-than-human way" or in ways "not fully our own," we must consider the meaning of the ends themselves: better children, superior performance, ageless bodies, and happy souls. Would their attainment in fact improve or perfect our lives as human beings? Are they—always or ever—reasonable and attainable goals?. . .

In many cases, biotechnologies can surely help us cultivate what is best in ourselves and in our children, providing new tools for realizing good ends, wisely pursued. But it is also possible that the new technological means may deform the ends themselves. In pursuit of better children, biotechnical powers risk making us "tyrants"; in pursuit of superior performance, they risk making us "artifacts." In both cases, the problem is not the ends themselves but our misguided idea of their attainment or our false way of seeking to attain them. And in both cases, there is the ubiquitous problem that "good" or "superior" will be reconceived to fit the sorts of goals that the technological interventions can help us attain. We may come to believe that genetic predisposition or brain chemistry holds the key to helping our children develop and improve, or that stimulant drugs or bulkier muscles hold the key to excellent human activity. If we are equipped with hammers, we will see only those things that can be improved by pounding.

The goals of ageless bodies and happy souls—and especially the ways biotechnology might shape our pursuit of these ends—are perhaps more complicated. The case for ageless bodies seems at first glance to look pretty good. The prevention of decay, decline, and disability, the avoidance of blindness, deafness, and debility, the elimination of feebleness, frailty, and fatigue, all seem to be conducive to living fully as a human being at the top of one's powers—of having, as they say, a "good quality of life" from beginning to end. . . . And, should aging research deliver on its promise of adding not only extra life to years but also extra years to life, who would refuse it?

But . . . there may in fact be many human goods that are inseparable from our aging bodies, from our living in time, and especially from the natural human life cycle by which each generation gives way to the one that follows it. Because this argument is so counterintuitive, we need to begin not with the individual choice for an ageless body, but with what the individual's life might look like in a world in which everyone made the same choice. We need to make the choice universal, and see the meaning of that choice in the mirror of its becoming the norm.

What if everybody lived life to the hilt, even as they approached an ever-receding age of death in a body that looked and functioned—let's not be too greedy—like that of a thirty-year-old? Would it be good if each and all of us lived like light bulbs, burning as brightly from beginning to end, then popping off without warning, leaving those around us suddenly in the dark? Or is it perhaps better that there be a shape to life, everything in its due season, the shape also written, as it were, into the wrinkles of our bodies that live it—provided, of course, that we do not suffer years of painful or degraded old age and that we do not lose our wits?. . .

Going against both common intuition and native human desire, some commentators have argued that living with full awareness and acceptance of our finitude may be the condition of many of the best things in human life: engagement, seriousness, a taste for beauty, the possibility of virtue, the ties born of procreation, the quest for meaning. . . .

What about the pursuit of [happiness], and especially of the sort that we might better attain with pharmacological assistance? Painful and shameful memories are disturbing; guilty consciences trouble sleep; low self-esteem, melancholy, and world-weariness besmirch the waking hours. Why not memory-blockers for the former, mood-brighteners for the latter, and a good euphoriant—without risks of hangovers or cirrhosis—when celebratory occasions fail to be jolly? For let us be clear: If it is imbalances of neurotransmitters that are largely responsible for our state of soul, would it not be sheer priggishness to refuse the help of pharmacology for our happiness, when we accept it guiltlessly to correct for an absence of insulin or thyroid hormone?

And yet, . . . there seems to be something misguided about the pursuit of utter and unbroken psychic tranquility or the attempt to eliminate all shame, guilt, and painful memories. Traumatic memories, shame, and guilt, are, it is true, psychic pains. In extreme doses, they can be crippling. Yet, short of the extreme, they can also be helpful and fitting. They are appropriate responses to horror, disgraceful conduct, injustice, and sin, and, as such, help teach us to avoid them or fight against them in the future. Witnessing a murder should be remembered as horrible; doing a beastly deed should trouble one's soul. Righteous indignation at injustice depends on being able to feel injustice's sting. And to deprive oneself of one's memory—including and especially its truthfulness of feeling—is to deprive oneself of one's own life and identity. . . .

Looking into the future at goals pursuable with the aid of new biotechnologies enables us to turn a reflective glance at our own version of the human condition and the prospects now available to us (in principle) for a flourishing human life. For us today, assuming that we are blessed with good health and a sound mind, a flourishing human life is not a life lived with an ageless body or an untroubled soul, but rather a life lived in rhythmed time, mindful of time's limits, appreciative of each season and filled first of all with those intimate human relations that are ours only because we are born, age, replace ourselves, decline, and die—and know it. It is a life of aspiration, made possible by and born of experienced lack, of the disproportion between the transcendent longings of the soul and the limited capacities of our bodies and minds. It is a life that stretches toward some fulfillment to which our natural human soul has been oriented, and, unless we extirpate the source, will always be oriented. It is a life not of better genes and enhancing chemicals but of love and friendship, song and dance, speech and deed, working and learning, revering and worshipping. If this is true, then the pursuit of an ageless body may prove finally to be a distraction and a deformation. And the pursuit of an untroubled and self-satisfied soul may prove to be deadly to desire, if finitude recognized spurs aspiration and fine aspiration acted upon is itself the core of happiness. Not the agelessness of the body, nor the contentment of the soul, nor even the list of external achievements and accomplishments of life, but the engaged and energetic being-at-work of what nature uniquely gave to us is what we need to treasure and defend.

PRESIDENT'S COUNCIL ON BIOETHICS is a presidential advisory body formed by President George W. Bush.

Ronald Bailey   → **NO**

The Case for Enhancing People

Does the enhancement of human physical and intellectual capacities undermine virtue?

In answering this question, we must first make a distinction between therapy and enhancement. Therapeutic technologies are meant to restore impaired or degraded human capacities to some more normal level. By contrast, any enhancements would alter human functioning beyond the normal.

We must also keep in mind that, whatever we think about them, enhancements are going to happen. Age-retardation or even age-reversal are prime targets for research, but other techniques aimed at preventing disease and boosting memory, intelligence, and physical strength will also be developed.

Much worried attention is focused particularly on the possibility of achieving these and other enhancements through genetic engineering; that will indeed one day happen. But the fastest advances in enhancement will occur using pharmaceutical and biomedical interventions to modulate and direct the activity of existing genes in the bodies of people who are already alive. These will happen alongside the development of human-machine interfaces that will extend and boost human capacities.

Contrary to oft-expressed concerns, we will find, first, that enhancements will better enable people to flourish; second, that enhancements will not dissolve whatever existential worries people have; third, that enhancements will enable people to become more virtuous; fourth, that people who don't want enhancement for themselves should allow those of us who do to go forward without hindrance; fifth, that concerns over an "enhancement divide" are largely illusory; and sixth, that we already have at hand the social "technology," in the form of protective social and political institutions, that will enable the enhanced and the unenhanced to dwell together in peace.

Strengthening Virtue

What is an enhancement? A good definition is offered by Sarah Chan and John Harris in a 2007 article in the journal *Studies in Ethics, Law, and Technology*: an enhancement is

"a procedure that improves our functioning: any intervention which increases our general capabilities for human flourishing." People will choose enhancements that they believe are likely to help them or their children to flourish. Of course, their knowledge of a benefit will be likely rather than certain because people choosing enhancements will recognize that there is always the risk that they are wrong about the benefit, or that the attempt at enhancement will go awry, such as with a treatment failure. After all, most medical and technological advances are riskier in their early stages.

Just as Dante found it easier to conjure the pains of Hell than to evoke the joys of Heaven, so too do bioethicists find it easier to concoct the possible perils of a biotech-nanotech-infotech future than to appreciate how enhancements will contribute to flourishing lives. One of the chief goals of this symposium is to think about the indispensable role that virtue plays in human life. The chief motivating concern seems to be the fear that biotechnologies and other human enhancement technologies will somehow undermine human virtue. As we will see, far from undermining virtue, biotech, nanotech, and infotech enhancements will tend to support virtue; that is, they will help enable people to be actually good.

Peter Lawler, in *Stuck With Virtue* (2005), agrees that "the unprecedented health, longevity, and other indispensable means for human flourishing will deserve our gratitude." So far, so good. Then he goes on to claim, "But the victories that will be won [over nature]—like most of the victories won on behalf of the modern individual—will also probably be, in part, at the expense of the distinctively human goods: love, family, friends, country, virtue, art, spiritual life, and, most generally, living responsibly in light of what we really know about what we have been given." In fact, according to Lawler, we don't have to wait for future enhancements; modern technology is already making people less virtuous: as he has argued in the pages of this journal, "one of the downsides of living in an increasingly high-tech society is that both virtue and opportunities to act virtuously seem to be in short supply" ["*Restless Souls*," Winter 2004].

Really? Thanks to modern technology, sanitation, better nutrition, and medical care, Americans are living much longer and healthier lives than people did just a century ago. Do longer lives mean that people today are less virtuous? Or, inversely, does this mean that when people lived shorter lives they were *more* virtuous? Harvard political philosopher Michael Sandel offered a tart and persuasive response to suggestions that enhancing life spans might result in a less virtuous world:

> Are the background conditions in human self-understandings for the virtues just about right now at 78 years of the average life span, or such that they would be eroded and diminished if we extend it to 120 or 150, or 180? . . . Is it the suggestion that back when it was 48, rather than 78, a century ago . . . that the virtues we prize were on greater display or more available to us? And if so, would that be reason to aim for, or at least to wish for or long for, a shorter life span, rather than a longer one? . . .

Further, on what grounds do Lawler and others suggest that smarter, stronger, healthier, longer-lived people will care less about human goods like friendship, art, and the pursuit of virtue? As Elizabeth Fenton argued in a 2008 article in the journal *Bioethics*, "none of these capabilities (bodily health, imagination, emotion, practical reason, friendship, etc.) are in fact threatened by, for example, enhanced intelligence or athleticism." Being stronger, healthier, and smarter would more likely aid a person in his pursuit of virtue and moral excellence. And the unspoken implication that the state should somehow aim at inculcating collective virtue is incoherent: the pursuit of virtue is what *individuals* do.

The Dangers of Immortality?

Age-retardation technologies are the "killer app" (so to speak) of enhancements—so deeply and self-evidently appealing that they would seem to sell the whole project of enhancement on their own. Nonetheless, there are those who oppose them. For example, Leon Kass, the former chairman of the President's Council on Bioethics (PCBE) under President Bush, has asserted, "the finitude of human life is a blessing for every individual, whether he knows it or not." And Daniel Callahan, co-founder of the Hastings Center, has declared, "There is no known social good coming from the conquest of death." Callahan added, "The worst possible way to resolve [the question of life extension] is to leave it up to individual choice." When asked if the government has a right to tell its citizens that

they have to die, Johns Hopkins University political scientist Francis Fukuyama answered, "Absolutely."

The PCBE's 2003 report *Beyond Therapy* raised concerns that a society of people with "ageless bodies" might have significant downsides. Much longer lives would weaken our "commitment and engagement," the Council fretted: Today, we live with the knowledge that we will soon die, and thus "aspire to *spend* our lives in the ways we deem most important and vital"; but this "aspiration and urgency" might flag because we would ask, "Why not leave for tomorrow what you might do today, if there are endless tomorrows before you?" Further, our "attitudes toward death and mortality" might shift dramatically because "an individual committed to the technological struggle against aging and decline would be less prepared for . . . death, and the least willing to acknowledge its inevitability." Finally, age-retardation might undermine "the meaning of the life cycle" so that we would not be able "to make sense of what time, age, and change should mean to us." The Council does admit that as "powerful as some of these concerns are, however, from the point of view of the individual considered in isolation, the advantages of age-retardation may well be deemed to outweigh the dangers." Indeed.

But what about the consequences of longer human life spans to society as a whole? *Beyond Therapy* highlights three areas of societal concern. Significant age-retardation would disrupt the succession of "generations and families." This succession "could be obstructed by a glut of the able," the report suggests, since cohorts of healthy geezers would have no intention of shuffling off this mortal coil to be replaced by younger people. Longer lives could also slow down "innovation, change, and renewal" since "innovation . . . is . . . often the function of a new generation of leaders." Finally, even if we are not aging individually, we will need to worry about "the aging of society" that would then result. Societies composed of people whose bodies do not age significantly might "experience their own sort of senescence—a hardening of the vital social pathways."

Let us address each of these concerns in turn. First, we must deal with the notion of a nursing-home world. The point of anti-aging research is not to make people older longer, but to make them younger longer. So what about the concerns raised by the PCBE? Political scientist Diana Schaub, who also served on the Council, has made similar points. For instance, in an article in *Cato Unbound*, she asked, if people lived for a thousand years, "how would human relations be affected? How would monogamy fare? . . . Would there be enough psychic energy for ever-renewed love?"

As we age today, our declining psychic energy correlates pretty well with our declining physical energy. Who is to say, then, that with renewed physical energy we would not have more psychic energy as well? Actually, a pressing current question is: why has monogamy already begun to fall apart in developed societies? The rise in life expectancy over the last century may have had a bit to do with it; but surely the advent of truly effective contraception and the entrance of women fully into the paid workforce are far more significant factors. Marriage based on romantic love is a relatively modern notion, after all. As some commentators have noted, marriage before the twentieth century was not often based on romantic love, but could well be described as an alliance in which a man and woman stood together back to back fending off attacks on their family. As the modern world became less economically and socially threatening, marriage partners began to turn toward each other seeking more emotional support and often found it lacking.

Schaub next asks, "What would the tally of disappointments, betrayals, and losses be over a millennium?" Try turning that question around: what would the tally of satisfactions, affections, and triumphs be over a millennium? Modern material and intellectual abundance has already offered many of us a way out of the lives of quiet desperation suffered by our impoverished ancestors. The twenty-first century will provide an ever-increasing menu of life plans and choices. Surely, exhausting the coming possibilities for intellectual, artistic, and even spiritual growth will take more time than a typical life span today.

Schaub also queries, "Would we love other people more or less than at present? Would we be better partners, parents, friends, and neighbors?" She does not offer any evidence that shorter-lived people in past centuries and societies loved more deeply or were better neighbors, friends, and parents. But as Steven Pinker has argued in *The New Republic*, it is very suggestive that as life expectancies increased over the past century, levels of domestic and international violence also declined: "When pain and early death are everyday features of one's own life, one feels fewer compunctions about inflicting them on others. As technology and economic efficiency lengthen and improve our lives, we place a higher value on life in general." More simply, perhaps empathy has more of an opportunity to flourish when we are not constantly in danger of our lives.

"What would it be like to experience the continued vitality of the body in conjunction with the aging of the spirit?" continues Schaub. She initially suggests that longer, healthier lives might happily unite the vitality of youth with the wisdom of maturity. But she then worries that, instead, longer lives would combine the "characteristic vices of age with the strength of will to impose them on others." What is meant by the phrase "aging of the spirit," and just what are the "characteristic vices of age" that trouble her? Which of the traditional vices—gluttony, anger, greed, envy, pride, lust, indifference, melancholy—does she expect will increase among hale near-immortals? As Georges Minois notes in his *History of Old Age*, avarice is among the vices of old age most commonly depicted in classical literature. Roman playwright Terence wrote, "A vice common to all mankind is that of being too keen after money when we are old." In Gulliver's Travels, Jonathan Swift warned, "avarice is the necessary consequence of old age." Swift was describing the immortal, but not ageless, people known as the Struldbrugs. There is little reason to doubt that material comfort and security grow in importance as physical vitality ebbs and mental acuity withers. But perpetually vital oldsters would have no need for such security, because they could count on having the mental and physical powers necessary to pursue new goals and possibilities. No failures would be permanent; they would instead become learning experiences.

In addition to these concerns, Schaub suggests that "a nation of ageless individuals could well produce a sclerotic society, petrified in its ways and views." Daniel Callahan makes a similar argument in a debate with life-extension advocate Gregory Stock, in which he claims, "I doubt that if you give most people longer lives, even in better health, they are going to find new opportunities and make new initiatives." Stock goes so far as to help his interlocutor with the hoary example of brain-dead old professors blocking the progress of vibrant young researchers by holding onto tenure. But that seems more of a problem for medieval institutional holdovers like universities than for modern social institutions like corporations. Assuming it turns out that even with healthy long-lived oldsters there is still an advantage in turnover in top management, then institutions that adopt that model will thrive and those that do not will be out-competed. Besides, even today youngsters don't simply wait around for their elders to die. They go out and found their own companies and other institutions. Bill Gates didn't wait to take over IBM; he launched Microsoft at age 19. Scott Harrison started a nonprofit to supply clean drinking water to poor people in developing countries at age 31. Larry Page and Sergey Brin were both 25 when they founded Google. Nor did human genome sequencer Craig Venter loiter about until the top slot at the National Institutes of Health opened up. In politics, we already solve the problem of entrenched oldsters by term-limiting the presidency, as well as many state and local offices.

In fact, the available evidence cuts against concerns about "a hardening of the vital social pathways." Social and technological innovation has been most rapid in those societies with the highest average life expectancies. Yale economist William D. Nordhaus estimates that increases in longevity in the West account for 40 percent of the growth in gross national product for the period 1975–1995. Why? Not only do people work longer, but they work smarter—long lives allow for the accumulation of human capital. Economists Kevin M. Murphy and Robert H. Topel have analyzed how much human capital was gained by overcoming the vagaries of nature, to the tune of $1.2 million in value per person over the course of the twentieth century, during which time life expectancy at birth for a representative American increased by roughly thirty years. In 1900, they note, "nearly 18 percent of males born in the United States died before their first birthday: today, cumulative mortality does not reach 18 percent until age 62." The economic and social dynamism of societies that already enjoy longer average life expectancies (such as ours) also cuts against fears that "urgency" and "engagement" might flag with increased life spans.

Schaub further conjures the possibility of near-immortal dictators—Stalin and Hitler, alive forever. The implied argument that everyone must continue to die before age 100 to avoid the possibility of thousand-year tyrants is not persuasive. Must we really surrender to the tyranny of aging and death in order to prevent human despotism? Wouldn't a better strategy be to focus on preventing the emergence of tyrants, either of the short- or long-lived variety?

Like the PCBE, Schaub also worries about decreased fertility—that healthy oldsters would be less interested in reproducing. The facts seem to support this view: already, countries with the highest life expectancies have the lowest levels of fertility. In a recent study published in the journal *Human Nature*, University of Connecticut anthropologists Nicola L. Bulled and Richard Sosis reported that total fertility rates (the number of children a woman will have over the course of her lifetime) drop by half in reaching a life expectancy threshold of 60. For example, they found that women who live in countries where life expectancy is below 50 years bear an average of 5.5 children. When life expectancy is between 50 and 60, they bear an average of 4.8 children. The big drop occurs when they can expect to live between 60 and 70 years, in which case women have about 2.5 children on average.

But so what? A lack of interest in progeny could have the happy side effect of addressing the possibility that radically increased human life spans might lead to overpopulation. On the other hand, it might turn out that bearing and rearing children would eventually interest long-lived oldsters who would come to feel that they had the time and the resources to do it right. Since assisted reproductive techniques will extend procreation over many decades, perhaps centuries, people who can look forward to living and working for hundreds of years will be able to delay and stretch out the period in which they can choose to become parents.

And again, what about love? Do people today love their children, their spouses, and their friends less than shorter-lived people did a century ago? Were our forebears who lived thirty fewer years on average more committed to their children than are twenty-first-century American parents? Do people today love their children less than nineteenth-century Americans did because, as Michael Haines of Colgate University reports, instead of having a one-in-five chance of dying in their first year of life, most American kids now face a roughly one-in-200 chance?

Then there is the allegedly special case of "manufactured children." Along with many other opponents of enhancement technologies, Peter Lawler darkly speculates in *Stuck With Virtue* that enhanced children will be less loved than those produced the old-fashioned way: "A world in which children are manufactured and sex and procreation are totally disconnected would surely be one without much love, one where one manufactured being would have little natural or real connection to other manufactured beings."

But Lawler and his *confrères* need not speculate on what happens to parental love in such cases, for we have actual data. As physician Sally Satel notes in the journal Policy Review, "For all the deference that conservative bioethics pays to the implicit wisdom of the ages, it rarely mines the recent past for lessons. Instead of concentrating on the ancients, why not also study the history of in vitro fertilization, paid egg donation, and surrogate motherhood to learn about cultural resistance and adaptation to such practices?" Indeed. Fears about waning parental love and loosening generational ties were expressed by many bioethicists when in vitro fertilization began to be used in the 1970s and 1980s. Forty years later, the evidence is that their worries were overblown. A recent study in the journal *Human Reproduction* finds that IVF children and their parents are as well-adjusted as those born in the conventional way. There are no good reasons to doubt that this will not be the case for enhanced children in the future as well. As Harvard philosopher Frances Kamm argues in an essay in the 2009 collection *Human Enhancement*: not accepting whatever characteristics nature will bring but altering them ex-ante does not show lack of love. . . . This is because no conscious being yet exists who has to work hard to achieve new traits or suffer fears of rejection at the idea that they should be changed. Importantly, it is rational and acceptable to seek good characteristics in a new person, even though we know that when the child comes to be and we love him or her, many of these characteristics may come and go and we will continue to love the particular person.

In fact, so many infertile people have wanted to have children to love that more than 4 million have been brought into the world using various reproductive technologies since the birth of the first test-tube baby back in 1978.

What about the PCBE's fears that age-retardation technologies would undermine "the meaning of the life cycle" so that we would not be able "to make sense of what time, age, and change should mean to us"? Left-leaning environmental writer Bill McKibben has also expressed this concern. "Without mortality, no *time*," he writes in *Enough: Staying Human in an Engineered Age* (2003). "All moments would be equal; the deep, sad, human wisdom of Ecclesiastes would vanish. If for everything there is an endless season, then there is also no right season. . . . The future stretches before you, endlessly flat." But that deep, sad wisdom of Ecclesiastes is a powerful human response of existential dread to the oblivion that stretches endlessly before the dead: "For the living know that they shall die: but the dead know not any thing, neither have they any more a reward; for the memory of them is forgotten. Also their love, and their hatred, and their envy, is now perished; neither have they any more a portion for ever in any thing that is done under the sun" (Ecclesiastes 9:5-6). Is there not in this an argument against death? If wisdom is lost in death, does it not follow that longer lives could lead to greater wisdom? And this is not to mention love and all the other good things that are snuffed out in that oblivion.

On the other hand, if the endless future turns out to be as horrible as McKibben imagines it to be, then people can still simply choose to give up their empty, meaningless lives. So if people did opt to live yet longer, would that not mean they had found sufficient pleasure, joy, love, and even meaning to keep them going? McKibben is right: We do not know what immortality would be like. But should that happy choice become available, we can still decide whether or not we want to enjoy it. Besides, even if the ultimate goal of this technological quest is immortality, what will be immediately available is only longevity. The experience of longer lives will give the human race an opportunity to see how it works out. If immortality is a problem, it is a correctable one. Death always remains an option. Let us turn on its head the notorious argument by

Leon Kass that our initial repugnance to biotechnological advances should make us wary of them. Put the other way around, the near-universal human *yearning for* longer, healthier lives should serve as a preliminary warrant for pursuing age-retardation as a moral good.

Inviolable Characteristics?

What other features of human life might ethically be altered by enhancements? Almost any, according to the argument of George Washington University philosophy professor David DeGrazia. Writing in the *Journal of Medicine and Philosophy*, he systematically examines several core human traits—internal psychological style, personality, general intelligence and memory, sleep, normal aging, gender, and being a member of the species *Homo sapiens*—that might be considered so fundamental that they cannot be ethically altered, but concludes that "*characteristics likely to be targeted or otherwise affected by enhancement technologies are not plausibly regarded as [ethically] inviolable.*"

Regarding psychological style, there is no ethical reason to require that a particular person remain worried, suspicious, or downbeat if he wants to change. As DeGrazia points out, psychotherapy already aims at such self-transformation. And what about the impact of education? Many people who come back from college or the military seem unrecognizable to their old friends. If a pill will make a person more confident and upbeat, then there is no reason for him not to use it if he so wishes. Personality is perhaps the external manifestation of one's internal psychological style, and here, too, it's hard to think of any ethical basis for requiring someone to remain, for example, cynical or excessively shy.

But what about boosting intelligence and memory? Of course, from childhood on, we are constantly exhorted to improve ourselves by taking more classes, participating in more job training, and reading good books. Opponents of biotech enhancements might counter that all of these methods of improvement manipulate our environments and do not reach to the genetic cores of our beings. But DeGrazia points out that the wiring of our brains is the result of the interaction between our genes and our environment. For example, our intellectual capacities depend on proper nutrition as well as on our genetic endowments. One's genome is not fundamentally more important than environmental factors, he concludes; rather, "they are equally important, so we should bear in mind that no one objects to deliberately introducing environmental factors [such as schools or diet] that promote intelligence." It does not matter ethically whether one's intellectual capacities are boosted by schooling, a pill, or a set of genes.

As for sleep: all vertebrates sleep. Sleep, unlike cynicism, does seem biologically fundamental—but again, so what? Nature is not a reliable source for ethical norms. If a person could safely reduce his need for sleep and enjoy more waking life, that wouldn't be at all ethically problematic. Our ancestors who lacked artificial light probably got a lot more sleep than we moderns do, yet history doesn't suggest that they were morally superior to us.

Then, again, there is the argument about normal aging. As everyone knows, the only inevitabilities are death and taxes. Death, however, used to come far more frequently at younger ages, but global average life expectancy has doubled in the past century. DeGrazia asks whether "normal aging" is "an essential part of any recognizable human life," and falters here, admitting, "frankly, I do not know how to determine whether aging is an inviolable characteristic." The question, then, is whether someone who does try to "violate" this characteristic by biotechnological means is acting unethically. It is hard to see why the answer would be yes. Such would-be immortals are not forcing other people to live or die, nor are they infringing on the rights or dignities of others. DeGrazia finally recognizes that biotech methods aimed at slowing or delaying aging significantly are not morally different from technologies that would boost intelligence or reduce the need for sleep. He concludes, "even if aging is an inviolable core trait of human beings, living no more than some specified number of years is not." . . .

DeGrazia convincingly argues that whatever it is that makes us fundamentally us is not captured by the set of characteristics he considers. The inviolable core of our identities is the narrative of our lives—the sum of our experiences, enhanced or not. If we lose that core (say, through dementia), we truly do lose ourselves. But whoever we are persists and perhaps even flourishes if we choose to use biotech to brighten our moods, improve our personalities, boost our intelligence, sleep less, live longer and healthier lives, change our gender, or even change species. . . .

Enhancement Wars?

Those who favor restricting human enhancements often argue that human equality will fall victim to differential access to enhancement technologies, resulting in conflicts between the enhanced and the unenhanced. For example, at a 2006 meeting called by the American Association for the Advancement of Science, Richard Hayes, the executive director of the left-leaning Center for Genetics and Society, testified that "enhancement technologies would quickly be adopted by the most privileged, with the clear intent of widening the divisions that separate them and their progeny from the rest of the human species." Deploying such enhancement technologies would "deepen genetic and biological inequality among individuals," exacerbating "tendencies towards xenophobia, racism and warfare." Hayes concluded that allowing people to use genetic engineering for enhancement "could be a mistake of world-historical proportions." . . .

In the same vein, George J. Annas, Lori B. Andrews, and Rosario M. Isasi have laid out a rather apocalyptic scenario in the *American Journal of Law and Medicine*:

> The new species, or "posthuman," will likely view the old "normal" humans as inferior, even savages, and fit for slavery or slaughter. The normals, on the other hand, may see the posthumans as a threat and if they can, may engage in a preemptive strike by killing the posthumans before they themselves are killed or enslaved by them. It is ultimately this predictable potential for genocide that makes species-altering experiments potential weapons of mass destruction, and makes the unaccountable genetic engineer a potential bioterrorist.

Let's take their over-the-top scenario down a notch or two. The enhancements that are likely to be available in the relatively near term to people now living will be pharmacological—pills and shots to increase strength, lighten moods, and improve memory. Consequently, such interventions could be distributed to nearly everyone who wanted them. Later in this century, when safe genetic engineering becomes possible, it will likely be deployed gradually and will enable parents to give their children beneficial genes for improved health and intelligence that other children already get naturally. Thus, safe genetic engineering in the long run is more likely to ameliorate than to exacerbate human inequality. . . .

The Necessity of Moral Toleration

People should not be forced to use medicines and technologies that they find morally objectionable. Take the case of the Amish. Amish individuals live in an open society—ours—and can opt out of our society or theirs whenever they want. As followers of a reasonable comprehensive doctrine, they have a system for voluntarily deciding among themselves what new technologies they will embrace. (For instance, despite their generally anti-technology stance, Amish practicality has caused them to embrace modern medicine when it comes to treating genetic maladies that plague their community.) The situation of the Amish demonstrates that technological choices don't have to involve everyone in a given society.

One can imagine that, eventually, different treatment and enhancement regimens will be available to accommodate the different values and beliefs held by citizens. Christian Scientists would perhaps reject most of modern biotechnology outright; Jehovah's Witnesses might remain leery of treatments that they consider akin to using blood products or blood transfusions; Catholics might refuse to use regenerative treatments derived from destroyed human embryos; and still others may wish to take the fullest advantage of all biomedical enhancements and treatments. In this way, members of a pluralistic society respect the reasonable comprehensive doctrines of their fellow citizens, thus enabling social peace among moral strangers.

Daniel Callahan, in an essay in *Cato Unbound*, writes: "I really wish we would be told, when the great day arrives and we have dozens, maybe hundreds of years ahead of us, exactly how it would all work." Well, I wish I knew too, but the fact of the matter is that humanity advances by trial and error. Even the smartest people cannot figure out how

scientific and technological advances will play out over the next few decades, much less centuries. In 1960, the optical laser was reputedly described as an invention looking for a job. In 2011, ubiquitous lasers routinely cut metal, play CDs, reshape corneas, carry billions of Internet messages, remove tattoos, and guide bombs. As age-retardation and other enhancement technologies are likely to develop incrementally, humanity will have lots of opportunities for course corrections as we go along.

The very good news is that the history of the last two centuries has shown that technological advance has been far more beneficial than harmful for humanity. The development of age-retardation and other enhancement technologies will be further steps along that encouraging progressive path. We should all have the right to choose to use or not use new technologies to help us and our families flourish. Is humanity ready for enhancements like radically longer life spans? We're about as ready as we'll ever be. In other words: yes. . . .

RONALD BAILEY is the science correspondent for *Reason* magazine and Reason.com.

EXPLORING THE ISSUE

Is the Use of Medical Tools to Enhance Human Beings Morally Troubling?

Critical Thinking and Reflection

1. How does the President's Council connect the idea of human happiness to human finitude? Do you find the Council's reflections about this connection plausible?
2. The Council holds that imperfection is an important part of human nature, but Bailey holds that it is human nature to make oneself ever better. Do you agree with either—or with both?
3. What is the proper human attitude toward nature generally, and does our attitude toward nature generally have anything to do with our attitude toward human nature?

Is There Common Ground?

Discussions of new technologies easily lead into flights of fancy, to descriptions of futuristic scenarios entirely unlike anything we are familiar with today, and the debate about human enhancement is no different. Some proponents of human enhancement identify themselves as "transhumanists," and they call for developing and using enhancement technologies that allow us to transcend the human condition, to develop new abilities, to achieve near-immortality, perhaps even to shuck off this mortal coil altogether and become, as it were, software-based beings, who can be periodically upgraded and uploaded to new hardware. On the other side of the debate about enhancement are the many dystopias of literature and film, from Frankenstein and Brave New World to Gattaca and Eternal Sunshine of the Spotless Mind.

None of the genetic enhancements that arouse either fear or anticipation are possible with current technologies. Some say that they will never be possible, since the most desired and most unwelcome characteristics are not well understood and result from an uncontrollable interaction of genes and environment. Still, the future may bring still-undreamed-of possibilities, and even a limited power to enhance human bodies may raise some troubling questions.

Additional Resources

There are many Internet resources available to explore transhumanism. The philosopher Nick Bostrom sets out his view in the article "Human Genetic Enhancements: A Transhumanist Perspective," at www.nickbostrom.com/ethics/genetic.html. The article was originally published in the *Journal of Value Inquiry*, vol. 37, no. 4 (2003). Bostrom's "A History of Transhumanist Thought," originally published in *Journal of Evolution and Technology* (vol. 14, no. 1, April 2005), is available at www.nickbostrom.com/papers /history.pdf. A variety of resources and documents can also be found at the web site of humanity plus, an organization dedicated to promoting enhancement technologies; http://humanityplus.org/.

The issue of *The American Journal of Bioethics* (vol. 5, no. 3, 2005), from which Howard Trachtman's essay is drawn, also contains several other articles on enhancement. The lead article by Frances M. Kamm, "Is There a Problem with Enhancement?" analyzes Sandel's article from a philosophical perspective.

Michael Sandel develops a book-length but accessible argument against enhancement in *The Case Against Perfection: Ethics in the Age of Genetic Engineering* (Belknap Press, 2007).

Allen Buchanan is skeptical of arguments against enhancement in *Beyond Humanity?* (Oxford University Press, 2011).

See Jonathan Glover, *Choosing Children: Genes, Disability, and Design* (Oxford University Press, 2008) for a perspective incorporating the viewpoints of people with disabilities.

Julian Savulescu argues that we have a moral obligation to enhance human beings and that "to be human is to strive to be better" ("New Breeds of Humans: The Moral Obligation to Enhance," *Reproductive Medicine Online* [March 2005]).

See also Erik Parens, "Authenticity and Ambivalence: Toward Understanding the Enhancement Debate," *Hastings Center Report* (May–June 2005).

On the Web: "Genetic Enhancement" from the National Human Genome Research Institute, www.genome.gov/10004767.

Internet References . . .

Presidential Commission for the Study of Bioethical Issues

www.bioethics.gov/

The Hastings Center

http://www.thehastingscenter.org/

World Anti-Doping Agency

https://www.wada-ama.org/

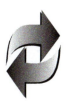

Selected, Edited, and with Issue Framing Material by:
Gregory E. Kaebnick, *The Hastings Center*

ISSUE

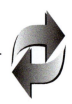

Should Research on Human Embryonic Stem Cells Be Halted, Given the Presence of Possible Alternatives?

YES: The Domestic Policy Council, Bush Administration, from "Advancing Stem Cell Science Without Destroying Human Life" (2007)

NO: Insoo Hyun, from "The Bioethics of Stem Cell Research and Therapy," *Journal of Clinical Investigation* (2010)

Learning Outcomes

After reading this issue, you will be able to:

- Discuss the prospects of regenerative cell-based medicine.
- Evaluate arguments for and against conducting research and developing medical treatments using human embryonic stem cells.

ISSUE SUMMARY

YES: The Bush Administration's Domestic Policy Council argues that advances with adult stem cells and alternative sources of pluripotent stem cells make it unnecessary to conduct stem cell research that destroys human embryos, and that if the research is unnecessary, then it should not be done.

NO: Insoo Hyun, past chair of the Ethics and Public Policy Committee of the International Society for Stem Cell Research, argues that the alternatives present their own ethical questions and do not eliminate the need to conduct research on embryonic stem cells.

Stem cells are cells that give rise to specialized cells found throughout the body. The stem cells found in early-stage embryos are capable of differentiating into all of the cells found in the body, and perhaps into the whole organism. Adult stem cells are cells that have partly but not fully differentiated and can give rise to specific types of tissue. Mesenchymal stem cells, for example, can produce new bone cells, muscle cells, fat cells, and other cells. Myosatellite cells produce muscle cells. They are found in a quiescent state in muscle fiber. Many other types of moderately differentiated stem cells are also found in the body.

What makes stem cells medically exciting is that they offer the prospect of harnessing the body's own mechanisms to repair injury. Perhaps, for example, stem cells

could be injected into the body to fix damaged heart tissue cell-by-cell, in situ, making heart transplantation and many kinds of open heart surgery unnecessary. Or perhaps neuronal stem cells could treat Parkinson's disease by generating new dopamine-producing cells in the brain. Parkinson's is caused by the loss of these cells. Perhaps injuries to the joints could be treated with appropriate stem cells.

Stem cell science is in a fairly early stage, although hopes for the science are so high—the hype surrounding possible stem cell treatments so strong—that waiting for the research to play out is difficult, and already commentators occasionally lament that the research has proved disappointing. Human embryonic stem cells were first isolated in 1998, and the years following have brought a steady stream of discoveries about how to obtain those cells, as well as about adult stem cells, other cells that have some of the properties of stem cells, and strategies for inducing differentiated cells to become stem cells.

The core ethical issue in research on human embryonic stem cells is about the status of the embryos from which they can be obtained, and perhaps about the status of the cells themselves, since if they are capable of producing a whole organism then they might be considered equivalent to embryos themselves. Removing cells from an embryo can destroy it, and even if it does not cause the embryo's destruction, discarding the embryo is usually considered necessary because of a risk that a child created from the embryo would have severe congenital abnormalities as a result of the cell extraction.

Recent discoveries concerning adult stem cells and other ways of producing entities similar to embryonic stem cells suggest that, if the alternative approaches lead to sufficiently good therapies, then research on embryonic stem cells could simply be set aside, and with it the difficult questions it raises. Exactly what lines of research will turn out to be productive, however, cannot be known in advance of actually carrying out the research. Research on embryonic stem cells has continued. During 2013 and 2014, three different teams of researchers in the United States reported that they had successfully created embryonic stem cell lines by means of somatic cell nuclear transfer.

It is easy to see the debate about embryonic stem cells as pitting an ethical question against science. Commentators who favor going forward with the research sometimes speak of advocating a "science-driven" agenda. But another way to understand the dilemma about whether to proceed with the research is to recognize that there are a variety of values on the other side of the question. First, there is whatever value might be found in the eventual medical treatments, some of which might address diseases that cause great human suffering. There is also the value of granting broad liberty to scientists to investigate whatever lines of research seem important to them. Scientific liberty might be justified partly by the benefits it can sometimes produce, or perhaps it is valued in its own right—perhaps this is what a "science-driven" agenda really means. The pursuit of human understanding of and mastery over the world might itself be considered good.

Mastery over the world is also connected with another ethical question about stem cell research. Stem cell treatments would be "regenerative" medicine: they would be treatments that allow the body to regenerate tissue, replacing damaged with new. In principle, regeneration could be put to use not only to treat injury but to "treat" the wear and tear of normal aging. It could lead to medical treatments that not only prevent premature death but also put off death somewhat indeterminately. Someday, maybe regenerative treatments will save a fifty-year-old patient from dying of heart disease, then save the same patient from dying of Parkinson's in his eighties, and then roll back the general wear and tear on body and brain as the patient advances into his nineties and beyond. Stem cell medicine is one potential route, therefore, to medical enhancement of human nature; it might allow for enhancement of life span. The prospect of these uses, in which medicine perhaps goes beyond ordinary therapeutic interventions into the body and begins to provide nontherapeutic treatments, raises broad questions about the desirability of enhancement.

Also, human embryonic stem cells are associated with somatic cell nuclear transfer, also known as cloning. Regenerative treatments would be most effective if the cells were genetically identical to the patient. One way of achieving that would be to create an embryo through cloning, by inserting the patient's genetical material into an egg and causing the egg to develop into an early-stage embryo. This would not be the only way of creating usable embryonic stem cells, but the mere prospect of producing the cells this way may have loaded some of the moral questions associated with cloning into the debate about embryonic stem cells.

Plainly, the debate about stem cells is rife with uncertainty. We do not yet know exactly what the benefits will be of embryonic stem cell research, and we do not know whether exactly the same benefits could be achieved with alternative kinds of stem cells. Perhaps embryonic stem cells are better than the existing alternatives, but maybe, especially if we push hard enough on developing alternatives, new approaches will emerge that are better than embryonic stem cells; we do not know. We also do not know quite what the eventual risks will be of these treatments. Current, still-experimental stem cell interventions appear to carry a risk of cancer; like cancer cells, stem cells do not senesce; they can continue to divide essentially forever. If the new cells generated by stem cell treatments cannot be forced to differentiate appropriately and turn into mature, nonproliferating cells, they might remain in the immature, proliferating mode, as if the treatment were a cell-generating machine that got stuck in the "on" position.

In the United States, the debate about whether to go forward with human embryonic stem cell research has ebbed and flowed with successive presidential administrations. In the 1990s, during the Clinton presidency, the National Bioethics Advisory Commission found that embryos have a special moral status but have less status than persons. It recommended that federal funding should not be provided for research that would create embryos expressly for the purposes of research, but should be available for research on embryos that had been created through in vitro fertilization for reproduction but had not been used for that purpose. The Bush administration adopted a more restrictive policy, which is described in the selections below. The Obama administration has adopted a more permissive policy, described below by Hyun.

The selections consider whether the availability of alternative sources of stem cells gives decisive reason to call a halt to human embryonic stem cell research. The Bush-era Domestic Policy Council argues clearly and strongly that it does. Insoo Hyun, a bioethicist who has taken a leading role in thinking about the ethical considerations that arise in moving stem cell research from basic science to trials with human subjects and eventually to clinical use, argues that ethical problems attend all forms of embryonic stem cell research—that they would not be avoided by avoiding stem cell research—and he calls for directing attention away from the question of whether to conduct research with embryonic stem cells and toward questions about how to move forward with any kind of stem cell research in a morally acceptable way.

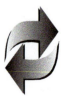

YES ⬅

**The Domestic Policy Council,
Bush Administration**

Advancing Stem Cell Science Without Destroying Human Life

1. Current Federal Law and Policy on Stem Cell Research

The Ethical Debate

Our nation has a long history of pioneering medical advances that improve life span and quality. We also have a deep tradition of protecting human life and dignity during scientific investigation.

Research on embryonic stem cells raises profound ethical quandaries. Most fundamentally, is an embryo a human life, and something therefore to be protected? This topic forces us to confront fundamental questions about the beginnings of life and the ends of science. These issues lie at a difficult moral intersection, where the desire to extend and improve life crosses the need to respect all human beings equally.

Embryos are humans in their earliest developmental stage. We do not have to think that human embryos are exactly the same in all ways as older humans to believe that they are entitled to respect and protection. Each of us originated as a single-celled embryo, and from that moment have developed along a continuous biological trajectory throughout our existence. To speak of "an embryo" is to designate a human being at a particular stage.

Our nation was founded on the principle that all of us are created equal, and endowed with a right to exist that is shared fully by all humans. There is no such thing as an excess life. And the fact that a human lacks some particular capacity, or even is going to die, does not justify experimenting on that individual, or exploiting him or her as a natural resource. That has long been the standard in medical ethics—as encoded in the Hippocratic Oath, as well as more modern codes like the Physician's Oath in the 1948 Declaration of Geneva, which states: "I will maintain the utmost respect for human life from the time of conception."

To think of other human beings (and especially the weakest and most vulnerable of us at the beginning or end of life) as potential spare parts for use by others is a profound threat to human dignity and our society's broader respect for its citizens. It is something the U.S. government has scrupulously avoided to this point.

The destruction of embryos for experimental purposes could also open the way to more general and profound manipulations and reengineerings of human life. Without an understanding that life begins at conception, and that an embryo is a nascent human being, there will always be arguments that other uses, takeovers, and makeovers of embryos are justified by potential scientific and medical benefits. Crossing this line would needlessly encourage a conflict between science and ethics that can only do damage to both, and to our nation as a whole.

This potentially dangerous opening would establish exactly the wrong tone as the era of biotechnology dawns. This emerging age has golden promise. But we must pursue its great hope in ways consistent with our principles. That will sometimes require saying no. To find the right paths for medical research, we must be willing to reject paths that are morally wrong.

A policy that defends the inviolability of human life does not preclude the hopeful possibilities of new findings and new therapies. It simply means we must harness the creative powers of our advancing knowledge only to humane and morally balanced means and ends. Amidst today's dizzying pace of technological innovation, it is worth taking care to make sure that our moral and ethical policies keep up. The biotechnology revolution will bring sound and wholesome human results over the long run only if it is sensibly governed.

The stem cell debate is only the first in what will be an onrushing train of biotechnology challenges in our future. We must establish a constructive precedent here for taking the moral dimensions of these issues seriously.

From Domestic Policy Council, Bush Administration, 2007.

We must make certain we don't force ourselves into a false choice between science and ethics—because we need both.

And there is good reason, and growing scientific evidence, to believe that we can have both.

2. Recent Developments in Non-Embryo-Destructive Stem Cell Research and Therapy

In January 2004, the President's Council on Bioethics published a report entitled "Monitoring Stem Cell Research." In the introduction, the report made the following comment:

Monitoring stem cell research can be a bit like watching Niagara Falls. Not only do scientific reports pour forth daily, as they do in many other areas of research, but a kind of mist rises up from the torrent of news flashes and editorials, making it difficult to separate knowledge from opinion and hope from hype. The underlying biology—whether viewed at the level of the gene, cell, tissue, organ, or organism—is dauntingly complex, as is all cell biology. At any of these levels, in this new and dynamic field, it is frequently difficult for even the most knowledgeable scientist to be truly certain of "what really causes what."[9]

The emotional appeal of stem cell research places further strains of exaggeration and misinterpretation on scientific claims. The cumulative effect is often a very foggy glass. In the two sections below—on developments in adult stem cell research, and on alternative sources of pluripotent stem cells—we offer a brief overview summarizing some significant recent research. Our aim is to build clearer public and legislative understanding that there are alternative scientific approaches which may be able to produce the functional equivalent of embryonic stem cells, but without harming embryos.

Advances in Adult Stem Cell Research

While research on adult stem cells began decades ago, important new discoveries have been made in just the past few years. Scientists have found adult stem cells in many more tissues than they once thought likely, including the brain, bone marrow, blood, blood vessels, skeletal muscle, skin, liver, and other body parts.[10] Given the right conditions, certain kinds of adult stem cells now seem to have the ability to differentiate into a number of different cell types. If this differentiation of adult stem cells can be controlled and sustained in the laboratory, these cells could become the basis of therapies for many serious common diseases and injuries. As examples of potential treatments,

an NIH list includes replacing the dopamine-producing cells in the brains of Parkinson's patients, developing insulin-producing cells for type I diabetes, and repairing damaged heart muscle with new cardiac muscle cells following a heart attack.[11]

Scientists have also reported that adult stem cells may, in some cases, exhibit the ability to form specialized cell types of other tissues, a characteristic known as transdifferentiation, or plasticity. Some experiments have even suggested that certain adult stem cell types may be pluripotent.[12] Over the past few years, several examples of adult stem cell plasticity have been reported.[13] Most evidence indicates that while embryonic stem cells are capable of becoming all of the cell types of the body, adult stem cells may be more limited. Adult stem cells can also be difficult to isolate, and methods of growing them in culture are still a work in progress.

Adult stem cells, however, do have some important scientific advantages as potential therapies. For one, since adult stem cells can be taken from the patient's own tissue, they are genetically matched, and would not be rejected by that patient's own immune system. This is one reason they have already been successful in treating many patients, while there are not yet any human clinical trials or successful therapies derived from embryonic stem cells.[14] As of April 2, 2007, there have been 1,373 publicly available clinical trials related to adult stem cells, including 671 that are currently recruiting patients.[15] Over the last couple of years, clinical trials using adult stem cells have produced encouraging improvements in patients suffering a range of diseases and disorders, including leukemia, lymphoma, diabetes, advanced kidney cancer, and several inherited blood disorders.[16]

It is important to note that in comparison to adult stem cell research, embryonic stem cell research is still in its infancy, and its potential should be understood in this context. Human embryonic stem cell studies are in early stages, and are currently being used to help understand the differentiation and functions of many human tissues, including neural, cardiac, vascular, pancreatic, hepatic, and bone. Embryonic stem cells have two properties that make them promising for research and cell therapy. First, they can be grown in tissue culture, and therefore provide an abundant, renewable source of cells. Second, they are pluripotent and can (theoretically) be directed to become virtually any cell type of the adult body.

But while much has been postulated about the ability of embryonic stem cells to generate transplantable cells for medical applications, many scientific hurdles remain before they could be used clinically in the United States.

One of the difficulties specific to embryonic stem cells is their propensity to form tumors. This dangerous property is the corollary to their extensive growth potential. Other issues needing solutions include questions of how to generate functional differentiated cells, and how to solve immune rejection issues. Although there is high potential for treatment of degenerative disease with human embryonic stem cells, development of practical applications lags behind adult stem cells, and indeed has been limited to animal studies thus far.[17]

Advances in Alternative Sources of Pluripotent Cells

Recent biological advances have raised encouraging possibilities for producing powerful stem cells without harming human embryos. What scientists value most about embryonic stem cells is their pluripotency and expandability—that they have the potential to be teased into many, and perhaps all, of the different cell types in the body. But scientists have begun to find that this potential may also exist in certain cells derived without embryos. New ways of producing pluripotent cells that don't require the destruction (or even endangerment) of human embryos are now being investigated.

In May 2005, the President's Council on Bioethics published Alternative Sources of Human Pluripotent Stem Cells, a White Paper which suggested four possible approaches for alternative sources: (1) by extracting viable cells from embryos already dead; (2) by non-harmful biopsy of living embryos; (3) by extracting cells from artificially created non-embryonic cellular systems or entities (engineered to lack the essential elements of an embryo); (4) by reprogramming (or de-differentiation) of adult cells back to pluripotency. Each of these methods carries its own scientific and ethical uncertainties, but one or more may ultimately offer a path toward an ethically responsible source of pluripotent stem cells.

In January 2007, landmark research from Wake Forest University has suggested yet another alternative: Amniotic fluid, investigators discovered, contains highly flexible stem cells shed by the fetus. These appear to have all the valuable qualities of embryonic stem cells, plus some advantages of their own—like greater ease and speed of culture, and no tendency to produce tumors. Meanwhile, they are comparatively easy to collect without harming human life.

We begin our review with the four methods identified by the Bioethics Council. Just in the short period since they were sketched out in May 2005, significant progress has been made on each of these techniques, as reported in a number of new, peer-reviewed research studies published in leading scientific journals. At this point, one of the most promising avenues appears to be somatic cell reprogramming, which uses chemical and genetic factors to reprogram an adult cell to function like an embryonic stem cell.

Each cell in an individual's body has the same DNA as every other cell. But in the course of developing into specialized adult tissues, different cells undergo different patterns of gene activation. Somatic cell reprogramming seeks to switch on or off the appropriate genes to transform an adult cell back into the equivalent of an embryonic stem cell. This might be accomplished by stimulating the adult cell with the right combination of chemicals and genes, or by exposing it to the cytoplasm of an existing line of stem cells. This method could, in theory, create stem cells in bulk while bypassing entirely the problem of creating and destroying embryos.

Two research teams that have demonstrated significant progress toward this sort of cell reprogramming are Kevin Eggan and Chad Cowan from the Harvard Stem Cell Institute, and Shinya Yamanaka and Kazutoshi Takahashi from the Department of Stem Cell Biology at Japan's Institute for Frontier Medical Science. In August of 2005 and August of 2006, respectively, each team published impressive results which seemed to produce pluripotent stem cells by reprogramming ordinary adult cells.

The project[18] conducted at the Harvard Stem Cell Institute fused a human adult cell with an embryonic stem cell. (These could come from one of the embryonic stem cell lines that President Bush has approved for use with federal funds.) That effectively turned back the clock on the adult cell such that it was reprogrammed to a pluripotent state. Eggan and Cowan believe that their research could lead to "an alternative route for creating genetically tailored human embryonic stem cells for use in the study and treatment of disease."[19]

Drs. Yamanaka and Takahashi published research based on mouse cells.[20] Their complex study produced stunningly simple results: They reprogrammed adult cells into a pluripotent state simply by bathing them in four genetic factors. "The finding is an important step in controlling pluripotency, which may eventually allow the creation of pluripotent cells directly from somatic cells of patients,"[21] comments Dr. Yamanaka. If successful, this could offer all the benefits of embryonic stem cells and more—these cells could be genetically matched to any prospective patient—without the ethical dilemmas of embryonic destruction.

Other promising avenues are likely to open in the future. The latest alternative, published[22] on January 7, 2007, in *Nature Biotechnology*, involves amniotic-fluid stem cells. Dr. Anthony Atala and a team from the Institute for Regenerative Medicine at Wake Forest University School of Medicine and the Harvard Medical School reported on a new category of readily available stem cells extractable from the waters cushioning babies in utero, as well as the placenta. While this very new research will need to be replicated and confirmed, Dr. Atala and colleagues have already managed to grow useful brain, bone, liver, muscle, and other replacement tissues using these stem cells.[23]

This discovery suggests that if all U.S. newborns had their amniotic stem cells frozen, they could be available for future tissue replacement without fear of immune rejection. Moreover, a bank of amniotic stem cells from the waters of 100,000 pregnancies could supply 99 percent of the U.S. population with genetically compatible stem cells for possible transplantation. More studies will be needed to confirm that amniotic stem cells can generate all other cell types, but so far every culture attempted has succeeded. It must also be determined that tests conducted in mice will translate to humans.

Meantime, that is but one of several promising glimmers in the latest research. What follows is a summary of the preliminary analysis from the Bioethics Council on the four alternative approaches they discussed in their May 2005 White Paper, supplemented by fresh additional findings from the most significant peer-reviewed studies published in each area since May 2005. It is important to note that while many of these alternative approaches show great promise, all of them are still being tested in animals and are thus in the early stages of development. The Bioethics Council has conducted only a preliminary analysis of the approaches, as used in animals. The Administration does not endorse any of these specific avenues of research in humans at this time. All new approaches will have to be carefully considered by scientists, regulators, and others as appropriate on a case-by-case basis, as further information and research becomes available. It may be that some of these research proposals could prove inconsistent with the Dickey-Wicker Amendment protections against creating, destroying, or harming human embryos, or they may fail some other test of ethical or scientific viability. But the cumulative weight of this emerging science is, as a *Washington Post* science journalist recently summarized, "adding credence to an emerging consensus among experts that the popular distinction between embryonic and 'adult' stem cells . . . is artificial."[24]

a. Pluripotent Stem Cells Derived from Dead Embryos

Under this proposal, viable cells would be derived from early in vitro fertilization (IVF) embryos (of roughly 4–8

cells) that have spontaneously died (as large percentages of early embryos do). Crucial to this approach is defining and verifying what represents organismic death in an early embryo, which represents an ongoing challenge for ethics and science. This would be a determining factor in whether this approach could ever be used in humans. Drs. Donald Landry and Howard Zucker of the Columbia University College of Physicians and Surgeons presented this proposal to the Council.

The preliminary evaluation from the Council in 2005 was that while it raised "some serious ethical questions," the Council found the proposal "to be ethically acceptable for basic investigation in humans" as long as "stringent guidelines like those proposed by Drs. Landry and Zucker were strictly observed." At the time, the proposal had not been tested, even in animals. The Council suggested that certain non-invasive studies to explore and define organismic death could be pursued immediately.

In June 2006, Dr. Landry published a peer-reviewed study[25] that proposed applying "the ethical framework currently used for obtaining essential organs from deceased persons for transplantation" to the harvesting of stem cells from dead human embryos. The study presented a history of the concept of embryonic death and compared the function of viable embryos with nonviable embryos. Dr. Landry's research suggested that an irreversible loss of function could be documented and thus used as criteria that would permit a determination of embryonic death. Using this criteria, Dr. Landry made the case that approximately a fifth of all embryos generated for in vitro fertilization could be re-classified as dead. This would enable thousands of new embryonic stem cell lines to be created without destroying a single living embryo.

In September 2006, scientists from the Centre for Stem Cell Biology and Developmental Genetics at the University of Newcastle in Britain published a peer-reviewed study[26] that described how embryos lacking essential function could be used as a source for the derivation of human embryonic stem cells.

Despite the promising work of Dr. Landry and the scientists at Newcastle, more work is required to address the concern that stem cells from dead embryos might not have the same pluripotent capacity as stem cells obtained from living embryos. In addition, more research is required on the concept and criteria that would permit determination of embryonic death in a way that is ethically unassailable for use in human embryos.

b. Pluripotent Stem Cells via Blastomere Extraction from Living Embryos

Under this proposal, pluripotent stem cells would be obtained through biopsy of an early human embryo. Crucial to this approach is finding a stage of early embryonic development at which one or a few cells can be removed without harming the embryo, with the removed cells being useable as a source of pluripotent stem cells.

The preliminary evaluation from the Council in 2005 was that this proposal was ethically unacceptable for humans. The Council stated that imposing "risks on living embryos destined to become children, for the sake of acquiring stem cells for research" could not be justified. While the approach could be attempted in animals, the Council did not anticipate that results from animal experimentation could alter its assessment that this method would be ethically unacceptable for humans.

In August 2006, Dr. Robert Lanza and a team at the firm Advanced Cell Technology (ACT) made widely reported[27] claims that human embryonic stem cells could be derived from blastomeres without requiring the blastomeres' destruction. However, once the details of the study's methodology were reported, it became clear that the techniques used by the researchers did in fact destroy every one of the human embryos used, a fact ACT did not make clear in its initial press releases. This work thus neither proved nor disproved that human embryonic stem cells could be derived from individual cells extracted from an embryo without harming it.

c. Pluripotent Stem Cells Derived from Biological Artifacts

Under this proposal, pluripotent stem cells lines would be derived from an engineered "biological artifact" that lacks the organismal character of a human embryo. Crucial to this approach is demonstrating both that the developing entity is truly not a human embryo and that the cells derived from it are normal human pluripotent cells. In addition, one must show that creating such biological artifacts does not itself introduce other ethical problems. One such proposal, Altered Nuclear Transfer (ANT), was presented to the Council by member Dr. William Hurlbut of Stanford University.

The preliminary evaluation from the Council in 2005 was that this proposal would need to be carefully tested in animals before human trials could be considered, but that there were no insuperable ethical objections that would preclude pursuing it. The possibility of any future endorsement for trying this approach in humans would depend upon a more thorough ethical analysis made possible in part by the animal experiments.

In October 2005, Rudolf Jaenisch and Alex Meissner, scientists at the Whitehead Institute for Biomedical Research at MIT, conducted a peer-reviewed study[28] of ANT in mice. "To assess the validity" of ANT, the researchers conducted a study that used a process of gene silencing and nuclear transfer to generate a laboratory-constructed biological entity that could not implant in a uterus and was morphologically unlike a natural embryo. This non-embryonic entity nonetheless yielded fully functional pluripotent stem cells with the same characteristics as those obtained from embryos. The study in mice noted that this approach could produce pluripotent stem cells genetically matched to patients (because the nucleus transferred could be from one of their own cells).

More recently, in November 2006 testimony[29] to the Bioethics Council, Dr. Hans Scholer, Director of Cell and Developmental Biology at the Max Planck Institute in Muenster, Germany, discussed further advances that support the scientific feasibility and moral acceptability of ANT. Dr. Scholer used ANT techniques to preemptively silence a key factor essential for defining an embryonic organism. Using this technique he was able to obtain pluripotent stem cell lines at an earlier stage and at a rate 50 percent higher than from direct destruction of IVF-created embryos.

d. Pluripotent Stem Cells via Somatic Cell De-differentiation

Under this proposal, adult cells would be reprogrammed to "de-differentiate" back into pluripotent stem cells. Crucial to this approach is discovering a way to reverse cell differentiation all the way to pluripotency, but without creating an organism capable of developing as nascent life.

The preliminary evaluation from the Council in 2005 was that this approach was ethically acceptable for use in humans, if and when it becomes scientifically practical, provided the line between pluripotent cell and living organism can be maintained. The Council noted that while this approach was scientifically and technically uncertain, there were encouraging results appearing in the scientific literature.[30]

In 2005, scientists from the Harvard Stem Cell Institute published a peer-reviewed study[31] in which a fusion of human embryonic stem cells with adult cells suggested that adult cells could be reprogrammed. If the remaining technical barriers are overcome—and some of them are significant—the approaches discussed in this study could circumvent societal concerns over cloning or the destruction of human embryos. A year later, Drs. Takahashi and Yamanaka of Japan published their peer-reviewed mouse study[32] examining 24 genes as candidates for conveying pluripotency.[33] They discovered that altering just four genetic factors proved sufficient to change adult cells into pluripotent stem cells. Scientists will now try to determine if human adult cells can be similarly reprogrammed using this method.

In November 2006, scientists from the School of Biosciences and Institute of Genetics, University of Nottingham, Loughborough, reviewed[34] the recent scientific advancements in reprogramming and concluded there is sufficient evidence demonstrating that adult cells can be reprogrammed and that cell-based approaches for therapeutics may be a realistic expectation in the future. The study reviewed nine reprogramming approaches that are commonly used today and commented on their respective advantages and limitations. While it is too early to tell which approaches may or may not work, the sheer number of methods makes clear that there may be several different ways to induce reprogramming of adult cells in the future.

Conclusion

As this report shows, there has been tremendous scientific progress of late in exploring methods of deriving pluripotent stem cells without destroying embryos. This groundbreaking alternative research has developed under President Bush's insistence on advancing stem cell research within clear ethical guidelines. With continued support for non-destructive alternatives, new developments will continue to unfold in this field in the years to come, holding the potential for innovative progress toward new medical cures, while at the same time upholding human dignity and the sanctity of innocent life.

Notes

1. President's Council of Bioethics, *White Paper: Alternative Sources of Human Pluripotent Stem Cells*, May 2005. (http://www.bioethics.gov/reports/white_paper/index.html)
2. Atala, A et al., Isolation of amniotic stem cell lines with potential for therapy, Nat Biotechnology. 2007 Jan 7; [Epub ahead of print].
3. Mary Carmichael, *New Stem-Cell Source Could Alter Debate*, Newsweek.com, January, 7, 2007.
4. Mary Carmichael, *New Stem-Cell Source Could Alter Debate*, Newsweek, Web Exclusive, January 8, 2007; Maggie Fox, Human stem cells found in amniotic fluid, Reuters, January 8, 2007; Breakthrough To Report In Stem Cell Research, The Discovery Of A New Source Of Stem Cells, NBC's Nightly News, January 7, 2007; Dan Harris, These Cells Can Be Gathered Without Hurting The Mother Or The Fetus, And Would Prove Much Less Controversial Than Research Done With Embryos,"ABC's World News Sunday, January 7, 2007.

5. Dan Harris, These Cells Can Be Gathered Without Hurting The Mother Or The Fetus, And Would Prove Much Less Controversial Than Research Done With Embryos, ABC's World News Sunday, January 7, 2007.
6. Rick Weiss, *Scientists See Potential in Amniotic Stem Cells*, Washington Post, January 8, 2007; Rick Weiss, Stem Cell Advances May Make Moral Issues Moot, Washington Post , June 6, 2005.
7. The full text of the Dickey Amendment can be found in each year's Labor/HHS Appropriations Bill. The law states that "None of the funds made available in this Act may be used for—(1) the creation of a human embryo or embryos for research purposes; or (2) research in which a human embryo or embryos are destroyed, discarded, or knowingly subjected to risk of injury or death greater than that allowed for research on fetuses in utero under 45 CFR 46.204 and 46.207, and subsection 498(b) of the Public Health Service Act (42 U.S.C. 289g(b)). (b) For purposes of this section, the term 'human embryo or embryos' includes any organism, not protected as a human subject under 45 CFR 46 as of the date of the enactment of the governing appropriations act, that is derived by fertilization, parthenogenesis, cloning, or any other means from one or more human gametes or human diploid cells."
8. Jason Woen-Smith and Jennifer McCormick, *An International gap in Human ES Cell Research*, Nature Biotechnology, 2006 Apr;24(4):391–2.
9. President's Council of Bioethics, *Monitoring Stem Cell Research*, January 2004, Pg. 15 (www.bioethics.gov/reports/stemcell/pcbe_final_version_monitoring_stem_cell_research.pdf)
10. http://stemcells.nih.gov/info/basics/basics4.asp
11. http://stemcells.nih.gov/info/basics/basics4.asp
12. http://stemcells.nih.gov/info/basics/basics4.asp
13. http://stemcells.nih.gov/info/basics/basics4.asp
14. http://www.clinicaltrials.gov/ct/search?term=stem+cell&submit=Search
15. http://www.clinicaltrials.gov/ct/search?term=stem+cell&submit=Search
16. http://stemcells.nih.gov/info/health.asp
17. http://stemcells.nih.gov/staticresources/info/scireport/PDFs/C.%20Chapter%201.pdf (Pg. 8)
18. Cowan, C.A., Eggan, Kevin, et al., Nuclear reprogramming of somatic cells after fusion with human embryonic stem cells, Science, 2005 Aug 26;309(5739):1369–73.
19. Cowan, C.A., Eggan, Kevin, et al., Nuclear reprogramming of somatic cells after fusion with

human embryonic stem cells, Science, 2005 Aug 26;309(5739):1369–73.

20. Takahashi, K. and S. Yamanaka, *Induction of Pluripotent Stem Cells from Mouse Embryonic and Adult Fibroblast Cultures by Defined Factors,* Cell, 2006 Aug 25;126(4):663–76. Epub 2006 Aug 10.

21. http://www.eurekalert.org/pub_releases/2006-08cp -wff080906.php

22. Atala, A et al., Isolation of amniotic stem cell lines with potential for therapy, Nat Biotechnology. 2007 Jan 7; [Epub ahead of print].

23. http://www.eurekalert.org/pub_releases/2007-01 /wfub-sdn010207.php

24. Rick Weiss, *Scientists See Potential in Amniotic Stem Cells,* Washington Post, January 8, 2007.

25. Don Landry et al., *Hypocellularity and Absence of Compaction as Criteria for Embryo Death,* Regenerative Medicine. Published in June 2006.

26. Zhang, X., P. Stojkovic, et al., *Derivation of human embryonic stem cells from developing and arrested embryos,* Stem Cells Express, 2006 Dec; 24(12):2669–76. Epub 2006 Sep 21.

27. Klimanskya, I., Y. Chung, S. Becker, et al., *Human embryonic stem cell lines derived from single blastomeres,* Nature, Advance online publication, August 23, 2006.

28. Meissner, A. and R. Jaenisch, *Generation of nuclear transfer-derived pluripotent ES cells from cloned Cdx2-deficient blastocyst,* Nature, 239: 212–5 (2006).

29. President's Council on Bioethics, Transcript from November 16, 2006. (http://www.bioethics.gov /transcripts/nov06/session1.html)

30. Guan K et al., *Pluripotency of spermatogonial stem cells from adult mouse testis,* Nature 440, 1199–1203, 27 April 2006; Kanatsu-Shinohara M & Shinohara T, *The germ of pluripotency,* Nature Biotechnology 24, 663–664, June 2006; Cyranoski D, *Stem cells from testes: could it work?* Nature 440, 586–587, March 30, 2006; Carlin R et al., *Reproductive Biology and Endocrinology* 4:8, doi:10.1186/1477-7827-4-8, 6 February 2006.

31. Cowan, C.A., Eggan, Kevin, et al., *Nuclear reprogramming of somatic cells after fusion with human embryonic stem cells,* Science, 309: 1369–1373, 2005 Aug 26;309(5739):1369–73.

32. Takahashi, K. and S. Yamanaka, *Induction of Pluripotent Stem Cells from Mouse Embryonic and Adult Fibroblast Cultures by Defined Factors,* Cell, 2006 Aug 25;126(4):663–76. Epub 2006 Aug 10.

33. http://www.eurekalert.org/pub_releases/2006-08cp -wff080906.php

34. Andrew Johnson et al., *Reprogramming Somatic Cells into Stem Cells,* Reproduction, November 2006.

THE DOMESTIC POLICY COUNCIL, part of the executive branch of the federal government, coordinates the domestic policy-making process in the White House.

Insoo Hyun   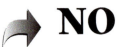 **NO**

The Bioethics of Stem Cell Research and Therapy

The main bioethical issues associated with human stem cells involve their derivation and use for research. Although there are interesting ethical issues surrounding the collection and use of somatic (adult) stem cells from aborted fetuses and umbilical cord blood, the most intense controversy to date has focused on the source of human embryonic stem (hES) cells. At present, new ethical issues are beginning to emerge around the derivation and use of other hES cell-like stem cells that have the capacity to differentiate into all types of human tissue. In the near future, as the stem cell field progresses closer to the clinic, additional ethical issues are likely to arise concerning the clinical translation of basic stem cell knowledge into reasonably safe, effective, and accessible patient therapies. This Review summarizes these and other bioethical issues of the past, present, and future of stem cell research.

The Past: Embryo Ethics

hES cells were first isolated and cultured in 1998 from embryos donated by couples no longer intending to use them for their own infertility treatment. From that point forward, hES cell research has been steeped in ethical controversy. Much of this controversy has been symptomatic of an ongoing public unease about the potential negative impacts of science on society. Since its inception, hES cell research has tapped into underlying dystopian fears about human cloning, the commodification of human biological material, the mixing of human and animal species, and the hubristic quest for regenerative immortality (1). While public concerns such as these about science and its implications are not in themselves new, hES cell research offered the opportunity for all of these inchoate worries to coalesce around a single, new scientific field.

Against this background dystopian view of science, a pro-life ideology rapidly emerged as a main driving force behind stem cell ethical debate and policy. It is safe to say that, despite a host of other concerns about where science

was leading us in the future, the ethical discourse over stem cell research for the past decade has been characterized predominantly by the debate over embryo destruction. In the United States, for example, a sizable minority has objected to the fact that five-day-old preimplantation human embryos are destroyed in the process of harvesting their stem cells (2). Those who oppose embryonic stem cell research believe for religious or other personal reasons that all preimplantation embryos have a moral standing equal to all living persons, regardless of whether they are located in a fertility clinic dish or in a woman's body. In this view, destroying preimplantation embryos during the course of research is akin to murder and therefore never acceptable, no matter how noble the aims of the research may be. On the other hand, supporters of embryonic stem cell research have pointed out that not all religious traditions grant full moral standing to early-stage human embryos. According to Jewish, Islamic, Hindu, and Buddhist traditions, as well as many Western Christian views, the moral standing of human beings arrives much later in the gestation process, with some religious views maintaining that the fetus must first reach a stage of viability outside the womb (1). Living in a pluralistic society such as ours, supporters argue, means having to tolerate differences in religious and personal convictions over such personally theoretical matters as when during the course of human biological development moral personhood first appears.

Other opponents of hES cell research have maintained that all preimplantation embryos have the potential to become full-fledged human beings and that it is always morally wrong to destroy this potential. In response to this potentiality argument, supporters of stem cell research have questioned whether it is true that all potential human life must be realized in every case. And even if the questionable assumption is granted that all potential life must be realized, it is simply false to claim that all early-stage embryos have the potential for complete human life, since many fertility clinic embryos are of poor quality and therefore not capable of producing a pregnancy, although they may yield stem cells. Potentiality is by no means guaranteed. For instance, developmental biologists have estimated that as many as 75%–80% of all embryos created through intercourse alone fail to implant and are naturally lost, many because of genetic abnormalities. In addition, some supporters of hES cell research have pointed out that no embryos eligible for hES cell research have an absolute, intrinsic potential for full human life, since the personal choice was made to not implant these excess fertility clinic embryos in a woman's uterus. And unless this essential step is taken, the potential of a preimplantation embryo for full human life exists only in the most abstract and hypothetical sense (3).

Despite this diversity of religious and philosophical views, it is well known that, over the past eight years, the Bush administration took an embryo protectionist position. It consequently put in place legislature, in the form of an executive order, that restricted federal funding for hES cell research to just those hES cell lines that were in existence on August 9, 2001. Scientists were quick to point out that the hES cell lines on the federal registry were insufficient to support the full range of stem cell research since they lacked genetic diversity, were beginning to accrue genetic mutations, and had been grown on mouse feeder layers (which introduce the threat of animal viruses). Scientists therefore believed that hES cell lines other than those on the federal registry would have to be studied. Other sources of hES cell research funding, notably state funding initiatives such as those in California, New York, and Massachusetts, began to emerge to help fill the void left by the Bush policy.

In order to bypass the ethical controversy surrounding embryo destruction and to help advance stem cell science, the President's Council on Bioethics recommended in 2005 that "alternative sources" of pluripotent stem cells be pursued that do not involve the destruction of or harm to human embryos (4). Four such approaches were identified as worthy of serious consideration: stem cells obtained from already-deceased embryos; stem cells obtained from living embryos by nondestructive biopsy; stem cells obtained from bioengineered embryo-like artifacts; and stem cells obtained from dedifferentiated somatic cells. Each of these approaches sought to generate the functional equivalent of hES cells derived from living blastocyst-stage embryos—pluripotent human stem cells that are genetically stable and long lived.

Two studies (5, 6) published soon thereafter in *Nature* pursued two of the President's Council's suggested alternative stem cell sources—live embryo biopsy and bioengineered embryo-like artifacts. In one of these studies (5), Robert Lanza and colleagues succeeded in deriving mouse embryonic stem cells from single blastomeres separated from eight-cell-stage mouse embryos. Since this technique sought to preserve the ability of the donor to implant and develop to birth, it theoretically could allow for the banking of autologous hES cell lines for children born from biopsied ex-corporeal embryos. In the other study (6), Alexander Meissner and Rudolf Jaenisch developed in mice a variation of somatic cell nuclear transfer (SCNT), a technique whereby the DNA of an unfertilized egg is replaced by the DNA of a somatic cell, by blocking the action of a gene (caudal type homeobox 2 [*Cdx2*]) that enables the developing embryo to implant into the uterus. By introducing this genetic defect in mouse somatic cells prior to nuclear transfer, they created cloned mouse embryos that generated pluripotent stem cells just before arresting developmentally.

This latter study was an early experimental realization of a concept called altered nuclear transfer (ANT), an idea that William Hurlbut had previously proposed to the President's Council (4). Research with mouse embryos carrying a mutation in the *Cdx2* gene showed that these embryos failed to form a trophectoderm and thus died at the blastocyst stage, but not before giving rise to mouse embryonic stem cells (7). Extrapolating from this mouse study, Hurlbut reasoned that a *CDX2* genetic mutation introduced into a human somatic cell prior to nuclear transfer might produce a blastocyst that could produce human pluripotent stem cells but lacked the biologic potential to develop into a complete human being (8). Hurlbut suggested that these possible ANT products should be viewed as complex tissue cultures (i.e., bioengineered embryo-like artifacts) rather than viable human embryos because of their limited cellular systems. Leon Kass, then chair of the President's Council and a vehement opponent of hES cell research, viewed Hurlbut's proposal as an ethically attractive alternative (4).

Unfortunately, there were many uncertainties surrounding ANT as a possible source for human pluripotent stem cells. In the conclusion of their study (6), Meissner and Jaenisch acknowledged that it was unknown whether *CDX2*-deficient human embryos would behave just like their mouse embryo counterparts, yielding pluripotent human stem cells just before arresting at the late blastocyst stage. And even if ANT were capable of generating human pluripotent stem cells, they noted that the additional manipulation of the donor cells to eliminate *CDX2* would complicate both the production and safety assessment of patient-specific stem cell lines. These scientific uncertainties called attention to the fact that ANT was motivated chiefly by political, not biomedical, utility. As George Daley and other stem cell scientists pointed out (9), determining whether ANT was feasible, efficient, and effective for research and clinical applications in humans would require significant amounts of time-consuming research and a considerable diversion of resources that could be used toward known methods for deriving hES cells.

There were also significant legal and practical challenges facing both ANT and live embryo biopsy. For instance, James Battey, then chair of the NIH Stem Cell Task Force, pointed out that these alternatives would require human embryo research at some point, either by involving live human embryo biopsy or the creation of human ANT embryos. As a result, the human equivalents of the two mouse studies just described would not be NIH-fundable under the Dickey-Wicker Amendment—a rider attached to a bill signed into law by President Clinton that prohibits federal funding for research that directly involves harm to embryos, including the derivation of new hES cell lines—which remains federal law today (10). Moreover, some observers at the time advanced the practical point that, with regard to live embryo biopsy for stem cell research, couples who want to support stem cell science may prefer to donate the embryos remaining after their course of in vitro fertilization (IVF) rather than consenting to "nondestructive" biopsies on those precious few embryos they plan to have implanted (11).

With the alternative strategies suggested by the President's Council for moving stem cell science forward stalled at the starting gate, and with limited federal funding for hES cell research, it was left to individual states and philanthropic organizations to rally behind stem cell progress for the duration of President Bush's tenure in office.

The Present: Beyond the Embryo

While the controversy over embryo destruction remains far from settled, two recent developments have helped reduce much of the heat behind the public debate over hES cell research. The first is the advent of human induced pluripotent stem (iPS) cells—dermal fibroblasts genetically engineered to behave like hES cells. The second is the far friendlier stance of the Obama administration toward hES cell research. At present, the main bioethical considerations tend to lean more toward *how* stem cell research ought to be conducted, rather than *whether* it ought to be conducted.

The iPS cell technique was pioneered in 2006 by Kazutoshi Takahashi and Shinya Yamanaka, in Kyoto,

Japan (12). Using retroviruses to insert four stem cell-associated genes (Octamer 3/4 [*Oct3/4*], SRY-box containing gene 2 [*Sox2*], *Myc*, and Kruppel-like factor 4 (gut) [*Klf4*]) into mouse dermal fibroblasts, they showed that these ordinary cells could be reprogrammed to behave like mouse embryonic stem cells and termed these reprogrammed cells *induced pluripotent stem cells* (iPS cells) (12). Later, Yamanaka's laboratory and an independent team of researchers were both able to show that human iPS cells could be created and that they behaved very much like hES cells (13, 14).

Predictably, opponents of hES cell research heralded the iPS cell revolution as marking the end of embryonic stem cells. However, most stem cell scientists do not believe that iPS cells (or indeed any other "alternative source" of stem cells) can obviate the need for ongoing hES cell research (15). For one thing, hES cells must be used as controls to assess the behavior and full scientific potential of iPS cells. In order to carry out these comparisons at the highest levels, scientists' knowledge of hES cells must continue to move forward. Furthermore, iPS cells may not be able to answer important questions about early human development; hES cells would have to be used in these studies instead. In addition, safety is a major issue for iPS cell research aimed at clinical applications, since the methods used in the process of generating iPS cells could cause harmful mutations later in the resulting cells. In light of these and other concerns, iPS cells may perhaps prove to be most useful in their potential to expand our overall understanding of stem cell biology, the net effect of which will provide the best hope of discovering new therapies for patients.

The relative ease with which new iPS cell lines can be derived means that new entrants into the stem cell field are now likely to emerge. However, while iPS cells do not require the use and manipulation of donated human embryos for their derivation, it would be a mistake to conclude that iPS cell researchers are free of their own set of ethical concerns. Unlike hES cells, iPS cells can be derived from the somatic tissues of a wide variety of living donors. Therefore, the prospect of having an iPS cell line derived from a living donor entails that familiar ethical issues come into play regarding, for example, the re-contacting and tracking of donors, what to do with incidental findings that may impact a living donor's health, and the extent and scope of donors' reach-through rights to the downstream research uses and commercial benefits of their genetically matched iPS cell lines (16, 17). The intersection of iPS cell research and these ongoing ethical questions in genetic and tissue research has yet to be fully explored (18). So, rather than avoiding ethical controversy altogether, researchers working with iPS cells will be effectively trading one set of ethical concerns for another.

Despite becoming connected to ongoing controversies in the biomedical sciences, the stem cell research field in the United States as a whole is likely to become much more active than it has ever been with the arrival of iPS cells and with expanded federal funding for hES cell research under the Obama administration. Perhaps the most important applications of stem cell research today lie in the areas of disease research and targeted drug development. By deriving and studying stem cells that are genetically matched to diseases such as Parkinson disease and juvenile diabetes, researchers hope to map out the developmental course of complex medical conditions to understand how, when, and why diseased specialized cells fail to function properly in patients. Such "disease-in-a-dish" model systems would provide researchers with a powerful new way to study genetic diseases not possible through animal research alone or by observing patients. Furthermore, researchers can aggressively test the safety and efficacy of new, targeted drug interventions on tissue cultures of living human cells derived from disease-specific hES cells and iPS cells, thus reducing the risks associated with research on human subjects.

To date, stem cell scientists have succeeded in producing a few disease-specific hES cell lines using unwanted fertility clinic embryos that had tested positive for serious genetic diseases, such as cystic fibrosis and fragile X syndrome (19, 20). However, no embryo genetic screening methods exist for complex diseases such as amyotrophic lateral sclerosis (also known as Lou Gehrig's disease) and Alzheimer disease; thus scientists have been using, with great success, the iPS cell technique to create disease-specific stem cell lines for these and many other diseases they wish to study (21).

However, questions still linger over whether iPS cells are absolutely identical to stem cells harvested from early-stage embryos. Another possible way of deriving disease-specific stem cells is through SCNT, otherwise known as "research cloning." Using this approach, researchers may be able to produce hES cells that are genetically matched to the patient and his or her particular disease. SCNT has worked recently in non-human primates to produce cell donor–matched primate stem cells, suggesting that human SCNT for disease research is, in principle, possible (22).

However, two realities appear to undermine the feasibility of SCNT as a widespread methodology in stem cell research. The first is that recently drafted NIH guidelines (23) only allow federal funds to be used for research on stem cell lines derived from excess IVF embryos, not embryos created specifically for research purposes (which includes those created via SCNT). The second is that, to date, women have been unwilling to donate their eggs for SCNT without any compensation for their efforts. Egg donor compensation for research is against the law in California and Massachusetts and is not recommended by the National Academy of Sciences' *Guidelines for human embryonic stem cell research* (24). The chief concern has been that compensation would undermine a woman's voluntary choice by creating an undue inducement to undergo hormonal induction to provide eggs for research (25). Bucking this trend, however, the State of New York has recently announced that it will allow donor compensation for providing eggs for research commensurate with what women typically earn for providing their eggs for infertility treatment.

Varying state and national stem cell research funding policies threaten to complicate attempts by researchers to collaborate across research locales, both nationally and internationally. For example, in the United States, the individual states have dramatically differing policies regarding the derivation and use of new hES cell lines, including divergent policies on the procurement of gametes, embryos, and other cells from donors (26). Some countries, such as Germany and Italy, permit hES cell research only with imported lines and prohibit the derivation of new hES cell lines from excess IVF embryos and SCNT. Other countries, such as Canada and Denmark, permit hES cell research and the derivation of new hES cell lines from donated IVF embryos but prohibit SCNT. Many other nations have no explicit laws governing hES cell research (27). Efforts to harmonize disparate standards have been undertaken by groups such as the Interstate Alliance on Stem Cell Research (IASCR) and the International Society for Stem Cell Research (ISSCR) and may blunt some of the potential sharp differences in research policies both in the United States and abroad.

Over the past few years, there has also evolved a new system of research oversight in stem cell research locales. Following professional guidelines issued by the National Academies and the ISSCR, all privately and publicly funded researchers working with pluripotent stem cells today are encouraged (and in most institutions required) to have their research proposals approved by a Stem Cell Research Oversight (SCRO) committee. SCRO committees include basic scientists, physicians, ethicists, legal experts, and community members and are designed to look at stem cell-specific issues relating to the proposed research. SCRO committees also work with local ethics review boards to ensure that the donors of embryos and other human materials are treated fairly and have given their voluntary, informed consent to stem cell research teams. Informed consent is especially important for somatic cell donors in iPS cell and SCNT studies, since the individuals represent a living genetic source of the resulting genetically matched stem cell lines. It is also crucial for patients donating somatic cells for disease-specific stem cell studies, as they might otherwise donate under a false expectation that they will benefit directly from eventual medical applications of their patient-specific stem cells.

The Future: Toward the Clinic

Perhaps the most exciting and vexing set of bioethical issues arising today involves the process of transitioning bench knowledge to the bedside. Emerging ethical issues of this clinical translational stage of stem cell research go far beyond the embryo debate, since they encompass all stem cell types, not just hES cells, and because they involve human subjects, who, despite what one may think about the moral status of embryos, are unequivocally moral persons with rights and interests that may be harmed.

Until very recently, there existed no professional guidance for researchers wanting to translate basic stem cell research into effective clinical applications for patients. This past year, the ISSCR released a set of international guidelines to fill this void (28). . . .

Currently, stem cell-based therapies are the clinical standard of care for a few conditions, such as hematopoietic stem cell transplants for leukemia and epithelial stem cell-based treatments for burns and corneal disorders. However, the public may not quite appreciate the many years of preclinical and clinical research that are required to establish new stem cell-based therapies. Unfortunately, there are some unscrupulous clinicians around the world exploiting the hopes of patients by purporting to provide effective stem cell therapies for large sums of money. These so-called "stem cell clinics" advance claims about their proffered stem cell therapies without credible rationale, transparency, oversight, or patient protections (29).

The administration of unproven stem cell interventions outside carefully regulated research protocols puts individual patients at risk and jeopardizes the legitimate progress of translational stem cell scientific research. Patients who travel for unproven stem cell therapies (this is colloquially referred to as "stem cell tourism") put themselves at risk of physical and financial harm. In condemning the fraudulent practices of these so-called stem cell clinics, however, we must be very careful not to squelch

simultaneously the possibility of responsible medical innovation outside the context of a clinical trial. Medically innovative patient care, in addition to regular clinical trials, can be a powerful route to the development of clinically established therapies, as has happened in other relevant areas of medicine, such as surgery (30). . . .

By moving forward from past debates about embryo status to issues concerning the uses of all varieties of stem cells, we can begin to focus the bioethical discourse on areas that have a much broader consensus base of shared values, such as patient and research subject protections and social justice. Looking to the future development of stem cell-based diagnostics and therapeutics, some commentators have wondered whether the potential for over-commercialization and restrictive patenting practices might delay or reduce the broad public benefit of stem cell research. As Patrick Taylor has forcefully argued (31), the promise of broad public benefit is one of the justifying conditions for conducting stem cell research; without the real and substantial possibility for public benefit, stem cell research loses one of its most important moral foundations. As stem cell-based clinical research advances, it is imperative that principles of social justice be taken proactively and seriously. This may include creatively reconfiguring existing models of intellectual property, licensing, product development, and public funding to encourage broad social access for stem cell-based therapies (18). Achieving social justice may also involve calling on regulatory and oversight agencies to include a greater involvement of community and patient advocates in the oversight of research. Dealing with the bioethics of *how* (rather than *whether*) to proceed with stem cell research demands that we wrestle with these and other tough questions. Much work lies ahead for the international community of researchers, clinicians, patient advocates, regulators, and bioethicists.

References

1. Cohen CB. *Renewing the Stuff of Life: Stem Cells, Ethics, and Public Policy*. New York, NY; Oxford University Press; 2007.
2. Nisbet MC. Public opinion about stem cell research and human cloning. *Public Opin Q.* 2004;68(1):131–154.
3. Hyun I, Jung KW. Human research cloning, embryos, and embryo-like artifacts. *Hastings Cent Rep.* 2006;36(5):34–41.
4. The President's Council on Bioethics. *White Paper: Alternative Sources of Human Pluripotent Stem Cells*. Washington, DC: National Academic Press; 2005.

5. Chung L, et al. Embryonic and extraembryonic stem cell lines derived from single mouse blastomeres. *Nature.* 2006;439(7073):216–219.

6. Meissner A, Jaenisch R. Generation of nuclear transfer-derived pluripotent ES cells from cloned Cdx2-deficient blastocysts. *Nature.* 2006; 439(7073):212–215.

7. Chawengsaksophak K, de Graff W, Rossant J, Deschamps J, Beck F. Cdx2 is essential for axial elongation in mouse development. *Proc Natl Acad Sci U S A.* 2004;101(20):7641–7645.

8. Hurlbut W. Altered nuclear transfer as a morally acceptable means for the procurement of human embryonic stem cells. *Perspect Biol Med.* 2005;48(2):211–228.

9. Melton DA, Daley GQ, Jennings CG. Altered nuclear transfer in stem cell research: a flawed proposal. *N Engl J Med.* 2004;351(27):2791–2792.

10. *Alternative Methods for Deriving Stem Cells: Hearing before a Subcommittee of the Committee on Appropriations, United States Senate* , 109th Cong, 1st Sess (2005) (testimony of James Battey, MD, PhD).

11. *Alternative Methods for Deriving Stem Cells: Hearing before a Subcommittee of the Committee on Appropriations, United States Senate*, 109th Cong, 1st Sess (2005) (testimony of George Q. Daley, MD, PhD).

12. Takahashi K, Yamanaka S. Induction of pluripotent stem cells from mouse embryonic and adult fibroblast cultures by defined factors. *Cell.* 2006;126(4):663–676.

13. Takahashi K, et al. Induction of pluripotent stem cells from adult human fibroblasts by defined factors. *Cell.* 2007;131(5):861–872.

14. Yu J, et al. Induced pluripotent stem cell lines derived from human somatic cells. *Science.* 2007;318(5858):1917–1920.

15. Hyun I, Hochedlinger K, Jaenisch R, Yamanaka S. New advances in iPS cell research do not obviate the need for human embryonic stem cells. *Cell Stem Cell.* 2007;1(1):367–368.

16. Aalto-Setälä K, Conklin B, Lo B. Obtaining consent for future research with induced pluripotent cells: opportunities and challenges. *PLoS Biol.* 2009;7(2):e42.

17. Wolf S, et al. Managing incidental findings in human subjects research: analysis and recommendations. *J Law Med Ethics.* 2008;36(2):219–248.

18. Hyun I. Stem cells from skin cells: the ethical questions. *Hastings Cent Rep.* 2008;38(1):20–22.

19. Pickering SJ, et al. Generation of a human embryonic stem cell line encoding the cystic fibrosis mutation deltaF508, using preimplantation genetic diagnosis. *Reprod Biomed Online.* 2005;10(3):390–397.

20. Eiges R, et al. Developmental study of fragile X syndrome using human embryonic stem cells derived from preimplantation genetically diagnosed embryos. *Cell Stem Cell.* 2007;1(5):568–577.

21. Park IH, et al. Disease-specific induced pluripotent stem cells. *Cell.* 2008;134(5):877–886.

22. Byrne JA, et al. Producing primate embryonic stem cells by somatic cell nuclear transfer. *Nature.* 2007;450(7169):497–502.

23. National Institutes of Health. Guidelines on Human Stem Cell Research. Stem Cell Information Web site. http://stemcells.nih.gov/policy/2009guidelines. Updated August 25, 2009.

24. National Research Council. *Guidelines for Human Embryonic Stem Cell Research.* Washington, DC: The National Academies Press; 2005.

25. Hyun I. Fair payment or undue inducement? *Nature.* 2006;442(7103):629–630.

26. Stayn S. A guide to state laws on hESC research and a call for interstate dialogue. *Medical Research Law & Policy Report.* 2006;5:718–725.

27. Caulfield T, et al. The stem cell research environment: a patchwork of patchworks. *Stem Cell Rev Rep.* 2009;5(2):82–88.

28. ISSCR Task Force for the Clinical Translation of Stem Cells. *Guidelines for the Clinical Translation of Stem Cells.* http://isscr.org/clinical_trans/pdfs/ISSCRGL ClinicalTrans.pdf. Published December 3, 2008.

29. Lau D, et al. Stem cell clinics online: the direct-to-consumer portrayal of stem cell medicine. *Cell Stem Cell.* 2008;3(6):591–594.

30. Cosgrove DM. Ethics in surgical innovation: vigorous discussion will foster future progress. *Cleve Clin J Med.* 2008;75(suppl 6):S6.

31. Taylor PL. Research sharing, ethics and public benefit. *Nat Biotechnol.* 2007;25(4):398–401.

INSOO HYUN is an associate professor in the Department of Bioethics and director of the Case Western Reserve University Stem Cell Ethics Center.

EXPLORING THE ISSUE

Should Research on Human Embryonic Stem Cells Be Halted, Given the Presence of Possible Alternatives?

Critical Thinking and Reflection

1. The Domestic Policy Council lays out a variety of alternatives, but it also leans heavily on the possibility that still more might be on the way. In choosing between pursuing human embryonic stem cells and developing alternative sources, should we look just to the science as it now stands, or should we bear in mind the possibility that still further advances in alternative source are possible in coming years?
2. Where would you draw the line with research on human embryonic stem cells? If most but not all of the medical benefits could be achieved with adult stem cells, would you conclude that the alternatives made embryonic cell research unnecessary? Do you think the research should go forward even if alternative approaches are likely to offer nearly all of the same benefits?
3. Does the choice depend just on the prospect of medical benefit, or are there other moral considerations as well? How important is scientific liberty and the pursuit of knowledge, wherever that search may lead?
4. Hyun suggests that the opposition to human embryonic stem cells is not just about the status of the cells, but also about "an ongoing public unease about the potential negative impacts of science on society." Do you agree? Would the Bush Domestic Policy Council have agreed?
5. Are you persuaded by Hyun's call to move past the debates about the status of the embryo and to turn from the question of whether to do human embryonic stem cell research to questions about how to do any kind of stem cell research?
6. To what degree is the choice to be settled by moral argument pro and con and to what degree should it be settled by public opinion? If public opinion is decisive, how should it be collected?
7. If public opinion is decisive, what is important about it: should the majority rule, or should the range of opinion be respected? What would respecting the range of opinion entail for stem cell research?

Is There Common Ground?

Hyun's argument that there are ethical problems associated with all forms of stem cell research is an attempt to find common ground: everyone doing stem cell research faces problems, he suggests, and instead of arguing about the status of the embryo, we should collectively turn our attention to the problems of moving from bench to bedside. Still, the core debate in embryonic stem cell research remains the vexed problem of the moral status of human embryos. This debate, the same problem that lies at the heart of the abortion debate, does not appear any closer to ending now than it did when embryonic stem cells were first cultured in 1998.

Additional Resources

M. Brown, "No Ethical Bypass of Moral Status in Stem Cell Research," *Bioethics* 27, no. 1 (2013): 12–19.

I. Hyun, W. Li, and S. Ding, "Scientific and Ethical Reasons Why iPS Cell Research Must Proceed with Human Embryonic Stem Cell Research," *Stanford Journal of Law, Science, and Policy* 3 (2010): 42–48.

I. Hyun, "Stem Cells from Skin Cells: The Ethical Questions," *Hastings Center Report* 38, no. 1 (2008): 20–22.

Internet References . . .

International Society for Stem Cell Research, Learn about Stem Cells

http://www.isscr.org/home/resources

National Academies of Science, Understanding Stem Cells

http://nas-sites.org/stemcells/

National Institutes of Health, Stem Cell Information

http://stemcells.nih.gov/info/basics/Pages /Default.aspx

Stanford Encyclopedia of Philosophy, Ethics of Stem Cell Research

http://plato.stanford.edu/entries/stem-cells/

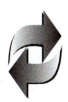

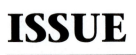

Selected, Edited, and with Issue Framing Material by:
Gregory E. Kaebnick, *The Hastings Center*

ISSUE

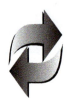

Should Governments Develop DNA Databanks to Support Law Enforcement?

YES: David H. Kaye and Michael E. Smith, from "DNA Identification Databases: Legality, Legitimacy, and the Case for Population-wide Coverage," *Wisconsin Law Review* (2003)

NO: Mark A. Rothstein and Meghan K. Talbott, from "The Expanding Use of DNA in Law Enforcement: What Role for Privacy" *Journal of Law, Medicine, and Ethics* (2006)

Learning Outcomes

After reading this issue, you will be able to:

- Discuss the pros and cons of creating a national DNA database for use in law enforcement.
- Discuss the value of privacy in a liberal society.
- Discuss the similarities and differences between genetic information and other information about people.

ISSUE SUMMARY

YES: David H. Kaye and Michael E. Smith, professors of law, argue that a population-wide DNA database could not only help solve crimes but would be fairer than more limited databases.

NO: Mark A. Rothstein, also a professor of law and a prominent advocate for maintaining genetic privacy, and his coauthor Meghan K. Talbott argue that DNA databases should be more limited in size and use.

Should information about our genotype be considered a private possession that is strictly off limits to the state except in special cases? This question raises further questions about the status of genetic information and about the value of privacy.

Genetic information has acquired a nearly exalted place in Western culture. People speak sometimes as if knowledge of genes is knowledge of the true nature and identity of a person or of an organism generally. To no small degree, this attitude has been encouraged, whether intentionally or not, by the way scientists speak of genes— as "the language of life," according to Francis Collins, director of the National Institutes of Health, and as the "software" that runs organisms, according to J. Craig Venter, president of the J. Craig Venter Institute. Genetic information can undoubtedly provide vital information

about a person. Genes sometimes play a significant role in the traits people possess and the diseases they acquire. Occasionally, genes solely determine an outcome. The vast majority of the time, however, genes interact with the environment in complex ways to determine outcomes.

The special status and mystery that surrounds genetic information has led to the coinage of a variety of new terms. "Genetic essentialism" is the idea that genes are the key to true nature and identity. "Genetic determinism" is the idea that genes always, not just occasionally, determine traits and diseases. "Genetic exceptionalism" is the idea that genetic information is inherently more important and morally special than other kinds of information about a person.

One could, however, reject the idea that there is anything morally unique about a person's genes while raising concerns about the possibility of "genetic discrimination"—that is, invidious action based on genetic information—and the importance of "genetic privacy"—that is, of the right to keep one's genetic information out of other people's hands in order to protect against genetic discrimination.

In health care, for example, genetic privacy has been considered important in order to ensure that health insurers cannot decide not to issue insurance policies to individuals who have genes associated with diseases that might require the insurer to pay for treatment. Because genes typically only raise the risk of disease rather than determining that a person will certainly get the disease, deciding whether to issue policies on the basis of a person's genetic profile has been considered unfair.

Genetic privacy has also been considered important in employment, on grounds that employers should not be making decisions about whom to hire and whom to fire, or what policies to enforce for its employers, on the basis of their genes. The most famous employment discrimination case in the United States involved the Burlington Northern Santa Fe Railway, which was accused of secretly conducting genetic tests on its employees in order to determine whether to deny claims filed by some employees for compensation for job-related carpal tunnel syndrome. The legal theory was that some employees might have a higher genetic risk of sustaining stress injuries, and that therefore their genes, rather than Burlington Northern Santa Fe Railway, might be the cause of their injury. The Equal Employment Opportunity Commission filed suit against the railroad in 2001. Later that year, the railroad agreed to stop its genetic testing program.

In 2008, then President Bush signed into law the Genetic Information Nondiscrimination Act in order to prohibit genetic discrimination in health insurance and employment. Senator Ted Kennedy hailed the bill as the "first major new civil rights bill of the new century."

The selections in this issue turn to another potential use of genetic information, namely, the use of genetic information to identify individuals who have been involved in a crime. As the selections detail, the federal government, states, and local authorities have developed DNA databanks (or databases) that store information about the genetic profiles of people who have been convicted of crimes as well as of DNA collected at crime scenes

or from unidentified human remains (that may be the result of crimes). Some state laws also permit police to collect samples from suspects. In 1994, the DNA Identification Act authorized creation of a system known as CODIS (the Combined DNA Index System) that links national, state, and local laboratories in order to facilitate searches for DNA. If DNA can be collected from a crime scene, law enforcement authorities can try to identify the perpetrator by searching for a match within CODIS. DNA can function in this regard exactly like fingerprints, and indeed this kind of use is known as DNA fingerprinting.

In recent years, DNA has also become an important tool for establishing innocence rather than guilt. If the DNA taken from a suspect is shown not to match the DNA believed to be from the perpetrator, a powerful piece of evidence is acquired that the suspect is innocent. Indeed, if the testing has been carried out well and the crime scene DNA is definitely from the perpetrator, then the suspect cannot be the perpetrator. Similar considerations apply to convicts, as well. A national endeavor known as the Innocence Project, founded in 1992 at Benjamin N. Cardozo School of Law with help from the genetic scientist Eric Lander, has become a leading force in using DNA to exonerate people who have been convicted of crimes and sentenced to prison, sometimes to death. Over 300 people have been exonerated in this fashion, including 18 who had been sentenced to death.

The selections here focus on the use of DNA fingerprinting to identify perpetrators and establish guilt, and they consider whether CODIS should be expanded to include all citizens, not just those who have been convicted and regardless of whether they want to have their genetic profile stored in a national database. The selections discuss the benefits to law enforcement of having such a system, and they also wrestle with the special value placed on privacy in U.S. law and culture. David Kaye and Michael Smith argue that the benefits would be considerable, the infringement on privacy minimal and appropriate, and the effects on racial justice superior to more limited databases. Mark Rothstein and Meghan Talbott argue that there are substantial risks, that the costs might not be justified by the benefits, and that to protect against authoritarianism, a firm line must be drawn to protect privacy.

YES ⟵

David H. Kaye and Michael E. Smith

DNA Identification Databases: Legality, Legitimacy, and the Case for Population-wide Coverage

Introduction

Over the past decade, law enforcement authorities have amassed huge collections of DNA samples and the identifying profiles derived from them. It is a development that has been greeted with ominous warnings[1] and extensive litigation. Large DNA databanks routinely help to identify the guilty and to exonerate the innocent, but as the databanks grow, so do fears about civil liberties. Slogans like "government-sponsored bioinvasion"[2] vie with reports of "cold hits" in cases of rape, murder, and theft that otherwise would go unsolved.

Perhaps, the most controversial policy issue in the creation of these databases is the question of coverage: whose DNA profiles should be stored in them? The possibilities extend from convicted violent sex offenders to all convicted felons, to everyone arrested, to the entire population. This article questions the rationales for drawing the line at all convicted offenders—which is fast becoming standard practice—or at all arrestees—which may be where we are headed. It suggests that such coverage results in sampling DNA disproportionately from racial minorities, which exacerbates racial tensions and undermines the preventative and investigative value of the databases. It argues that a population-wide database with strict privacy protections may supply the better answer to the coverage question, and to the privacy concerns raised by any government program to take and analyze individuals' DNA. . . .

I. Which Offenses Should Trigger Inclusion?

DNA profiles of convicted sex offenders are obvious candidates for inclusion in DNA databases. Indeed, most states began by authorizing databases limited to sex-offender profiles as part of their general effort to better protect women and children from sexual assault. Databases of convicted sex-offender records were not especially controversial given the general abhorrence of sex offenders,

with the popular image of rapists as sexual predators who strike again and again, and the ubiquity of potentially incriminating biological evidence in most rape cases.[3] However, it soon became difficult to confine to this group the statutory authority to take DNA samples. First, the data never supported the view that recidivism was dramatically higher for sex offenders in general than for other categories of offenders. To the contrary, recidivism rates were and still are similar or even higher for other offender groupings. Second, potentially incriminating DNA evidence is hardly peculiar to sex crimes. Traces of blood, saliva, hair, and other DNA-bearing material are left at the scene of many types of crimes. Finally, although sexual assault is among the most detested of crimes, the public does not have high regard for murderers, burglars, and petty thieves either.

The result is pressure to extend the coverage of the databases to all violent felons; and then to all felons and many misdemeanants. Defining the point at which the collection of DNA profiles should stop requires a theory for including profiles in the database in the first place. Two such theories can be found in case law on the constitutionality of offender databases. One we call the forfeiture theory. It holds that upon criminal conviction, individuals forfeit any right they might otherwise enjoy to be free from having their DNA typed and the resulting profile placed on file. But this notion of "forfeiture" is a conclusion in search of an argument. To be sure, a conviction at a trial where the defendant is afforded due process of law may trigger the most serious of punishments—from deprivation of life, to loss of liberty, to loss of property. The Constitution explicitly countenances these punishments.[4] But there are limits to what other deprivations of liberty or property are constitutionally permissible. As the Supreme Court explained in *Hudson v. Palmer*, "prisoners [must] be accorded those rights not fundamentally inconsistent with imprisonment itself or incompatible with the objectives of incarceration." . . .

Kaye, D.H.; Smith, Michael E. "DNA Identification Databases: Legality, Legitimacy, and the Case for Population-Wide Coverage," *Wisconsin Law Review*, 2003. Copyright © 2003 by The Board of Regents of the University of Wisconsin System. Reprinted by permission of the Wisconsin Law Review.

How, then, could the bare fact of conviction work a forfeiture of the right to be free from unreasonable searches and seizures? . . .

Thus, a second justification for convicted-offender DNA databases is woven through the court opinions that find them permissible in the face of Fourth Amendment challenges. This is a predictivist theory: if persons convicted at least once are more likely to commit future crimes for which DNA evidence might be found than are those with no such criminal histories, then including DNA profiles of samples taken when these offenders are convicted would be expected to help—perhaps substantially—to deter and solve crimes.

The logic of the predictivist theory for limiting DNA databases to some subset of convicted offenders can be stated neatly, but it is difficult to apply. The justification turns on (1) the likelihood of future crimes, by category of current conviction, as well as (2) the likelihood that the scenes of future crimes committed by offenders of any given type will present investigators with incriminating DNA evidence. Currently available data on these probabilities are sketchy, and it proves difficult to limit the sweep of the predictivist argument to convicted offenders. A later arrest, upon probable cause to believe the arrestee has committed a crime, is more likely among those who have been arrested at some point in the past, and prior arrest generally has some predictive value, whether or not a conviction follows.

But there are many predictors of who will engage in future crimes—some of them more powerful than prior arrest or prior conviction. Dysfunctional family or neighborhood, disengagement from the labor market or school, past antisocial acts, age, gender, and a host of other personal and environmental factors are, particularly in combination, statistical predictors of future criminal conduct. Thus, the predictivist theory offers no satisfactory basis for separating people who have been convicted of crimes, or who have been arrested, from other people who carry comparable or even greater probabilities of leaving incriminating traces of DNA behind in the commission of future crimes. . . .

II. The Prospect of Universality

A. One Possible Path to a Population-wide Database
Creating a national identification database all at once would be prohibitively expensive today, even if we had the laboratory capacity to do it. But DNA typing technology is advancing at a pace reminiscent of Moore's Law for microprocessor capacity that has made the "personal computer" a fixture on every desk. Soon it will be feasi-

ble to create a DNA identification record for everyone, at least prospectively. For example, it would be easy to extract identification profiles as an adjunct to public health programs that for many years have screened blood samples from almost all newborns, to identify infants with treatable genetic diseases. The identification profiles could be transmitted to a single, secure, national database. To the extent that additional sampling would be necessary—to include immigrants or citizens born abroad, for example—these samples could be destroyed after they are typed. In fact, an instrument could be built that would extract an identifying profile and destroy the sample at the same time. Proper procedures for sampling the DNA, extracting the identifying profile, and immediately destroying the sample would protect everyone's genetic privacy.

The loci used for those identification profiles would be limited to sequences that have no relationship to health or other physical or mental traits and propensities. As discussed above, each profile would be a set of digits devoid of any special meaning, comparable to a social security or passport number. Access to the database would be limited to law enforcement personnel investigating specific crimes in which DNA trace evidence already has been found. Law enforcement agencies would not need—and should not be permitted—to handle, much less retain, the samples.

A system of this sort would resemble, to the greatest extent possible, a digitalized collection of identifying features very much like ordinary fingerprints. However, it would be far more useful in deterring potential offenses, in generating investigative leads, and in exonerating the innocent. There would be no need to resort to inefficient "DNA dragnets" of entire neighborhoods, as have been conducted in California, Florida, Louisiana, Michigan, New York, and elsewhere or to infer probable racial or ethnic status, as some observers fear. Not only would a comprehensive database be valuable for public safety purposes but it also could also be useful in identifying bodily remains in mass disasters or other tragedies and in returning missing persons to their families.

Despite the understandable concerns over the privacy implications of all DNA databases, we believe that a properly designed and administered national database might well be the best solution to the coverage question. It would entail but a limited intrusion on individual freedom and privacy while advancing both public safety and racial evenhandedness in the criminal justice system and serving as a firewall against far greater intrusions on privacy by law enforcement authorities pawing through medical and other records looking for a "match" to DNA found at the scenes of notorious crimes. We began with no enthusiasm for the idea of an inclusive national database, but the more we considered the drawbacks of the likely alternatives and the plausibility of procedures for database creation that would limit the government's access to sensitive genetic information, the more we found it to be a viable policy choice.[5] To explain our conclusion, we survey the arguments that have been made against a national database, then consider in more detail the advantages it offers over the current system.

B. Opposition to a Population-wide Database

1. Public acceptance

Opponents of broad DNA databases sometimes suggest that it is pointless to consider a population-wide database because the public opposes it. They note that in the 1940s, Congress did not adopt proposed legislation providing for universal fingerprinting and identity cards. Since the American public today regards DNA with a mixture of suspicion, horror, and awe, it is said a population-wide DNA database is too far from popular acceptance to be worth considering. However, a database constructed in the manner we have described offers pronounced advantages over the present system of incremental expansions of law enforcement databases. . . .

2. Constitutionality

A second argument against pursuit of a population-wide database is that even if it were popular, it would be unconstitutional. The most powerful constitutional challenge flows from the Fourth Amendment requirement that government "searches" be "reasonable," which the Supreme Court has interpreted to require a judicial warrant based on probable cause, unless the search lies within one of the "specifically established and well-delineated exceptions" to the warrant requirement.[6] Yet, in some respects, a population-wide database such as we have described would be easier to defend under Supreme Court precedent than conventional convicted-offender databases.

For both practices, a threshold question is whether the acquisition of DNA would even amount to a "search" within the meaning of the Fourth Amendment. There is no doubt that blood samples taken from infants by governmental edict would "constitute searches of 'persons', and depend antecedently upon seizures of 'persons.'"[7] But what if the DNA were acquired by applying a sticky pad to the infant's skin to acquire some exfoliating, epidermal cells without even a scratch? Would the reduced level of bodily invasion and the fact that these cells are constantly exposed to the public and being shed from the surface of the body lead a court to hold that no search is involved? . . .

3. Nation of suspects

A third objection is that a universal database would constitute a "step toward an Orwellian society"[8] that will make "us a 'nation of suspects', and radically alter the relationship between the citizen and government."[9] "Storing information on otherwise unsuspected individuals," it is said, "expresses an ethos of suspicion."[10] As rhetoric, this is powerful stuff, but its substance is fluffier. Privacy is an important value, but the privacy threat from digital records of DNA types that reveal nothing about a person's nature or status is not self-evident. Certainly, it bears no resemblance to George Orwell's dystopia in which the state monitored every conversation and action, and responded to mere thoughts of disloyalty with profound "reeducation." Establishing a system that has the ability to link individuals to crime scenes to the greatest possible extent without probing their minds or invading their homes or possessions does not make everyone a "suspect" in any meaningful or problematic sense. Indeed, a population-wide database should quickly limit the number of suspects—typically to a single person—in many crimes. By promptly eliminating everyone else as a viable suspect, it would reduce the burden on many individuals who would have been primary suspects.

4. Loss of anonymity

"Privacy" is a protean term that encompasses a heterogeneous set of interests. It is not privacy in general that is put at risk when the state has an ability to match found DNA with a profile retained in an identification database. It is not even autonomy. Rather, DNA databases threaten three forms of anonymity.

a. Temporal anonymity. There is a largely unspoken assumption, deeply rooted in American history and culture, that if we are moved to do so, it is possible for us to leave the past behind and to reinvent ourselves in another place. But this seems a romantic, unrealistic prospect today. The lives we lead leave a trail in medical records, in credit card records, in school records, in employment files—in any records that link to our social security numbers, drivers' license numbers, and the like. We can be found if the state, or anyone with means, really cares to find us. No doubt, biometric identifiers, from fingerprints to facial recognition systems, iris scans to DNA profiles, make it harder to transform one's identity. But anonymity in the sense of recreating one's identity—of riding into town, as it were, to start a new life without carrying the weight of the past—is a quixotism.[11]

b. Conduct anonymity. There is a second sense of anonymity that is often worth protecting—the anonymity of those engaged in certain types of desirable conduct. The ability to act anonymously may be personally or socially valuable in contexts such as making charitable donations, expressing unpopular opinions, or informing authorities of wrongdoing or dangerous situations. . . . But a population-wide DNA identification database maintained for law enforcement purposes would not interfere with those protections.

In other situations, conduct anonymity is an enemy of public safety. It is a rare offender who expects to be identified and apprehended when he or she commits a crime. If witnesses to offenses do not recognize the offenders, the offenders will likely elude apprehension. Knowing this, a person bent on crime who is anonymous in a place where the opportunity presents itself is undeterred. Conversely, there is no special trick to apprehending a burglar, a robber, or a hit-and-run driver (or deterring an otherwise motivated offender) whose name can be given to police by a passerby. To the extent that a comprehensive DNA identification database merely reduces anonymity for criminal conduct, it infringes no interest worthy of protection.

c. Spatial anonymity. There is a particular form of conduct anonymity that is valued by nearly everyone in our culture, and is likely to remain so. It is spatial anonymity—the ability to keep one's movements and location confidential. Spatial anonymity is not threatened by all biometric identification systems, but it is threatened by systems that can link individuals to particular locations. The shadowy figure disappearing into the London fog and the nondescript face lost among many in the crowd are anonymous. The ability to be at a particular place and time without revealing one's identity is vital to criminal enterprises; but ordinary individuals want to be free to visit a friend, enter a store, or take a drive into the country without being tracked by the government. Pervasive government surveillance that tracks one's locations at all times of the day and night would strip us of the "breathing room" in which our liberty takes shape—we require a private sphere of action in which to be ourselves, free from observation.

Nevertheless, a population-wide DNA identification database would not destroy all spatial anonymity—the confidentiality of one's movements could be preserved—since it is not feasible to reconstruct a person's travels by looking at DNA molecules. A comprehensive DNA identification database would not present the potential "abuse" of "24-hour surveillance of any citizen" that gave the Supreme Court momentary pause in the course of holding that the use of a radio beeper to track a car to the defend-

ant's house did not even rise to the level of a search within the meaning of the Fourth Amendment.[12] Still, the fact remains that it is technologically possible for a determined search for remnants of hair, saliva, or other DNA-bearing material to uncover traces of many peoples' DNA at crime scenes or other locations. For instance, there will be a loss of anonymity if and when police are able to deduce, from these biological traces, all the people who frequented the bedroom of the deceased. This power to reconstruct past events, however partially, will be invaluable to criminal investigators, but it must be recognized that it diminishes our spatial anonymity—the privacy of our movements—by reducing our ability to enter bedrooms or other embarrassing locations without risk of our presence there later being discovered. . . .

C. Advantages of a Population-wide Database

The current approach to creating law enforcement databases focuses exclusively on individuals' contacts with the criminal justice system. When a criminal conviction, an arrest, or a stop by traffic or foot patrol is the trigger for sampling a person's DNA, profiling it, and retaining that profile in a database for use in future criminal investigations, the database will be racially skewed and will fall far short of the full potential of this technology to exonerate innocent suspects, to identify the guilty, to protect victims of crime, and to assist in the identification of missing persons.

1. Efficacy

Those who insist that it is sufficient to record the DNA profiles of felons are, perhaps without realizing it, proposing to sacrifice most of the preventative and investigative force of the technology. As explained in Part I, the justification put forward for making felony conviction the threshold for amassing DNA profiles is that the likelihood of further felony offenses is especially elevated among those once before convicted of a felony. However, 62 percent of those arrested and prosecuted for a felony have no prior felony conviction.[13] Furthermore, among those arrested and prosecuted for serious felonies, those arrested and prosecuted for rape are the least likely to have a prior felony conviction of any kind—only about 30 percent have such a prior record, as compared to almost 50 percent for burglary.[14] A DNA database cannot deter or lead to apprehension before a profile is included in the database. Therefore, a convicted-felon database is of no help in deterring or investigating felonies committed by persons not previously convicted of a felony—and they are a majority of those now arrested on felony charges. . . .

Racial justice and the legitimacy of law

There can be no doubt that any database of DNA profiles will be dramatically skewed by race if the sampling and typing of DNA becomes a routine consequence of criminal conviction.[15] Without seismic changes in Americans' behavior or in the criminal justice system, nearly 30 percent of black males, but less than 5 percent of white males will be imprisoned on a felony conviction at some point in their lives.[16] Arrest, prosecution, and conviction are so pervasive in black communities that, on any given day, a black American is five times more likely to be in jail than is a white.[17] An adult black male is four times more likely to be under some form of correctional supervision,[18] six-and-a-half times more likely to be incarcerated somewhere,[19] and eight times more likely to be in prison[20] than his white counterpart.

Racial skewing of the DNA databases will be reduced somewhat if the legal authority to sample and type offenders' DNA continues to expand and comes to include the multitudes convicted of lesser, but more numerous, felonies and misdemeanors. Racial imbalance in the databases would be further reduced if, as leading law enforcement leaders have urged,[21] arrest rather than conviction becomes the occasion for sampling DNA and including profiles in the database. But the decrease in racial disparity would come not come from a racial parity in arrest rates—the annual arrest rate among blacks is more than two and a half times the white rate,[22] and a black man's lifetime chances of being arrested are more than double a white man's.[23] Rather, expanding DNA databases to include arrestees would diminish the racial disparity by bringing many more whites into the databases—about half of all males experience at least one misdemeanor or felony arrest in their lifetimes.[24]

Thus, although a black man's relative chance of being included in the database would be reduced from at least four times that of a white man's in a convicted offender database to roughly twice a white man's in an arrestee database, about 90 percent of urban black males would be included if DNA were routinely sampled on arrest. Such an "arrest-only" database would have the look and feel of a universal DNA database for black males, whose already jaundiced view of law enforcement's legitimacy[25] is itself a threat to public safety.[26] White men would not likely be pleased either. Some would surely be offended by the racial imbalance in their favor—particularly one so redolent of past genetic discrimination—and many white males would be distressed to learn that, absent dramatic change in their behavior or in police practices, at least half of them would have their DNA profiles entered into the database, following arrest for a felony or misdemeanor. If legislation were to authorize DNA sampling for traffic offenses as well, then a majority of the entire population might eventually find its way into the database.

If arresting officers were given discretion not to sample DNA, this fraction might well be reduced, but there is little comfort in the prospect of individual officers on the highways sampling DNA from those who strike them as likely perpetrators of other crimes, while sending the rest on their way. Under those conditions, racial conflict in police encounters with civilians and racial disparities in the database would be likely to grow considerably worse. Neither are state legislatures likely to make parsimonious decisions about which arrests permit or require DNA sampling. As is happening with convictions, if arrest becomes the threshold for inclusion in the databases, then the pressure for comprehensive coverage is likely to be nearly irresistible.

The likely reach of an arrest-based database should give pause to anyone hoping to limit database coverage to a small fraction of the population. Inclusion in a DNA identification database of half or more of the male population and nearly all African American men is an odd result for a policy intended to limit government's control of samples and profiles of our DNA—and it is one that would further damage the legitimacy of the criminal law and of law enforcement agencies in areas where public safety is most in disrepair. Finally, the data on prevalence of arrest in the population should provoke skepticism about two propositions often advanced in opposition to a comprehensive identification database: (1) that it is financially and logistically feasible to sample DNA on arrest, but not feasible to sample everyone; and (2) that privacy interests will be substantially protected if DNA is taken and typed "only" from those who have been arrested.

In contrast, a population-wide DNA database could serve as at least a partial, much-needed antidote for the racial distortions that plague the criminal justice system. DNA evidence does not care about race. A database profile either does or does not match a crime scene sample. With a population-wide database, the identity of any matching individual would be known—no matter what the race. Routine production of a short list of people whose DNA matches samples found at a crime scene thus could help counteract the presence or perception of racism in the investigation of crime. When a person is arrested and incriminating crime scene DNA evidence points to the guilt of another person whose DNA profile is in the database, prompt exoneration and release of the innocent is likely to follow—regardless of the initial suspect's race or status. If an innocent defendant does go to trial in such a case, the crime scene DNA evidence and the results of the database search would be available, regardless of the defendant's race, to raise reasonable doubt about guilt.

This is not to say that a population-wide database would eliminate all racial inequities in law enforcement. Obviously, it would not. For instance, even the most inclusive database will not cure the racial distortions that result from selectively enforcing drug laws against African Americans or from enforcing evenhandedly drug laws that have a disparate impact on these citizens. But to concede that a comprehensive DNA identification-only database is no panacea for the racial ills that beset the criminal justice system is not to deny its power to mitigate what has become a crippling problem. It is simply more fair and more useful to include DNA identification profiles from all whites as well as from all other groups than it is to amass databases predominantly consisting of the DNA profiles of African Americans and other minorities.

Conclusion

The current debate over the scope of DNA databases for law enforcement is myopic in its focus on which crimes should be collection offenses and at which stage in the criminal process DNA samples should be taken. In principle, it is not at all why the obligation to provide personally identifying DNA data should be restricted to those individuals who are swept into the criminal justice system. In practice, settling for a DNA identification database restricted to convicts, or to convicts and arrestees, is sure to aggravate racial polarization in society, undermine the legitimacy of law and law enforcement, and further compromise public safety by halting far short of the deterrent and investigative capability that a population-wide database would afford. Like the double helix of the DNA molecule, privacy and equality are intertwined in complex ways. When they are untangled and evaluated, the case for a population-wide DNA database is strong.

Notes

1. See D. H. Kaye, The Constitutionality of DNA Sampling on Arrest, 10 Cornell J. L. & Pub. Pol'y 455, 456–57 (2001) (citing examples).
2. Paul R. Billings, Editorial, DNA Data Banks Would Taint Justice, Boston Globe, Jan. 14, 1999, at A19.
3. But see DNA on Trial: Genetic Identification and Criminal Justice (Paul R. Billings ed., 1992) (criticizing the creation of sex-offender databases).
4. See U.S. Const. amends. V & XIV.
5. We find it impossible to be anything but appalled at the prospect of government or others—perhaps others, more than government—possessing everyone's genome, and able to peer into and analyze at leisure the genetic code that can give up secrets we do not

even know we have. This is the prospect that turns debate from the method of DNA sample collection to the uses made of the samples. We could not favor authorizing a more inclusive DNA database, much less a comprehensive one, unless its creation were coupled with transparent procedures to assure destruction of whatever tissue samples are used, once the nonphenotypic loci useful only for identification have been typed and their profile has been recorded. But we foresee technology soon being available that would permit destruction of a sample almost simultaneously with its profile being recorded, and we can specify procedures that would keep whole DNA out of law enforcement control when only an identification profile is transmitted to an identification database by a hospital or other agency which routinely analyzes samples for health or other nonlaw enforcement purposes. Similarly, we could not favor secondary analysis for the identification loci, of DNA sampled for other purposes—by health authorities, for example—unless transparent procedures assured that the samples themselves would be kept out of law enforcement's control.

6. See, e.g., *Florida v. White*, 526 U.S. 559, 568 (1999).
7. See *Schmerber v. California*, 384 U.S. 757, 767 (1966)....
8. Jean E. McEwen, Sherlock Holmes Meets Genetic Fingerprinting, Boston Coll. L. Sch. Mag., Spring 1994, at 44, 49.
9. George Annas, Privacy Rules for DNA Databanks: Protecting Coded 'Future Diaries', 270 JAMA 2346, 2347 (1993); Jean E. McEwen, DNA Databanks, in Genetic Secrets: Protecting Privacy and Confidentiality in the Genetic Era, *supra* note 56, at 236 ....
10. Jonathan Kimmelman, The Promise and Perils of Criminal DNA Databanking, 18 Nature Biotech. 695, 696 (2000); cf. Kimmelman, *supra* note 10, at 215....
11. Witness protection programs are an exception, but the government's ability to protect witness from retaliation by offering them new identities would not be compromised by a governmental database of DNA profiles.
12. *United States v. Knotts*, 460 U.S. 276, 283 (1983)....
13. This is usually stated the other way: "more than half" of felony defendants have prior "felony records" and "two-thirds have prior arrests." See, e.g., Brian A. Reaves, Bureau of Justice Statistics, Felony Defendants in Large Urban Counties, 1994, Executive Summary, at 2 (1998)....
14. See id. at 1 tbl. (Felony arrest and conviction record of felony defendants in the 75 largest counties 1994.) Not surprisingly, in light of those data, half of those imprisoned after felony conviction are going to prison for the first time. Id.

16. See Thomas P. Bonczar & Allen J. Beck, Bureau of Justice Statistics, Lifetime Likelihood of Going to State or Federal Prison (1997. . . .

17. Allen Beck & Jennifer C. Karberg, Bureau of Justice Statistics, Prison and Jail Inmates at Midyear 2000, at 7 (2001) (reporting 132 whites per 100,000 whites in the population were in local jails at midyear 2000, compared to 736 blacks per 100,000 blacks).

18. See Allen J. Beck, Trends in U.S. Correctional Populations, in The Dilemmas of Corrections: Contemporary Readings (K.C. Haas & G.P. Alpert eds., 4th ed. 1999). . . .

19. The Bureau of Justice Statistics reports the following data on the total incarceration, including both jail and prison, of blacks and whites: . . . Beck & Karberg, *supra* note 17, at 9 tbl.13. . . .

20. Allen J. Beck, Prisoners in 1999, Bureau of Justice Statistics 9 tbl.14 (2000). . . .

21. See Kaye, *supra* note 1, at 458 n.12; Howard Safir, New York City Police Commissioner, Presentation to the National Commission on the Future of DNA Evidence (March 1, 1999) (transcript available at http://www.ojp.usdoj.gov/nij/dnamtgtrans4/trans-n.html). . . .

22. Bureau of the Census, Statistical Abstract of the Unites States: 2000, 12 tbl.10 . . . ; Federal Bureau of Investigation, Crime in the United States 1999, 230 tbl.43 . . . .

23. The lifetime likelihood of arrest cannot be drawn directly from routinely collected data, but it can be projected from annual arrest statistics and from cohort studies, in which a jurisdiction's police records are combed for contacts with anyone born in that jurisdiction in a given year. See Alfred Blumstein, Systems Analysis and the Criminal Justice System, 374 Annals Am. Acad. Pol. & Soc. Stud. 92, 99 (1967) . . .; Alfred Blumstein & Elizabeth Graddy, Prevalence and Recidivism Index Arrests: A Feedback Model, 16 L. & Soc'y Rev. 265, 279–280 (1981–1982). . . .

24. That a majority of males will be arrested for a non-traffic offense, at some point in their lives, is evident from the studies described *supra* note 20; . . .

25. See Randall Kennedy, Race Crime and the Law 24-26 (1997); Michael Tonry, Malign Neglect: Race, Crime and Punishment in America (1995). . . .

26. See Tom Tyler, Why People Obey the Law (1990) (finding that compliance with the criminal law is secured not so much by the threat of punishment as by perceptions that the laws are congruent with moral obligations, or at the least enacted properly by legitimate authority, and that they are executed fairly).

DAVID H. KAYE is an associate dean for research and a professor of law at Pennsylvania State's Dickinson School of Law.

MICHAEL E. SMITH is a professor emeritus at the University of Wisconsin School of Law.

Mark A. Rothstein and Meghan K. Talbott

➡ **NO**

The Expanding Use of DNA in Law Enforcement: What Role for Privacy?

DNA identification methods are such an established part of our law enforcement and criminal justice systems it is hard to believe that the technologies were developed as recently as the mid-1980s, and that the databases of law enforcement profiles were established in the 1990s. Although the first databases were limited to the DNA profiles of convicted rapists and murderers, the success of these databases in solving violent crimes provided the impetus for Congress and state legislatures to expand the scope of the databases with little critical examination of each expansion's value to law enforcement or cost to privacy and civil liberties.

We are now entering a new stage of DNA forensics, in which successive database expansions over the last decade have raised the possibility of creating a population-wide repository. In addition, new applications of DNA profiling, including familial and low stringency searches, have been added to DNA dragnets, the use of medical samples for forensic analysis, and other measures to create a series of crucial, yet largely unexplored, second-generation legal and policy issues. In this article, we assess these emerging issues and conclude that limits must be placed on the use of DNA in law enforcement and that privacy considerations must play an important part in the development of policies for the use of DNA profiling.

The Expanding Use of DNA

Scope

State DNA databases, which began almost exclusively as collections of adult sexual offenders' DNA profiles, have now expanded to include many or all convicted felons, juvenile offenders, those convicted of certain misdemeanors, and even arrestees.[1] In 2004, California voters approved Proposition 69, expanding the state database of felons convicted of serious, violent crimes, to include

samples from *all* felons and individuals with past felony convictions. The state will expand its database in the future to include profiles from individuals arrested for felonies and even individuals detained as mere suspects.[2] Laws in Louisiana,[3] Texas,[4] and Virginia[5] also authorize collecting DNA samples from arrestees. Recently, the DNA Fingerprinting Act of 2005 was signed into law, authorizing the expansion of the federal DNA database to include DNA collected from "individuals arrested, and from non-United States persons who are detained under the authority of the United States."[6]

The prevailing view among law enforcement officials is that more profiles included in a database allow a greater chance that a profile will match evidence found at a crime scene.[7] The promise of increased efficacy has some members of law enforcement and legal academia advocating for the expansion of criminal DNA databases to include DNA samples from the entire population.[8] Proponents of expansion argue that reducing the social cost of crime justifies the creation of a population-wide database, and that a universal database is necessary to maximize the utility of DNA profiling.[9] Although a few countries, such as Iceland and Estonia, are establishing national DNA databases for research purposes,[10] no country has implemented a population-wide database for forensic purposes.[11] Yet such an endeavor may not be far off. In 2005, the Portuguese government announced its intention to create a DNA database including the DNA profiles of all its approximately ten million inhabitants.[12]

A variety of practical and policy issues need to be addressed before a population-wide DNA forensic database can be seriously considered in the United States. On the practical side, virtually every state reports a substantial backlog in the analysis of extant samples collected under current laws, including crime scene evidence.[13] There are too few trained laboratorians, and nearly all states lack the equipment and storage facilities to support a major increase in the scope of the databases. Cost is also an issue. At a time of budgetary constraints, new DNA forensic expenses would likely consume a substantial percentage of new funds that could be allocated to law enforcement.[14] It is an open question whether the cost of a database expansion would deter crime and thus justify foregoing expenditures for additional front-line personnel, other forensic equipment, new vehicles, weapons and protective equipment, or crime control programs.

Assuming that the practical issues can be overcome, we are left with the policy question concerning whether we ought to develop a universal database. Notwithstanding civil liberties issues (discussed below), it is essential to have a clear picture of the expected law enforcement benefits. To justify a database expansion, even from a purely financial standpoint, there must be convincing evidence of the likelihood that databases of increased scope would be significantly more effective than the current databases in solving and preventing crimes in absolute terms and relative to other possible law enforcement expenditures. What is the evidence?

The Combined DNA Index System (CODIS), started by the Federal Bureau of Investigation (FBI) as a pilot program in 1990, was formally established in 1994.[15] Through its tiered system of databases, CODIS enables federal, state, and local crime laboratories to exchange and compare DNA profiles electronically, thereby linking crimes to each other and to convicted offenders. Over a decade of experience with DNA databases in most states supports the following two conclusions. First, DNA databases have had many spectacular successes in connecting seemingly disparate crimes and in identifying probable perpetrators in the absence of any other leads. Second, including "lesser offenses" in the databases helps to solve an indeterminate number of later, more serious crimes. For instance, yesterday's burglar may be today's rapist,[16] and having the DNA from a previously convicted burglar may help in solving a subsequent rape case.

Although recognizing these points, we note that there is virtually no scientific, comprehensive, independent, peer-reviewed analysis quantifying the overall effectiveness of DNA databases in solving or preventing crimes. The only quantitative measure used to assess the value of DNA databases is the total number of "cold hits" or "investigations aided."[17] These totals make for good headlines and legislative testimony, but their use raises a number of serious methodological and policy concerns. To begin with, there is no clear definition of the terms "cold hits" or "investigations aided," and thus the inclusion criteria vary widely among jurisdictions or even individual reporters. There is also no comparative information available to estimate the likelihood that other forensic techniques or additional investigation would have identified the suspect.

It is also not clear how many of the "investigations aided" actually result in conviction. Based on the claims of increased efficacy in solving crimes, one might expect that the percentage of crimes being solved or "cleared" would have increased as DNA databases expanded. However, while the crime rate has dropped over the past ten years, clearance rates have changed very little during that period. Moreover, the clearance rates for crimes typically associated with the availability of perpetrator DNA, homicide and forcible rape, were actually lower in 2004 than in 1995, meaning that law enforcement actually solved fewer of the reported crimes than it did when DNA databases were still in their infancy.[18]

A match between crime scene DNA and an individual's database profile does not necessarily mean that the individual is guilty. For example, a murder suspect might have acted in self-defense or there maybe some other reason to account for the presence of DNA found at the crime scene. Indeed, according to one study in Virginia, DNA matches resulted in convictions in less than thirty percent of the cases.[19] Case resolution, not conviction, maybe a more accurate measure of the effectiveness of DNA databases. For example, a suspect identified by DNA may have subsequently died without a conviction, yet in another case, a single DNA match may lead to multiple convictions where a suspect identified by his or her DNA confesses to other crimes without DNA evidence.

Finally, virtually all of the data are compiled and released by crime laboratories and other entities with an interest in promoting the maintenance or expansion of DNA databases. Unfortunately, a series of scandals throughout the country in which DNA evidence has been negligently (and even worse, intentionally) misidentified,[20] must give one pause before accepting at face value any claims by interested parties about the effectiveness of the DNA forensic identification system. In the absence of rigorous, independent, scientific studies of the efficacy of DNA databases of varied scope in helping to solve a range of crimes, it is foolish to consider further expansion of the current system.

Even without adequate data, it is still possible to compare, from a policy standpoint, today's typical state DNA database (restricted to most or all felons) with a universal database. The two compelling justifications for establishing a forensic DNA database of sex offenders, violent felons, or all felons is that these individuals are likely to engage in repeated criminal activity, and their conviction of a serious crime forfeits certain rights of bodily integrity and privacy relative to the law enforcement system.[21] With a more comprehensive database, however, especially one in which the entire population is included, neither of these justifications apply. Adding more law-abiding citizens to the database will result in an ever-diminishing percentage of matches relative to the total database. Furthermore, law-abiding citizens have done nothing that could be considered a forfeiture of their right to be outside of the law enforcement system.

The argument has been made that a population-wide database will promote "racial justice" because it will eliminate the current overrepresentation of minority groups in offender DNA databases and the increased overrepresentation of minorities if arrestees are added.[22] The overrepresentation of minorities in offender DNA databases reflects the overrepresentation of minorities in the criminal justice and correctional systems, and this overrepresentation is caused by sentencing policies that disparately impact minorities as well as gross disparities in education, employment, housing, health care, and other essential life opportunities. The overrepresentation of minorities among arrestees is caused by "racial profiling" and other dubious law enforcement practices. Having a disproportionate number of minority criminals and suspects is a social problem; it is not a DNA database problem. The solution is *not* a more egalitarian, universal database in which the entire population shares the indignity of inclusion in the DNA database while simultaneously giving greater power to the police.

Sociologist Troy Duster makes a more practical argument in opposition to the claim that a universal database will help eliminate racial bias.

> If the lens of the criminal justice system is focused almost entirely on one part of the population for a certain kind of activity (drug-related, street crime), and ignores a parallel kind of crime (fraternity cocaine sales a few miles away), then even if the fraternity members' DNA samples are in the databank, they will not be subject to the same level of matching, or of subsequent allele frequency profiling research to "help explain" their behavior.[23]

Thus, it is unrealistic to expect that a "neutral" database policy, layered over an unequal criminal justice system, will eliminate the systemic bias. . . .

Balancing Privacy and Law Enforcement

We have noted that the expanded use of DNA in law enforcement raises numerous concerns: (1) increasing the number of individuals from whom a DNA sample may be required on a routine basis; (2) coercing large numbers of individuals to submit samples as part of a DNA dragnet;

(3) obtaining DNA samples from close relatives, including children, as a way of indirectly searching the DNA of a suspect; (4) performing low-stringency searches to identify the close relatives of the alleged perpetrators of a crime; (5) accessing biological specimens in health care institutions for DNA testing; (6) using DNA samples for research without the consent of the sample donor; (7) using behavioral genetic forensic profiling based on crime scene DNA; and (8) retaining non-crime scene DNA samples indefinitely.

Each of these uses involves different ethical and legal issues, each has a different significance, and each demands a somewhat different method of analysis. Nevertheless, for simplicity, they may be considered to implicate a similar interest of individuals to be free from having their DNA profile used for law enforcement.

Privacy Interests

The interests of individuals in DNA identification relate to privacy, autonomy, anonymity, secrecy, freedom, and liberty. For ease of discussion, we will call all of these interests privacy. They all deal with the conditions under which law enforcement agencies may require information from or impose other conditions on individuals (e.g., submission of a biological sample) in connection with a criminal investigation or the criminal justice system.

In general, legal limitations on law enforcement activities depend on the nature of the intrusion upon individuals. Because of the varied levels of intrusiveness, law enforcement officers must meet a different legal and evidentiary standard to make an arrest, conduct a nonconsensual search, or obtain confidential information, such as bank records or medical records. What law enforcement standard should apply to individuals' interest in being free from having their DNA analyzed by the police?

To answer this question, we must first consider the issue of genetic exceptionalism, which refers to the treatment of genetic information separately from other forms of health (or in this context, forensic) information. Although legislatures have frequently enacted genetic-specific laws (for reasons beyond the scope of this article), the overwhelming majority of scholars to consider the issue in the context of genetic privacy and genetic nondiscrimination have argued against genetic exceptionalism.[24] The reasoning is as follows. Scientifically, it is questionable whether health information can be meaningfully divided into genetic and non-genetic information; practically, it is unlikely that health information can be segregated to permit the disclosure of only one type of information; and from a policy standpoint, genetic exceptionalism may make matters worse by reinforcing notions of stigma.

These arguments against genetic exceptionalism all have been made in the context of privacy and nondiscrimination. To our knowledge, the issue has not been considered in the context of criminal justice. Do these arguments apply here as well?

Suppose that police are investigating a series of murders at pharmacies in a certain area. All of the murders occurred in the course of an armed robbery in which the robber only took large quantities of an expensive and relatively rarely used prescription drug. Police theorize that the robber is someone who is dependent on the medication. They want to conduct a dragnet in the area to ask people to submit to a blood test or saliva test to check for the presence of the drug. Leaving aside the logic or the likely success of such an investigatory measure, would the public and legal scholars have the same objections to the drug test dragnet as they do to DNA dragnets? It should be noted that the hypothetical drug test will reveal more personal health information about the individual than a DNA test of the thirteen CODIS loci. The DNA profiling is more limited, but more specific. It might provide a match with the crime scene evidence, whereas, in this example, the drug test will only indicate whether the person is among an unknown number of individuals taking a certain medication.

It seems to us that the privacy and civil liberties analysis surrounding expanded use of DNA forensics in law enforcement should not be based on whether the test performed is "genetic." The justification for, the intrusiveness of, and the procedures surrounding a test are at least as important as the type of test performed on a sample. Thus, the legal and policy question should concern the legal basis on which law enforcement personnel require or "encourage" individuals to submit to a biological test of an invasive nature, or infringe upon an individual's dignity. It seems paradoxical that if the police seek to obtain a court order directing a particular individual to submit a DNA sample or to undergo a medical test, the order would not be granted in the absence of probable cause. On the other hand, if police strongly encourage all individuals in a certain area to "voluntarily" submit a sample as part of a dragnet, then a different standard will be applied and the requirement will be generally upheld. Furthermore, some legal scholars have argued that even a statute establishing a universal database would be constitutional.[25]

The prospect of expanded use of DNA forensics needs to be placed in context. In a world in which personal privacy is difficult to maintain against an onslaught of computer file sharing, surveillance cameras, biometric imaging, thermal imaging, and other technological "advances," for many people, the last "off limit" area for access to personal information is law enforcement. Millions of people enthusiastically send their credit card information via computer to unknown merchants and other users. If a police officer asked someone for credit card information however, we doubt there would be the same eager response.

The leading privacy concerns about more inclusive DNA forensic databases are that this powerful information (and the biological samples from which it is obtained) would be collected on a routine basis without any individualized suspicion of wrongdoing, that individuals would be coerced to provide samples in dragnets, that relatives of potential suspects would be tested, and that the original specimens would be retained indefinitely.

Assume that a hypothetical country routinely required all of its residents to submit the following items to the police: a DNA sample, a yearly photograph, handwriting exemplar, voiceprint, fingerprints, hair samples, retinal scans, bank statements, credit card information, health records, and other details of their personal life. Obviously, ready access to this information by police would help solve crimes. Nevertheless, such comprehensive information submission to law enforcement would be widely viewed as hallmarks of a repressive, totalitarian state, quite different from the United States, with our libertarian tradition and Bill of Rights protecting citizens against unreasonable governmental interference with our lives. We are concerned that the United States not heedlessly proceed in this direction. Fingerprints already are widely available to police and photographs appear on drivers' licenses and passports. Each individual intrusion is easier to defend than the sum of government demands. At what point is the cumulative intrusion by the government unacceptable?

In *Osborn v. United States*,[26] Justice Douglas warned what can happen when technology is utilized without an assessment of its true value to or effect on society:

> [T]he privacy and dignity of our citizens is being whittled away by sometimes imperceptible steps. Taken individually, each step may be of little consequence. But when viewed as a whole, there begins to emerge a society quite unlike any we have seen—a society in which government may intrude into the secret regions of man's life at will.[27]

Our concern is not that expanded DNA databases would transform our country into a "nation of suspects."[28] Our concern is that we would become a nation with unfettered police powers. Moreover, once greater information about individuals is in the possession of police, it will be difficult to prevent other uses of the information by the government.

We recognize the difficulty of deciding when to oppose intrusions by the government undertaken in the name of protecting the public. It is easy to object to outrageous conduct, but, as with DNA forensics, it is harder when there is a seemingly compelling justification for the intrusion on privacy. In the landmark 1886 case of *Boyd v. United States*,[29] in which the Court spelled out the scope of Fourth Amendment protections, Justice Bradley wrote: "It may be that it is the obnoxious thing in its mildest and least repulsive form; but illegitimate and unconstitutional practices get their first footing in that way, namely, by silent approaches and slight deviations from legal modes of procedure."[30] We believe that in the absence of probable cause or prior conviction, individuals have legitimate interests in not submitting their DNA to law enforcement officials for profiling and retention.

Law Enforcement Interests

The public's interests in law enforcement are more concrete than its privacy interests, and perhaps this is one reason law enforcement interests have tended to prevail in the area of DNA identification. Members of the public—and not just law enforcement officials—are justifiably concerned about crime. Although we have previously noted our discomfort with the use of "cold hits" and "investigations aided" as the sole measures of the efficacy of DNA databases, we do not question that DNA databases work. DNA databases have helped to solve numerous crimes, including heinous crimes that were unlikely to have been solved without them. To the extent they result in the incarceration of criminals, the DNA databases also prevent crimes by known criminals and serve as a general deterrent. In getting violent criminals off the streets, DNA databases also help ease the psychological burden from crime victims and their families.

We believe that the crime solving and prevention benefits of DNA databases justify the establishment, continuation, and funding of the CODIS system. These benefits, however, do not constitute a blanket justification for the use of DNA in unlimited ways. It is not necessarily the case that if a DNA database containing profiles of rapists and murderers is valuable, then a DNA database with all felons, misdemeanants, juvenile offenders, arrestees, or the entire population will produce significantly more hits and therefore be positive for society. It is also not necessarily the case that if the public supports and benefits from DNA forensics that any expansion, including indirect, low stringency, and

dragnet searches, also will have the same level of public support. Each new application and extension of DNA forensics must be independently assessed and weighed against the substantial privacy interests implicated.

Whenever there are any restraints placed on law enforcement, the argument is raised that some criminals will escape detection or go free. Certainly, this has been the argument surrounding the exclusionary rule, where the issue is whether the criminal should go free because "the constable has blundered." In *Mapp v. Ohio*,[31] in which the Supreme Court held that the exclusionary rule applies in state criminal cases, Justice Clark responded to this argument by stating: "The criminal goes free, if he must, but it is the law that sets him free. Nothing can destroy a government more quickly than its failure to observe its own laws, or worse, its disregard of the charter of its own existence."[32]

Law enforcement is essential to the public and an important responsibility of government. Nevertheless, our government was founded on the principle that privacy, dignity, due process, and liberty serve to constrain law enforcement activity. These values are embodied not only in the Fourth Amendment prohibition on unreasonable search and seizure, but also in the Fifth Amendment guarantees of due process, equal protection, and freedom from self-incrimination; in the Sixth Amendment right to counsel; and the Eighth Amendment ban on cruel and unusual punishment. Undoubtedly, there would be more convictions if police could enter homes without warrants and seize contraband and instrumentalities of crime, if they could wiretap and electronically intercept telephone calls without a warrant, if they could coerce confessions, if they could set up roadblocks for any reason at any time, if they were not required to give *Miranda* warnings to suspects, and if they could engage in myriad other practices that are antithetical to our way of life. The golden gift of preventing and solving crime is not worth the price of our liberty.

Conclusion

In writing about the importance of privacy, especially in the context of search and seizure law, the temptation to quote from Justice Brandeis' legendary dissent in *Olmstead v. United States*[33] is irresistible. In this, the sesquicentennial of his birth, resistance is futile. In *Olmstead*, the majority rejected a Fourth Amendment challenge to wiretapping on the ground that there was no physical invasion. In his dissent, Justice Brandeis captured the essential nature of privacy, and he provided a moving and compelling explanation of why protecting privacy is so fundamental to freedom.

The makers of our Constitution undertook to secure conditions favorable to the pursuit of happiness. They recognized the significance of man's spiritual nature, of his feelings and of his intellect. They knew that only part of the pain, pleasure and satisfactions of life are to be found in material things. They sought to protect Americans in their beliefs, their thoughts, their emotions and their sensations. They conferred, as against the Government, the right to be let alone—the most comprehensive of rights and the right most valued by civilized men. To protect that right, every unjustifiable intrusion by the Government upon the privacy of the individual, whatever the means employed, must be deemed a violation of the Fourth Amendment.[34]

In probably the most frequently quoted passage of his dissent, Justice Brandeis alerted us not to let the exigencies of the day and the beneficent intent of governmental actions weaken our resolve in defending privacy and safeguarding liberty.

Experience should teach us to be most on guard to protect liberty when the Government's purposes are beneficent. Men born to freedom are naturally alert to repel invasion of their liberty by evil-minded rulers. The greatest dangers to liberty lurk in insidious encroachment by men of zeal, well-meaning but without understanding.[35]

DNA databases and their forensic applications must be assigned their proper place in law enforcement. New expansions of DNA technology should not be considered until scientifically rigorous, independent studies demonstrate that the new application would have significant utility to law enforcement. Even then, the expanded use of DNA should be adopted only if it would be consistent with fundamental privacy and civil liberties interests.

Acknowledgments

The authors are indebted to Lori Andrews and Fred Bieber for helpful comments on an earlier draft of this article.

References

1. See T. Simoncelli and B. Steinhardt, "California's Proposition 69: A Dangerous Precedent for Criminal DNA Databases," *Journal of Law, Medicine & Ethics* 33 (2005): 279–293, at 282; Reprinted in *Journal of Law, Medicine & Ethics* 34 (2006): 199–213; M. Ballve, "DNA Fingerprinting Trend Threatens Genetic Privacy," Pacific News Service, July 14, 2004, *at* <http://www.alternet.org/rights/19234/> (last visited February 6, 2006). This article points out that in 2003 alone, over a dozen states changed their laws to expand the scope of their DNA collection.

2. Cal. Pen. Code § 296 (West Supp. 2005); T. Simoncelli and B. Steinhardt, *supra* note 1, at 279.

3. La. Rev. Stat. Ann. §15.609.

4. Tex. Gov't Code Ann. §411.1471.

5. Va. Code Ann. §19.2–310.2:1.

6. Title X of the Violence Against Women and Department of Justice Reauthorization Act of 2005, Pub. Law No. 109–162, 119 Stat. 2960 (2006).

7. See National Institute of Justice, *National Commission on the Future of DNA Evidence*, "The Future of Forensic DNA Testing: Predictions of the Research and Development Working Group," (2000): at 35 [hereinafter "The Future of DNA Tasting"].

8. See A. R. Amar, "A Search for Justice in Our Genes," *New York Times,* May 7, 2002, *available at* <http://www.law.yale.edu/outside/html/Public_Affairs/246/yls_article.htm> (last visited February 6, 2006); D. H. Kaye, et al., "Is a DNA Identification Database in Your Future?" *Criminal Justice* 16 (2001): 4–11.

9. D. H. Kaye, *supra* note 8, at 19.

10. C. Rosen, "Liberty, Privacy, and DNA Databases," *The NewAtlantis* 1 (2003): 37–52.

11. M. J. Boavida, "Portugal Plans a Forensic Genetic Database of its Entire Population," *Newropeans Magazine,* April 11, 2005, *at* <http://www.newropeans-magazine.org/index.php?option=com_content&task=view&id=2063&Itemid=121> (last visited February 6, 2006).

12. *Id.*

13. S. Ailing, P. S. Lane, Division of Governmental Studies and Services, Washington State University, "National Forensics DNA Study Report," (2003): Appendix 3d, at 46, *available at* <http://www.dna.gov/pubs/gen_interest> (last visited February 15, 2006).

14. These expenses could vary depending on how the samples are collected, analyzed and stored, but would conceivably include the cost of devices and materials for collecting, analyzing, storing, and accessing the data, as well as the cost of training and labor cost of personnel needed to run the system. Although there have been no estimates of the cost of a universal database in the U.S., estimates done in Europe and per person profile costs can serve as a basis for a rough estimate. Based on the con-

servative estimate of $60 per person it would cost approximately $18 billion for the profiles. Based on the £5.5 billion estimate made by the British government for its 60 million inhabitants, it would cost $50 billion to create a national database in the U.S. (Government estimate of £5.5 billion, others up to £20 billion, for a universal database involving the approximately 60 million people in the U.K.) A. Deane, "Identity Cards in Britain," *Contemporary Review* 286, no. 11672 (2005): 268–270, at 269; M. J. Boavida, *supra* note 11 (estimate of Portugal universal database made at 40–80 euros per person); American Society of Law, Medicine & Ethics, "DNA Fingerprinting and Civil Liberties," *Project Description,* at <http://www.aslme.org/dna_04/description.php> (last visited February 7,2006), estimating $50 to $100 per profile.

15. CODIS Program, *Mission Statement & Background,* Federal Bureau of Investigation (FBI) website, *at* <http://www.fbi.gov/hq/lab/codis/program.htm> (last visited February 7,2006).

16. According to Dr. Paul Ferrara, Director of the Virginia Division of Forensic Science, more than half the violent crimes solved by the use of the state database involved DNA samples obtained from convicted burglers. R. Willing, "DNA Links Burglars to Harder Crime," *USA Today,* December 7,1998.

17. CODIS Program, *Measuring Success,* Federal Bureau of Investigation (FBI) website, *at* <http://www.fbi.gov/hq/Iab/codis/success.htm> (last visited February 7,2006).

18. FBI, *Uniform Crime Reports, Crime in the United States,* 1995, 2004, *available at* <http://www.fbi.gov/ucr/ucr.htm> (last visited February 7, 2006).

19. R. Willing, "DNA Matches Win Few Convictions in Va.," *USA Today,* November 7, 2005.

20. See S. McVicker, "More DPS Labs Flawed: DNA Testing Woes Across State Threaten Thousands of Cases," *Houston Chronicle,* March 28, 2004, at Al; K. Herbert, "Crime-lab Mistakes Spark Alert: Hundreds of Pa. Cases May Be Reexamined," *Philadelphia Inquirer,* June 19, 2003, at A01; R. Willing, "Mueller Defends Crime Lab After Questionable DNA Tests," *USA Today,* May 1, 2003, at A03; L. Hart, "DNA Lab's Woes Cast Doubt on 68 Prison Terms: Forensic Science at a Houston Police Unit Was Plagued by Problems. The inmates for Whom Retesting is Ordered Include 17 on Death Row," *Los Angeles Times,* March 31, 2003; R. Stutzman, "State DNA Analyst's Data: Forgeries Could Result in New Trial for Rapist," *Orlando Sentinel,* July 25,2002; D. Baldwin, "Gilchrist Faces More Scrutiny: Review Ordered in Three Death-row Cases," *Daily Oklahoman,* July 17, 2001; L. Gorman, "The Brady Solution: A Due Process Remedy for those Convicted with Evidence from Faulty Crime Labs," *University of San Francisco Law Review* 39 (2005): 725–727.

21. *Willis v. Artuz,* 301 F.3d 65, 66 (2d Cir. 2002); *Jones v. Murray,* 962 F.2d 302, 306 (4th Cir. 1992).

22. See D. H. Kaye and M. E. Smith, "DNA Databases for Law Enforcement: The Coverage Question and the Case for a Population-Wide Database," in D. Lazer, ed., *DNA and the Criminal Justice System: The Technology of Justice* (Cambridge, MA: MIT Press, 2004): 247–284, at 269–271.

23. T. Duster, "Behavior Genetics and Explanations of the Link Between Crime, Violence, and Race," in E. Parens, A. R. Chapman and N. Press, eds., *Wrestling with Behavioral Genetics: Science, Ethics and Public Conversation* (Baltimore, MD: Johns Hopkins University Press, 2006): 150–175, at 168.

24. M. A. Rothstein, "Genetic Exceptionalism and Legislative Pragmatism," *Hastings Center Report 35,* no. 4 (2005): 27–33.

25. See D. H. Kaye and M. E. Smith, *supra* note 22.

26. 385 U.S. 323 (1966).

27. *Id.,* at 343.

28. See D. H. Kaye & M. E. Smith, *supra* note 220.

29. 116 U.S. 616 (1886).

30. *Id., at 635.*

31. 367 U.S. 643 (1961).

32. *Id., at 659.*

33. 277 U.S. 438 (1928).

34. *Id.,* at 478.

35. *Id.,* at 479.

MARK A. ROTHSTEIN holds the Herbert F. Boehl Chair of Law and Medicine and directs the Institute for Bioethics, Health Policy and Law at the University of Louisville School of Medicine.

MEGHAN K. TALBOTT is a lawyer and has served as research associate at the Institute for Bioethics, Health Policy and Law at the University of Louisville School of Medicine.

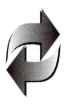

EXPLORING THE ISSUE

Should Governments Develop DNA Databanks to Support Law Enforcement?

Critical Thinking and Reflection

1. Rothstein and Talbott put a lot of emphasis on the idea that citizens have a strong interest in being free from having their DNA profile used for law enforcement. Do you agree with Rothstein and Talbott about the value of being free of law enforcement mechanisms, and if you do, do you find the response from Kaye and colleagues helpful?
2. Kaye and Smith try to deflect the concern about privacy by drawing a distinction between three different kinds of privacy. Summarize their account and explain whether you find it persuasive.
3. These two selections offer very different views of how forensic DNA databanks will affect racial injustices in law enforcement. Which position is the more convincing, in your view?
4. Both selections also address the usefulness of creating a national DNA database. Kaye and colleagues assert that the incremental costs are modest, Rothstein and Talbott that more evidence is needed. What values, in your view, should drive the decision on usefulness.

Is There Common Ground?

These selections set out similar views on the moral exceptionalness of genetic information. Neither supposes that genetic information needs to be thought of as inherently different from other kinds of information. Both agree that a DNA database of some sort may be appropriate. Both also agree that it should be racially just. Nor, probably, do they disagree about whether privacy is important.

Where they disagree may simply be on how privacy is best defended. Can a slight infringement of privacy be tolerated, or will slight infringement tend to lead to serious erosion? Kaye and Smith see a slight infringement as both necessary and inevitable in the modern world; Rothstein and Talbott argue strenuously that even small incursions on privacy must be avoided in order to protect liberty.

The battle lines for access to genetic information for forensic uses may well be fully drawn in the selections in this unit. For other kinds of uses, the debate about genetic privacy will probably grow ever more heated and complicated, as ever more genetic information is acquired and as more is learned about the significance of that information. Currently, we still know very little about how genes contribute to complex behavioral traits such as intelligence and honesty, but eventually, we will probably begin to build our understanding of how sets of genes interact

with different kinds of environmental circumstances to produce behavioral traits. Many of the claims we make about how genes contribute to behavior may turn out to be overly simplistic, even inaccurate. Whether we accurately map genes onto behavior or draw wildly mistaken connections between genes and behavior, the extent of appropriate access to that information will be an important topic of debate.

Additional Resources

H. T. Greely, "Time to Raise Some Hell," *GeneWatch* 24, no. 1 (2011): 4–5.

J. J. Koehler and M. J. Saks, "What DNA 'Fingerprinting' Can Teach the Law about the Rest of Forensic Science," *Cardozo Law Review* 13 (1991): 361–72.

Osagie K. Obasogie and Troy Duster, "All That Glitters Isn't Gold," *Hastings Center Report* 41, no. 5 (2011): 15–18.

National Institute of Justice, "The Future of Forensic DNA Testing: Predictions of the Research and Development Working Group" (Washington, D.C.: U.S. Department of Justice, 2000).

Internet References . . .

DNA and Law Enforcement

http://www.thehastingscenter.org/Publications
/BriefingBook/Detail.aspx?id=2168

Genetic Testing, Privacy, and Discrimination

http://www.councilforresponsiblegenetics.org
/projects/PastProject.aspx?projectId=1

Innocence Project

http://www.innocenceproject.org/

Genetic Privacy Network

http://geneticprivacynetwork.org/

NCSL Forensic Science Laws Page

http://www.ncsl.org/research/civil
-and-criminal-justice/dna-laws-database.aspx

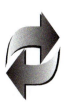

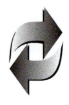

Selected, Edited, and with Issue Framing Material by:
Gregory E. Kaebnick, *The Hastings Center*

ISSUE

May Doctors Offer Medical Drugs and Surgery to Stop a Disabled Child from Maturing?

YES: **Sarah E. Shannon**, from "In Support of the Ashley Treatment," *Pediatric Nursing* (2007)

NO: **Teresa A. Savage**, from "In Opposition of the Ashley Treatment," *Pediatric Nursing* (2007)

Learning Outcomes
After reading this issue, you will be able to: • Evaluate the kinds of considerations that parents and physicians should weigh in thinking about how to use medical technology to care for children with disabilities.   • Outline some of the social issues that should be borne in mind when developing public policy concerning the treatment of people with disabilities.   • Discuss some of the concerns that disability advocates have about the treatment of cognitively disabled people.

ISSUE SUMMARY

YES: Nurse Sarah E. Shannon believes that ethically and legally parents have the right and duty to make decisions and to care for their family members who are unable to do so themselves and that we should not abandon parents of severely developmentally disabled children to the harsh social and economic realities that are barriers to good care.

NO: Nurse Teresa A. Savage believes that children like Ashley should have independent advocates, preferably persons with disabilities, to weigh the risks and benefits of proposed interventions.

Ashley (her real name) was born in 1997 with a severe brain impairment condition called static encephalopathy. She will never progress beyond the developmental level of an infant. At the age of 7, she was already showing signs of early puberty. Her parents wanted to keep her at home, but felt that as she grew older and bigger, and matured physically, it would be difficult to manage. They were concerned that the quality of life of the child they called their "pillow angel" would be diminished. In 2004, the parents and doctors at the Children's Hospital in Seattle devised a new treatment, which came to be called the "Ashley treatment."

This treatment included the administration of high-dose estrogen (sex steroid) therapy, which would stunt her growth; a hysterectomy (removal of her reproductive organs), which would prevent menstruation and make her infertile; and removal of her breast buds to prevent normal breast development. Before embarking on this treatment, the doctors consulted the hospitals' ethics committee, which met with the parents, Ashley herself, and her physicians. The committee agreed that the requests for estrogen therapy and hysterectomy were ethical in this case but should be considered in future patients only after review by an interdisciplinary panel.

This was not the first time that medical technology had been used to alter children's bodies. In "Tall Girls: The Social Shaping of a Medical Therapy," Joyce M. Lee and Joel D. Howell describe the practice in the second half of the twentieth century of prescribing estrogen therapy to otherwise healthy girls to keep them from growing too tall (*Archives of Pediatric and Adolescent Medicine*, October 2006). The definition of "too tall" was determined by societal beliefs about what it meant to be tall and female—not a good thing in those days.

As early as the 1940s, scientists observed that abnormal hormone levels influenced growth patterns both by prematurely closing long-bone growth plates (leading to short stature) and by keeping growth plates open over a prolonged time (leading to acromegaly, or extreme height). Through the 1950s and 1960s, articles appeared in medical journals attesting to the success of estrogen therapy in preventing girls from growing too tall, a condition that made them "self-conscious" and "embarrassed."

Lee and Howell assert that parents wanted to keep their girls shorter in order to improve their marriage prospects, since marriage was at that time thought to be a prerequisite for a successful life for a woman. As social norms changed toward the end of the twentieth century, scientific and medical interest in keeping girls from growing to their natural height diminished. And even among doctors who continued to treat girls, the expected height to which they might grow also increased. In 1956, a girl expected to reach 5'9" might be offered treatment, while by 1999 only girls who might grow to 6'2" would be in that category.

On the other hand, the use of growth hormone for very short but otherwise healthy boys has increased. The reasons are also socially determined. Tall men achieve more in society, it is believed, and have a greater choice of mates.

Ashley's treatment raises somewhat different questions. She has an underlying medical condition that means she will always be dependent on caregivers. In modifying her body, too, the goal was not to keep her normal, but to make her more abnormal—to prevent her from becoming fully adult. Ashley's parents hoped that, by preventing her from becoming sexually mature and from reaching a normal adult height, they could make it easier to care for her. They also thought that it would be easier for her not to have a mature woman's body.

In 2007, her parents created a blog (www.pillowangel.org) in order to tell her story. They believed parents of other children in similar circumstances should be able to consider using the "Ashley Treatment" for their children.

The YES and NO selections lay out the issues. Nurse Sarah E. Shannon believes that Ashley's parents' desire to care for her at home is their ethical and legal right, and that they should be able to make decisions in what they understand as Ashley's best interest. Nurse Teresa A. Savage argues that children like Ashley should have independent advocates to weigh the risks and benefits so that perceptions of "quality of life" from a disability perspective are included.

YES ⤶

Sarah E. Shannon

In Support of the Ashley Treatment

The news about Ashley, a severely cognitively and developmentally delayed child whose parents chose to medically limit her physical size, grabbed the attention of all of us. What if this was my child? Would I want to make my child smaller so that she would always be able to be cared for in a home, by family members? Growth attenuation treatment for children such as Ashley challenges us to think beyond our initial reactions. Ashley has the developmental and cognitive capacity of a young infant (Gunther & Diekema, 2006). She cannot hold up her head, roll or otherwise change her body position. She moves her arms and legs but cannot sit unsupported. Ashley responds positively to music and is able to vocalize but cannot talk (Parents' blog, 2006). She is alert to her environment but it is not clear that she recognizes people, including her own family. Ashley cries to express her frustration or discomfort. Currently, she lives at home with her parents and two siblings and is cared for by extended family.

Ashley's parents chose to attenuate Ashley's growth—to make her smaller—through the use of high dose estrogen therapy. In addition, Ashley's parents requested, and her physicians agreed, to remove her uterus and breast buds (Gunther & Diekema; Parents' blog; 2006). These three choices were made for separate therapeutic reasons. Growth attenuation through high dose estrogen therapy hastens the normal impact of puberty on girls' height. With puberty, estrogen levels rise and growth plate maturation occurs (Gunther & Diekema, 2006). High dose estrogen therapy takes advantage of this normal effect by stimulating growth plate maturation to occur prematurely. Therapy usually lasts for several years and, while data in developmentally delayed young children is sparse, the major risks appear similar to those for birth control pills, including uterine bleeding, breast development, and a small increased risk of deep vein thrombosis (DVT). Once puberty begins or growth attenuation is achieved, estrogen is stopped. The younger the child, the greater will be the effect on height. Ashley's physicians predict that "treatment beginning in a 5-year-old boy of average height and weight might result in a reduction in final length of as much as 24 inches (60 cm) and in weight of more than 100 pounds (45 kg)." (Gunther & Diekema, 2006, p. 1015).

Hysterectomy raises the issue of sterilization and whether this procedure was done primarily for birth control. Ashley has the mental capacity of an infant however making any possibility of consensual sex or parenthood impossible. Conversely, there are several health benefits resulting from removal of the uterus. First, it allows the high dose estrogen therapy to be administered without progesterone, reducing the risk of DVT (Gunther & Diekema, 2006). Second, hysterectomy avoids future hormone therapy to control menses. Menses can be a significant source of discomfort and a hygiene challenge that can aggravate skin breakdown when mobility is already impaired. For these reasons, a significant number of disabled women receive depot medroxyprogesterone acetate (DepoProvera) to suppress menstrual bleeding. However recent research has found that this increases their fracture risk 2.4 times above disabled women not on this medication (Watson, Lentz, & Cain, 2006). Hence, hysterectomy is being reconsidered as a more appropriate treatment for long-term control of menses. Third, a hysterectomy removes the cervix, alleviating the need to do routine PAP smears for health maintenance. For a woman as profoundly disabled as Ashley, the personal invasion and discomfort of a routine PAP smear can be intolerable (Brakman & Amari-Vaught, 1999).

The third procedure was breast bud removal, done while Ashley was under anesthesia for the hysterectomy. Was this cosmetic? An effort on the part of Ashley's parents to keep her child-like? How could removal of her breasts possibly benefit Ashley? Ashley's maternal lineage includes large and often, fibrocystic breasts, a painful condition (Parents' blog, 2006). Due to her profound developmental disability, Ashley is unable to sit up without chest support such as a chest strap, which puts pressure

From *Pediatric Nursing Journal,* vol. 33, no. 2, April 2007, pp. 175–178. Reprinted with permission of the publisher, Jannetti Publications, Inc., East Holly Avenue, Box 56, Pitman, NJ 08071-0056; (856) 256-2300; fax: (856) 589-7463; Web site: www.pediatricnursing.net; for a sample copy of the journal, please contact the publisher.

on breast tissue. This is a potential source of skin break-down and discomfort aggravated by large breasts. Breast bud removal is a relatively simple procedure to remove the small subcutaneous breast tissue while retaining the nipple and areola. It is true that if Ashley's breast size becomes problematic later, she could have breast reduction surgery done. However, this is a much more complicated, painful and risky procedure.

Ashley's parents believe that the two biggest challenges Ashley faces in life are discomfort and boredom (Parents' blog, 2006). Avoiding discomfort in persons such as Ashley is a complex goal involving the entire multidisciplinary team. Ashley is fortunate to not suffer from any chronic health problems. However, persons with profound limitations in mobility have a lifetime risk of increased skin breakdown, a major cause of discomfort and morbidity. This risk is increased through factors that include increased body weight, body morphology (such as large breasts), and poor nutritional status and is decreased through actions such as frequent repositioning, optimal hygiene, and good nutritional status. Having a smaller body size minimizes the potential for skin breakdown. A smaller size also increases the opportunity that caregivers can reposition a person more frequently and effectively. Ashley's parents have argued that having Ashley remain small affords other benefits to her. Her grandparents can physically continue to provide care for her. She can continue to use a stroller that she seems to prefer and allows her to be moved around the home to hear and watch family activities, as is often done with an infant. She will continue to fit into a standard bathtub. She will be able to be picked up and held on a parent's lap. She will be kept at home to be cared for within a family environment.

Yet should we change Ashley to fit the home, or change the home to fit Ashley? We could insure that caregivers who are large and strong be available to families to provide care for profoundly disabled persons. We could redesign homes to accommodate persons with disabilities so that their wheelchairs could fit through doorways, their bodies into bathtubs. Yet this utopian view of care would require a level of public financing that is currently unavailable. Americans currently tolerate having 46 million of their neighbors, co-workers, and the strangers they walk past on the sidewalk living without heath care insurance (Hoffman, 2007). Custodial care, such as Ashley needs, is not covered by even the most generous of health care plans. After a few weeks, care at home must be provided by non-paid family caregivers, or helpers paid out-of-pocket, or those paid for through long-term care insurance that the adult person obtained prior to the event, or paid for by public assistance through the Medicaid program after the person (and their spouse) have exhausted their personal finances (U.S. Department of Health and Human Services, 2007). For the elderly who require assistance with activities of daily living, for example after suffering a stroke, finding homecare is difficult. For disabled infants and children it may be nearly impossible. Catlin (2007) described the plight of parents who are trying to secure home health nursing for fragile children. Pediatric-trained caregivers willing to work for the low wages paid in home care settings are in short supply. Reimbursement is nearly non-existent. Equipment for pediatric patients is in short supply. Ashley does not live in a utopian world. By allowing parents of severely developmentally disabled children to have access to growth attenuation treatment, we do not abandon them to these harsh social and economic realities.

The last criticism to address is that Ashley's parents have attenuated her growth for their own convenience. We are disquieted by the thought that Ashley's parents might have decided to keep her small, a 'pillow angel' as they call her, without regard for her dignity or safety. Perhaps it is this last point that disturbs us most deeply. Yet in most healthcare settings, across all age groups, we are witnesses to family decision-making for loved ones who lack decision-making capacity: the distraught family in the intensive care setting making choices for a seriously ill or injured loved one, the exhausted family in mental health making choices for the acutely mentally ill person, the young parents in the NICU making choices for the babies who came too soon and too small. Families approach these decisions without medical training, often in crisis, and with multiple demands on their care giving and financial means. Ethically and legally, we invest in the family the right and duty to make decisions and to care for family members who are unable to do so themselves. Why? Because families do the best they can and it is better than we, as professionals, could do for them. Sometimes we are called upon to protect our patients in situations of abuse or neglect. But most often, we are asked to simply bear witness to the daily sacrifices and acts of love that constitute family caregiving and to humbly guide these families in their decision-making. Ashley's parents, physicians and the multidisciplinary ethics committee have allowed us to share, and judge, their thoughtful deliberations (Gunther & Diekema; Parents' blog; 2006). Each of us can learn from their decisions and benefit from their generosity. So ask yourself again, what if this were my child—who I loved dearly and desperately wanted to ensure would always be able to be cared for in a home setting, by family members? What would I do?

References

Brakman S.V., & Amari-Vaught E. (1999). *Resistance and refusal. Hastings Center Report, 29*(1), 22.

Catlin A.J. (2007). Home care for the high-risk neonate: success or failure depends on home health nurse funding and availability. *Home Healthcare Nurse, 25*(2), 1–5.

Gunther D.F., & Diekema D.S. (2006). Attenuating growth in children with profound developmental disability: A new approach to an old dilemma. *Archives of Pediatrics & Adolescent Medicine, 160*(10), 1013–1017.

Hoffman C.B. (2007). Simple truths about America's uninsured. *American Journal of Nursing, 107*(1), 40–3, 46–47.

Parents' Blog: Ashley's Mom and Dad. (2006). The "Ashley Treatment", toward a better quality of life for "Pillow Angels." . . .

U.S. Department of Health and Human Services, *Medicare: The Official U.S. Government Site for People with Medicare. Long-term Care.* . . .

Watson K.C., Lentz M.J., & Cain K.C. (2006). Associations between fracture incidence and use of depot medroxyprogesterone acetate and anti-epileptic drugs in women with developmental disabilities. *Womens Health Issues 16*(6), 346–52.

Sarah E. Shannon is an associate professor, biobehavioral nursing and health systems, University of Washington, Seattle.

Teresa A. Savage

➡ **NO**

In Opposition of the Ashley Treatment

Ashley, at age 6 years, had surgery to remove her uterus and breast buds and after recovering from surgery, was placed on high doses of estrogen for 3 years to permanently stunt her linear growth; her parents refer to the surgeries and hormonal medication as the "Ashley treatment." Her parents believed the surgery and medication would improve their daughter's quality of life by keeping her from reaching adult growth in height and weight. Ashley is permanently disabled from a static encephalopathy. She is reported to have the cognitive abilities arrested at a 3-month level. She is unable to move out of the position in which she is placed and prefers not to be in a sitting position but in a lying position. Her parents are devoted to their daughter and say that they made the decision for the "Ashley treatment" in order to keep her at home. They fear that if she grew an anticipated adult height of 5'6" and adult weight, they would be unable to move and carry her and include her in family gatherings.

Her parents described their reasoning in choosing the "Ashley treatment" in their blog (http://ashleytreatment .spaces.live.com/). Within their blog, there are certain assumptions that underlie their reasoning. I challenge these assumptions.

Assumption 1: Keeping Ashley small will improve her quality of life. Her parents listed "bedsores," "pneumonia," and "bladder infection" as reasons for keeping her small and therefore less likely to be "bedridden" and susceptible to those three complications of immobility.

In my experience in caring for premature infants, who are the smallest human beings ex utero, if you do not re-position them, they will get skin breakdown. If you do not use appropriate bedding, they will get skin breakdown. If you do not re-position them and perform pulmonary hygiene, they will get pneumonia. If you do not keep them adequately hydrated with appropriate nourishment, they are at risk for bladder infections. Size is less important as attention to positioning, bedding materials, pulmonary hygiene, nutrition, and elimination.

Ashley will still require total care and keeping her smaller will make it easier to provide her care. Keeping her small makes it physically easier to care for her, which will positively impact the quality of her life. If she was not kept small, she could still have a "good" quality of life, but her care may require more effort. Caregiver effort is no minor factor in Ashley's quality of life; it is perhaps the most critical factor in her quality of life, so I don't think her parents should deny that it was a motivating factor in the decision to use high dose estrogen to stunt her growth.

Assumption 2: Ashley will never bear children so she doesn't need her uterus. It is anticipated that menstrual hygiene will pose a caregiver problem and she may have menstrual cramps.

Do the risks of a hysterectomy outweigh the potential for monthly cramps and bleeding? One might argue that she will be wearing diapers all her life, so what difference does it make if there is urine, stool, or blood in the diaper? She may have discomfort with her periods or she may not. Do the known and real risks of a hysterectomy outweigh the potential risks of her monthly periods?

If she does have skin problems associated with her menses, or she has discomfort that cannot be relieved with medication, she can be treated as any woman is treated— with hormonal therapy to relieve symptoms or to reduce or eliminate menstrual flow. If conservative therapy fails, she could have endometrial ablation or a hysterectomy. Why is it necessary to make this decision at age 6?

Some parents believe that a hysterectomy will protect their child from sexual abuse. A hysterectomy will protect against pregnancy but not molestation, rape, or sexually transmitted diseases.

Assumption 3: Ashley will have large breasts because there is a family history of large breasts, fibrocystic disease, and breast cancer. [It is unclear if she tested positive for the BRCA 1/2 gene. If she has the gene, she's at a greater than average risk for ovarian cancer, so why weren't her ovaries removed too?] Therefore, she is better off having her breast buds removed.

From *Pediatric Nursing Journal*, vol. 33, no. 2, April 2007, pp. 175–178. Reprinted with permission of the publisher, Jannetti Publications, Inc., East Holly Avenue, Box 56, Pitman, NJ 08071-0056; (856) 256-2300; fax: (856) 589-7463; Web site: www.pediatricnursing.net; for a sample copy of the journal, please contact the publisher.

Large breasts can be uncomfortable, although there are many women with large breasts who do not choose to have them removed or even reduced. Her parents worry that her breasts will create difficulties in strapping her into her adaptive seating. A penis and scrotum may present difficulties when positioning boys with the same type and degree of disability as Ashley's, but it has not been suggested that the penis and scrotum be removed because of ease in positioning. A boy with the same disability will not reproduce and can void through a shortened urethra, much like a girl's urethra, and surgery may require minimal cutting. So the same argument about justifying removal of the uterus and breasts could be made to remove a disabled boy's penis and scrotum, but that sounds more like mutilation.

Her parents' blog also maintained that large breasts could "invite" abuse. Parents of children with this level of disability worry about vulnerability to sexual molestation. No surgery or hormonal medicating can prevent molestation, and large breasts do not "invite" abuse. Opportunity and lack of supervision invite abuse. Only close supervision of anyone coming in contact with the vulnerable person can protect against abuse.

Assumption 4: High dose estrogen will cause the growth plates to close, thereby stopping linear growth and concomitant weight gain.

Are the long-term risks of high dose estrogen in a 6-year old girl known? Is it known whether or not the high dose estrogen will reduce growth to the degree that is desired? (Were the breast buds removed because of the possibility for breast cancer with high dose estrogens?) Again, it is disturbing to have healthy tissue removed in anticipation of a problem.

Assumption 5: Adults with a mental age of an infant are undignified.

Adults with profound intellectual disability often do not look like the rest of the population. Their features may be coarse; they may have open mouths, protruding tongues, and drooling. They are often the subject of ridicule by unkind, cruel people. Do the attitudes and behavior of uncouth people warrant surgery and hormonal medicating of the recipient of the bad behavior? The stigma toward people with disabilities has persisted despite community integration, mainstream education, independent living, and the Americans with Disabilities Act. The parents' view of dignity, keeping Ashley's appearance more consistent with her intellectual level, differs from the view of dignity from people in the disability communities. The parents quote a passage in their blog that says "The estrogen treatment is not what is grotesque. Rather, it is the prospect of having a full-grown and fertile woman endowed with a

mind of a baby." It is regrettable if her parents capitulate to the stigma and believe growth attenuation is necessary to preserve their daughter's dignity.

Disability groups have responded to the "Ashley treatment" with a fervor. They view the choices these parents made as a failure of society to provide the support to people with disabilities and their families (American Association on Intellectual and Developmental Disabilities, 2007; Disability Rights Education & Defense Fund, 2007; Not Dead Yet, 2007; Dick Sobsey [parent of a child with a disability and Director of the John Dossetor Health Ethics Centre, University of Alberta], 2007; Feminists Response in Disability Activism, 2007; ADAPT Youth, 2007r; TASH, 2007). They criticize the medical establishment for offering drastic interventions with unknown long-term risks instead of advocating for social changes that would support Ashley and her family.

I have a colleague who talks about "holding families hostage to the revolution." It's unfair to malign this family who acted with medical endorsement in choosing interventions that many people in the disability community find repugnant. They were doing what they thought was best for Ashley and their family and were extremely brave in publicly sharing their experience. However, before the revolution is over, and to afford children like Ashley all the protections that a human being should have, due process should occur when interventions like the "Ashley treatment" is recommended. The child should have an independent advocate to weigh the risks and benefits of the proposed intervention. Preferably, the advocate should be a person with a disability who is better able to envision from a disability perspective what able-bodied parents can never know—what it is like to live with a disability. Albrecht and Devlieger (1999) describe the disability paradox where people with moderate to severe disabilities report a good or excellent quality of life. The parents' projection of Ashley's quality of life may be conflated with the projection of their own or their family's quality of life. They fear the effects of the "unending work" (to borrow from Corbin and Strauss, 1988) on their lives and, in turn, believe it will adversely affect Ashley's quality of life. It seems the vast majority of disability activists strongly oppose the "Ashley treatment." I wonder if her parents viewed it as the lesser of two evils.

References

ADAPT Youth. (2007). ADAPT Youth appalled at parents surgically keeping disabled daughter childlike. . . .

Albrecht, G. L., & Devlieger, P. J. (1999). The disability paradox: High quality of life against all odds. *Social Science & Medicine, 48,* 977–988.

American Association on Intellectual and Developmental Disabilities. (2007). Unjustifiable non-therapy: A response to Gunther & Diekema (2006), and to the issue of growth attenuation for young people on the basis of disability. . . .

Corbin, J., & Strauss, A. (1988). *Unending work and care: Managing chronic illness at home.* San Francisco: Jossey-Bass publishers.

Disability Rights Education and Defense Fund. (2007). Modify the system, not the person. . . .

Feminists Response in Disability Activism (FRIDA). (2007). FRIDA demands ethics and accountability from the AMA. . . .

Gunther, D. F., & Diekema, D. S. (2006). Attenuating growth in children with profound developmental disability: A new approach to an old dilemma. *Archives of Pediatric & Adolescent Medicine, 160,* 1013–1017.

Not Dead Yet. (2007). *Not Dead Yet statement on "Growth Attenuation" experimentation.* . . .

Sobsey, D. (2007). Growth attenuation and indirect-benefit rationale. *Ethics and Intellectual Disability: Newsletter of the Network on Ethics and Intellectual Disability, 10*(1), 1–2, 7–8.

TASH. (2007). Attenuating growth. . . .

Turnbull, R., Wehmeyer, M., Turnbull, A., & Stowe, M. (2007). *KU experts examine issues in surgery to halt girl's growth.* . . .

Teresa A. Savage is an associate director, Donnelley Family Disability Ethics Program, Rehabilitation Institute of Chicago, and the assistant professor—research, Department of Maternal-Child Nursing, University of Illinois at Chicago College of Nursing.

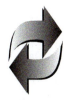

EXPLORING THE ISSUE

May Doctors Offer Medical Drugs and Surgery to Stop a Disabled Child from Maturing?

Critical Thinking and Reflection

1. What would be the best way, in your view, of helping a family care for a severely disabled child? Is the strategy chosen by Ashley's parents an acceptable strategy, in your view, given the help available to them?
2. Dignity is invoked in two different ways by Theresa Savage—as one of the possible reasons for offering the Ashley treatment, and as a reason for prohibiting the treatment. Explain these two uses, and explain which you find more persuasive, if you are drawn to one or the other side.
3. Are there policy options in between banning this kind of intervention and doing nothing to limit its use?

Is There Common Ground?

Ashley is now 14 years old and according to a blog her parents keep about her development and their family life (www.pillowangel.org/), she is happy and doing well. (An earlier blog at http://ashleytreatment.spaces.live.com/blog/ has been discontinued.) The blog contains pictures of Ashley, interviews with the family, and stories about children who have undergone versions of "the Ashley treatment."

Most of the commentaries on the "Ashley treatment" have acknowledged the parents' deep love for their child and their good intentions but have criticized the treatment on several grounds: unknown risks, the possibility of abuse in other cases; focus on the parent's convenience rather than benefit to Ashley; and failure to consider the rights of persons with disabilities.

Edwards, a British philosopher, develops a theme that was common in the initial reaction in 2007 to news about the Ashley treatment. He argues that the treatment sets a worrisome precedent that could be used to justify even more radical interventions. Another kind of reaction, however, is articulated by the bioethicist Erik Parens, who argues that parents' wishes—as well as those expressed by people with disabilities themselves, when they are able to express them—should be respected, as long as their assumptions can be discussed to ensure that they are truly informed.

Additional Resources

Daniel F. Gunther and Douglas A. Diekema, physicians involved in the case, describe their decision-making process in "Attenuating Growth in Children with Profound Developmental Disability: A New Approach to an Old Dilemma," *Archives of Pediatric and Adolescent Medicine* (October 2006).

S.D. Edwards discussion is in "The Ashley Treatment: A Step Too Far, or Not Far Enough?" *Journal of Medical Ethics* (May 2008).

Erik Parens's discussion of the Ashley treatment is "Respecting Children with Disabilities—and Their Parents," *Hastings Center Report* (January–February 2009). It is part of a set of essays on the use of medical technologies to alter children's bodies.

Heather T. Battles and Lenore Manderson emphasize the importance of medical anthropological research on the meanings of personhood and childhood disability, autonomy, and the ethics of body modification surgery ("The Ashley Treatment: Furthering the Anthropology of/on Disability," *Medical Anthropology* [vol. 27, no. 3, July 2008]).

N. Tan and I. Brassington look at the Ashley treatment from the viewpoint of professional responsibilities and find worrisome aspects ("Agency, Duties, and the 'Ashley Treatment,'" *Journal of Medical Ethics* [vol. 35, 2009]).

After weighing all the arguments, Peter A. Clark and Lauren Vasta conclude that "When solutions exist that allow individuals with severe brain impairments to be cared for without interfering with their natural developmental patterns, then these solutions should always take priority." They recommend a moratorium on the Ashley treatment ("The Ashley Treatment: An Ethical Analysis," *The Internet Journal of Law, Healthcare and Ethics* [vol. 5, no. 1, 2007]).

See also S. Matthew Liao, Julian Savulescu, and Mark Sheehan, "The Ashley Treatment: Best Interests, Convenience, and Parental Decision-Making," *Hastings Center Report* (March–April 2007).

Internet References . . .

Ashley's Blog

http://www.pillowangel.org/

Disability Rights Washington, Ashley treatment: The investigation

http://www.disabilityrightswa.org/ashley-treatment
-investigation

The Hastings Center

http://www.thehastingscenter.org/

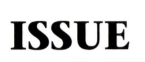

Selected, Edited, and with Issue Framing Material by:
Gregory E. Kaebnick, *The Hastings Center*

ISSUE

Should Scientists Create Artificial Living Things?

YES: The President's Commission for the Study of Bioethical Issues, from "New Directions: The Ethics of Synthetic Biology and Emerging Technologies" bioethics.gov (2010)

NO: Friends of the Earth et al., from "The Principles for the Oversight of Synthetic Biology," foe.org (2012)

Learning Outcomes

After reading this issue, you will be able to:

- Discuss "synthetic biology" and the ethical questions it raises.
- Explain and begin to evaluate the idea of a precautionary approach to new technologies and other endeavors.
- Identify regulatory strategies for limiting the risks of emerging technologies.

ISSUE SUMMARY

YES: The President's Commission for the Study of Bioethical Issues, a bioethics commission created by President Obama, calls for developing the field of synthetic biology, a branch of biological science that aims at genetically modifying organisms to carry out medical, industrial, and other tasks, with "prudent vigilance."

NO: Friends of the Earth, International Center for Technology Assessment, and the ETC Group, leading a group of civil society organizations, counter by recommending a "precautionary" approach and calling for a moratorium on the release and commercial use of synthetic organisms.

On May 20, 2010, the J. Craig Venter Institute (JCVI) announced that it had engineered the "first self-replicating synthetic bacterial cell." This achievement was described in some media reports as "creating life" or "playing God." Although the achievement was indeed significant, the self-replicating cell involved the complete replacement of genetic material, including more than one million base pairs of DNA and almost 1,000 genes. Most careful commentators held that JCVI had not created life; it had instead synthesized a cell's genome and inserted it into an existing cell. Possibly, however, researchers following in JCVI's footsteps will someday manage to do something that looks more like creating life.

JCVI's "synthetic cell" represents one of several lines of work in a field called "synthetic biology." JCVI

is working on synthesizing whole cellular genomes. Others in synthetic biology are working on creating short, standardized genetic sequences that can be put together in various combinations and inserted to do useful or interesting things. Others start with existing organisms such as *Escherichia coli* and modify their metabolisms. Still others are intent on creating living organisms using entirely new kinds of materials, rather than borrowing from existing life forms.

Much work in synthetic biology can also be viewed as essentially an extension of genetic engineering, that is, of the modification of biological systems by inserting genes from other sources and combining them in new ways. But if scientists succeed in creating new kinds of living organisms, it seems to bring biotechnological control over life to a whole new level. As Joachim Boldt and Oliver

Müller from Freiburg University explain, "If we look at nature through the glasses of genetic engineering, we see a world filled with entities that are already useful to us in many respects and that just need some reshaping here and there to perfectly match our interests. In contrast, synthetic biology does not soften edges, but creates life-forms that are meant not to have any edges from the start. . . . Nature is a blank space to be filled with whatever we wish" (*Nature Biotechnology*, April 2008, p. 388).

These new microorganisms will be designed to serve a specific purpose, such as creating new biofuels or clean water. There are potential medical uses as well, such as developing new medications or destroying cancer cells. Synthetic biology has accelerated in recent years because of the increased sophistication and power of genetic sequencing technologies. At the same time, these technologies have become much cheaper. The basic components are readily available.

The introduction of a new technology raises both hopes and fears. While many scientists see enormous possibilities in synthetic biology, others worry about the risk that the engineered cell will escape the laboratory, cause environmental havoc, or be used by terrorists. Other worries are more philosophical—that the very enterprise will somehow imperil other important societal values, such as environmentalism and protection of nature.

This discussion has historical roots. In the early 1970s, when genetic engineering was introduced, the scientists who had developed the ability to splice and combine genes were themselves concerned about the implications, primarily risk to laboratory workers. They agreed on a voluntary moratorium on conducting the most dangerous experiments and convened a conference at Asilomar in Pacific Grove, California, in 1975 to discuss the potential hazards. They lifted the moratorium but established safety guidelines, including containment standards and a review system. Over the years, with the benefit of extensive experience, scientists and government agencies have modified the restrictions. One of the current questions is whether existing government oversight for genetic engineering is adequate for synbio. The President's Commission for the Study of Bioethical Issues acknowledges the unknowns but concludes that on balance the potential benefits of synthetic biology outweigh the risks and that the risks are manageable. A coalition of civil society groups led by Friends of the Earth, International Center for Technology Assessment, and the ETC Group argues that the risks require strong oversight, and that a moratorium on the release and commercial use of synthetic organisms is appropriate until the oversight mechanisms are in place. Underlying these contrasting recommendations are opposed views about how to assess risks and potential benefits, with the President's Commission recommending "prudent vigilance" and the civil society groups calling for "precaution."

YES ↵

The President's Commission for the Study of Bioethical Issues

New Directions: The Ethics of Synthetic Biology and Emerging Technologies

The 21st century is widely heralded as the century of biology. Building on the fundamental understanding achieved in the second half of the last century, revolutionary advances are expected to improve many aspects of our lives, from clean energy and targeted, safer medicines to new industries. Prominent among emerging technologies is "synthetic biology," which aims to apply standardized engineering techniques to biology and thereby create organisms or biological systems with novel or specialized functions to address countless needs.

The idea of managing or manipulating biology to identify or develop specific characteristics is not new. Scientists have used DNA to create genetically engineered cells and organisms for many years; the entire biotechnology industry has grown around our expanding abilities in this area. The shelves of grocery stores across the United States are stocked with genetically engineered foods. Medical testing for genetically linked diseases is widely used by people across society.

By contrast, the idea of assembling living organisms wholesale from non-living parts has intrigued human imagination for centuries with no success outside of fiction. For some, that possibility came one step closer last May with the announcement that scientists at the J. Craig Venter Institute had created the world's first self-replicating synthetic (human-made from chemical parts) genome in a bacterial cell of a different species. Intense media coverage followed, and the announcement ricocheted across the globe within hours as proponents and critics made striking claims about potential risks and benefits of this discovery and whether it amounted to an early-stage example of "creating life."

In response, President Barack Obama asked the Presidential Commission for the Study of Bioethical Issues (the Commission) to review the developing field of synthetic biology and identify appropriate ethical boundaries to maximize public benefits and minimize risks. The

Commission approached this task through inclusive and deliberative engagement with a wide variety of sources, including scientists, engineers, faith-based and secular ethicists, and others who voiced, as expected, sometimes conflicting views on the science, ethics, and social issues surrounding synthetic biology. Through public meetings in Washington, D.C., Philadelphia, and Atlanta, the Commission created a forum for open dialogue to hear and assess competing claims about the science, ethics, and public policy relating to synthetic biology.

What the Commission found is that the Venter Institute's research and synthetic biology are in the early stages of a new direction in a long continuum of research in biology and genetics. The announcement last May, although extraordinary in many ways, does not amount to creating life as either a scientific or a moral matter. The scientific evidence before the Commission showed that the research relied on an existing natural host. The technical feat of synthesizing a genome from its chemical parts so that it becomes self-replicating when inserted into a bacterial cell of another species, while a significant accomplishment does not represent the creation of life from inorganic chemicals alone. It is an indisputable fact that the human-made genome was inserted into an already living cell. The genome that was synthesized was also a variant of the genome of an already existing species. The feat therefore does not constitute the creation of life, the likelihood of which still remains remote for the foreseeable future. What remains realistic is the expectation that over time research in synthetic biology may lead to new products for clean energy, pollution control, and more affordable agricultural products, vaccines, and other medicines. The Commission therefore focused on the measures needed to assure the public that these efforts proceed with appropriate attention to social, environmental, and ethical risks.

President Obama gave the Commission a rare and exceptional opportunity in the world of presidential bioethics commissions to be forward looking instead of

Presidential Commission for the Study of Bioethical Issues, December 2010. Web site: "http://www.bioethics.gov"

reactive. We are ahead of the emerging science, and this unique opportunity underscores the need for the government to act now to ensure a regular, ongoing process of review as the science develops. The Commission calls on the government to make its efforts transparent, to monitor risks, to support (through a peer-review process) the most publicly beneficial research, and to educate and engage with the public as this field progresses. The government must regularly review risk assessment and other issues as the science of synthetic biology progresses. Only through openness and active engagement with all the relevant communities will the government ensure ongoing public support and appropriate oversight. The Commission emphasizes the need to engage the public over time through improved science education, a publicly accessible fact-checking mechanism for prominent advances in biotechnology, and other efforts promoting clearer communication on the state of science.

Basic Ethical Principles for Assessing Emerging Technologies

To reach its recommendations, the Commission identified five ethical principles relevant to considering the social implications of emerging technologies: (1) public beneficence, (2) responsible stewardship, (3) intellectual freedom and responsibility, (4) democratic deliberation, and (5) justice and fairness. The principles are intended to illuminate and guide public policy choices to ensure that new technologies, including synthetic biology, can be developed in an ethically responsible manner.

The ideal of *public beneficence* is to act to maximize public benefits and minimize public harm. This principle encompasses the duty of a society and its government to promote individual activities and institutional practices, including scientific and biomedical research, that have great potential to improve the public's well-being. Public beneficence requires that when seeking the benefits of synthetic biology, the public and its representatives be vigilant about risks and harms, standing ready to revise policies that pursue potential benefits with insufficient caution.

The principle of *responsible stewardship* reflects a shared obligation among members of the domestic and global communities to act in ways that demonstrate concern for those who are not in a position to represent themselves (e.g., children and future generations) and for the environment in which future generations will flourish or suffer. Responsible stewardship recognizes the importance of citizens and their representatives thinking and acting collectively for the betterment of all. Importantly, it calls

for *prudent vigilance*, establishing processes for assessing likely benefits along with assessing safety and security risks both before and after projects are undertaken. A responsible process will continue to assess safety and security as technologies develop and diffuse into public and private sectors. It will also include mechanisms for limiting their use when necessary.

Democracies depend on *intellectual freedom* coupled with the *responsibility* of individuals and institutions to use their creative potential in morally accountable ways. Sustained and dedicated creative intellectual exploration begets much of our scientific and technological progress. While many emerging technologies raise "dual use" concerns—when new technologies intended for good may be used to cause harm—these risks alone are generally insufficient to justify limits on intellectual freedom. As a corollary to the principle of intellectual freedom and responsibility, the Commission endorses a principle of *regulatory parsimony*, recommending only as much oversight as is truly necessary to ensure justice, fairness, security, and safety while pursuing the public good. This is particularly important in emerging technologies, which by their very definition are still in formation and are not well suited for sharply specified limitations. While clear guidelines to protect biosecurity and biosafety are imperative, undue restriction may not only inhibit the distribution of new benefits, but it also may be counterproductive to security and safety by preventing researchers from developing effective safeguards.

The principle of *democratic deliberation* reflects an approach to collaborative decision making that embraces respectful debate of opposing views and active participation by citizens. It calls for individuals and their representatives to work toward agreement whenever possible and to maintain mutual respect when it is not. Public discussion and debate with open interchange among all stakeholders can promote the perceived legitimacy of outcomes, even if those outcomes are unlikely to satisfy all interested parties. An inclusive process of deliberation, informed by relevant facts and sensitive to ethical concerns, promotes an atmosphere for debate and decision making that looks for common ground wherever possible and seeks to cultivate mutual respect where irreconcilable differences remain. It encourages participants to adopt a societal perspective over individual interests.

The principle of *justice and fairness* relates to the distribution of benefits and burdens across society. Biotechnology and emerging technologies such as synthetic biology, for good or ill, affect all persons. Emerging technologies like synthetic biology will have global impacts. For this reason, every nation has a responsibility to champion fair and just systems to promote wide availability of information and fairly distribute the burdens and benefits of new technologies.

Recommendations

With these guiding principles in mind, the Commission considered the array of public policy issues surrounding the emerging science of synthetic biology and makes the following recommendations. The reasons behind each recommendation are provided in the body of the report, and all readers are urged to consider carefully this more comprehensive account. In the cases of recommendations 1, 3, 5, 9, 11, 12, and 17, the Commission recommends ongoing review by the government, in consultation with the relevant scientific, academic, international, and public communities, with initial action completed within 18 months and made public. Some of these actions could easily be completed sooner, and the government is encouraged to do so and make its progress public.

Promoting Public Beneficence

Under the principle of public beneficence, the Commission recommends that the government review and make public findings regarding the scope of its research funding, especially for risk assessment and ethical and social issues raised by synthetic biology. This will promote public engagement and ensure needed transparency regarding federal efforts in the field of synthetic biology.

Recommendation 1: Public Funding Review and Disclosure

Through a central body such as the Executive Office of the President, the federal government should undertake a coordinated evaluation of current public funding for synthetic biology activities, including funding for research on techniques for risk assessment and risk reduction, and for the study of ethical and social issues raised by synthetic biology. This review should be completed within 18 months and the results made public.

Most potential products of synthetic biology are in very early stages of development. Therefore, basic research is critical to further expansion of this science and its effective translation into useful products. Necessary funding decisions should be made with the goal of advancing the public good, whether these decisions support synthetic biology research or other fields. The Commission does not offer an opinion on the relative merits of particular

research directions, but recommends that such decisions receive ongoing evaluation as to the state of the science and its potential applications.

Recommendation 2: Support for Promising Research

Advancing the public good should be the primary determinant of relative public investment in synthetic biology versus other scientific activities. The National Institutes of Health, the Department of Energy, and other federal agencies should continue to evaluate research proposals through peer-review mechanisms and other deliberative processes created to ensure that the most promising scientific research is conducted on behalf of the public.

Information sharing is a critical mechanism for promoting scientific progress and innovation. The principle of public beneficence requires researchers, inventors, patent holders, and others to work together to develop creative strategies to maximize opportunities for innovation. The government should consider best practices and other policy guidance, if needed, to ensure that access to basic research results and tasks is not unduly limited.

Recommendation 3: Innovation Through Sharing

Synthetic biology is at a very early stage of development, and innovation should be encouraged. The Executive Office of the President, as part of the coordinated approach urged in Recommendation 4, should lead an effort to determine whether current research licensing and sharing practices are sufficient to ensure that basic research results involving synthetic biology are available to promote innovation, and, if not, whether additional policies or best practices are needed. This review should be undertaken with input from the National Institutes of Health, other agencies funding synthetic biology research, such as the Department of Energy and the National Aeronautics and Space Administration, the U.S. Patent and Trademark Office, industry, academia, and public civil society groups. The review should be completed within 18 months and the results made public.

Promoting Responsible Stewardship

The Commission endorses neither a moratorium on synthetic biology until all risks are identified and mitigated, nor unfettered freedom for scientific exploration. Instead, the Commission believes that the field of synthetic biology can proceed responsibly by embracing a middle ground—an ongoing process of prudent vigilance that carefully monitors, identifies, and mitigates potential and realized harms over time. Responsible stewardship requires clarity, coordination, and accountability across the government. While new agencies, offices, or authorities are not necessary at this time, the Executive Office of the President should lead an interagency process to identify and clarify, if needed, existing oversight authorities and ensure that the government is informed on an ongoing basis about developments, risks, and opportunities as this field grows. This process must be undertaken by an office with sufficient authority to bring together all parts of the government with a stake in synthetic biology and be sufficiently authoritative to effectively engage or oversee engagement with foreign governments.

Recommendation 4: Coordinated Approach to Synthetic Biology

The Commission sees no need at this time to create additional agencies or oversight bodies focused specifically on synthetic biology. Rather, the Commission urges the Executive Office of the President, in consultation with relevant federal agencies, to develop a clear, defined, and coordinated approach to synthetic biology research and development across the government. A mechanism or body should be identified to: (1) leverage existing resources by providing ongoing and coordinated review of developments in synthetic biology, (2) ensure that regulatory requirements are consistent and non-contradictory, and (3) periodically and on a timely basis inform the public of its findings. Additional activities for this coordinating body or process are described in other recommendations.

Because synthetic biology poses some unusual potential risks, as "amateur" or "do-it-yourself" (DIY) scientists and others outside of traditional research environments explore the field, these risks must be identified and anticipated, as they are for other emerging technologies, with systems and policies to assess and respond to them while supporting work toward potential benefits.

Recommendation 5: Risk Assessment Review and Field Release Gap Analysis

Because of the difficulty of risk analysis in the face of uncertainty—particularly for low-probability, potentially high-impact events in an emerging field—ongoing assessments will be needed as the field progresses. Regulatory processes should be evaluated and updated, as needed, to ensure that regulators have adequate information. As part

of the coordinated approach urged in Recommendation 4, the Executive Office of the President should convene an interagency process to discuss risk assessment activities, including reasons for differences and strategies for greater harmonization across the government. It should also identify any gaps in current risk assessment practices related to field release of synthetic organisms. These reviews should be completed within 18 months and the results made public.

Coordination and careful risk analysis are essential steps for responsible stewardship, but they are not sufficient. There are several additional approaches, which are known today and continue to evolve as our abilities in this field grow, to limit uncertain risks in synthetic biology. Technology can be harnessed to build in safeguards. A number of safety features can be incorporated into synthetic organisms to control their spread and life span. Surveillance or containment of synthetic organisms is a concrete way to embrace responsible stewardship.

Recommendation 6: Monitoring, Containment, and Control

At this early stage of development, the potential for harm through the inadvertent environmental release of organisms or other bioactive materials produced by synthetic biology requires safeguards and monitoring. As part of the coordinated approach urged in Recommendation 4, the Executive Office of the President should direct an ongoing review of the ability of synthetic organisms to multiply in the natural environment and identify, as needed, reliable containment and control mechanisms. For example, "suicide genes" or other types of self-destruction triggers could be considered in order to place a limit on their life spans. Alternatively, engineered organisms could be made to depend on nutritional components absent outside the laboratory, such as novel amino acids, and thereby controlled in the event of release.

The timing of deliberate release of synthesized organisms into the environment and the need to analyze risks prior to release raises special concern. We must proceed carefully, particularly when the probability or magnitude of risks are high or highly uncertain, because biological organisms may evolve or change after release. For any field release, there must be adequate consideration of risk.

Recommendation 7: Risk Assessment Prior to Field Release

Reasonable risk assessment should be carried out, under the National Environmental Policy Act or other applicable law, prior to field release of research organisms or commercial products involving synthetic biology technology. This assessment should include, as appropriate, plans for staging introduction or release from contained laboratory settings. Exceptions in limited cases could be considered, for example, in emergency circumstances or following a finding of substantial equivalence to approved products. The gap analysis described in Recommendation 5 should determine whether field release without any risk assessment is permissible and, if so, when.

Synthetic biology is an international enterprise. Oversight and regulatory mechanisms should adopt an analogous approach, so that the United States is involved in regular discussions with other national and transnational organizations so they may seek coordination and consistency when possible.

Recommendation 8: International Coordination and Dialogue

Recognizing that international coordination is essential for safety and security, the government should act to ensure ongoing dialogue about emerging technologies such as synthetic biology. As part of the coordinated approach urged in Recommendation 4, the Executive Office of the President, through the Department of State and other relevant agencies such as the Department of Health and Human Services and the Department of Homeland Security, should continue and expand efforts to collaborate with international governments, the World Health Organization, and other appropriate parties, including international bioethics organizations, to promote ongoing dialogue about emerging technologies such as synthetic biology as the field progresses.

Responsible conduct of synthetic biology research, like all areas of biological research, rests heavily on the behavior of individual scientists. Creating a culture of responsibility in the synthetic biology community could do more to promote responsible stewardship in synthetic biology than any other single strategy. There are actors in the world of synthetic biology, namely engineers, chemists, materials scientists, computer modelers, and others, who practice outside of conventional biological or medical research settings. These groups may not be familiar with the standards for ethics and responsible stewardship that are commonplace for those working in biomedical research. This poses a new challenge regarding the need to educate and inform synthetic biologists in all communities about their responsibilities and obligations, particularly with regard to biosafety and biosecurity.

Recommendation 9: Ethics Education

Because synthetic biology and related research cross traditional disciplinary boundaries, ethics education similar or superior to the training required today in the medical and clinical research communities should be developed and required for all researchers and student-investigators outside the medical setting, including in engineering and materials science. As part of the coordinated approach urged in Recommendation 4, the Executive Office of the President, in consultation with the National Academy of Sciences, the National Academy of Engineering, the scientific community, and the public, should convene a panel to consider appropriate and meaningful training requirements and models. This review should be completed within 18 months and the results made public.

Additionally flowing from the principle of responsible stewardship, the Commission observed that careful and deliberate attention should be paid to discussions of potential moral objections as the field advances. Such moral objections include concerns that synthetic biology may conflict with essential conceptions of human agency and life; that its overall impact may be harmful to biodiversity, ecosystems, or food and energy supplies; and that it may fail to respect the proper relationship between humans and nature. The Commission devoted particular time and attention to discussing these possible moral objections during its deliberations. It heard relatively few objections from religious or secular ethicists concerning the present status of the field. Although the field currently is capable of significant but limited technical achievements, potential developments might raise further moral objections—for example, applications relying on the synthesis of genomes for higher order or complex species. Current objections to synthetic biology on moral grounds are often based on concerns regarding activities that the field is currently incapable of carrying out. however, continued evaluation and efforts to reach and maintain consensus will be needed as this field develops.

Recommendation 10: Ongoing Evaluation of Objections

Discussions of moral objections to synthetic biology should be revisited periodically as research in the field advances in novel directions. Reassessment of concerns regarding the implications of synthetic biology for humans, other species, nature, and the environment should track the ongoing development of the field. An iterative, deliberative process, as described in Recommendation 14, allows for the careful consideration of moral objections to synthetic biology, particularly if fundamental changes occur in the capabilities of this science and its applications.

Promoting Intellectual Freedom and Responsibility

The principle of intellectual freedom and responsibility asserts that restrictions on research, whether by self-regulation by scientists or by government intervention, should limit the free pursuit of knowledge only when the perceived risk is too great to proceed without limit. A moratorium at this time on synthetic biology research would inappropriately limit intellectual freedom. Instead, the scientific community—in academia, government and the private sector—should continue to work together to evaluate and respond to known and potential risks of synthetic biology as this science evolves. This effort may require the government to expand current oversight or engagement activities with non-institutional researchers. National Institutes of health or the Department of Energy, for example, could be charged to sponsor education programs and workshops that bring together these groups. They could fund training grants or related programs to promote a culture of responsibility among this community. To exercise the appropriate level of oversight, the government will need to monitor the growth and capacity of researchers outside of institutional settings.

Recommendation 11: Fostering Responsibility and Accountability

The government should support a continued culture of individual and corporate responsibility and self-regulation by the research community, including institutional monitoring, enhanced watchfulness, and application of the *National Institutes of Health Guidelines for Recombinant DNA Research*. As part of the coordinated approach urged in Recommendation 4, the Executive Office of the President should evaluate, and re-evaluate periodically, the effectiveness of current research oversight mechanisms and determine what, if any, additional steps should be taken to foster accountability at the institutional level without unduly limiting intellectual freedom. Academic and private institutions, the public, the National Institutes of Health, and other federal funders of synthetic biology research should be engaged in this process. An initial assessment should be completed within 18 months and the results made public.

The norms of safe and responsible conduct that have evolved over time for many researchers in institutional settings may not be understood or followed by those new to the field or outside of these settings. It is important to note that presently there appears to be no serious risk of completely novel organisms being constructed in non-institutional settings including in the DIY community. Scrutiny is required to ensure that DIY scientists have an adequate understanding of necessary constraints to protect public safety and security, but at present the Commission sees no need to impose unique limits on this group.

Recommendation 12: Periodic Assessment of Security and Safety Risks

Risks to security and safety can vary depending on the setting in which research occurs. Activities in institutional settings, may, though certainly do not always, pose lower risks than those in non-institutional settings. At this time, the risks posed by synthetic biology activities in both settings appear to be appropriately managed. As the field progresses, however, the government should continue to assess specific security and safety risks of synthetic biology research activities in both institutional and non-institutional settings including, but not limited to, the "do-it-yourself" community. As part of the coordinated approach urged in Recommendation 4, the Executive Office of the President, working with the Department of Homeland Security, the Federal Bureau of Investigation and others, should undertake and periodically update this assessment. An initial review should be completed within 18 months and the results made public to the extent permitted by law.

Certain risks—generally involving national security—often warrant additional protections. Completely free exchange of data and materials might endanger public safety, but unilateral action to limit exchange could damage American research efforts in synthetic biology if U.S. scientists and students are excluded from full collaboration with the international community. Several recent advisory groups have recommended ongoing discussions among research universities, industry, and government on this topic. The Commission agrees that scientists should be actively engaged in these debates.

Recommendation 13: Oversight Controls

If the reviews called for in Recommendation 12 identify significant unmanaged security or safety concerns, the government should consider making compliance with certain oversight or reporting measures mandatory for all researchers, including those in both institutional and non-institutional settings, regardless of funding sources. It may also consider revising the Department of Commerce's export controls. Any such change should be undertaken only after consultation with the scientific, academic, and research communities and relevant science and regulatory agencies such as the National Institutes of Health, the Department of Homeland Security, and the Environmental Protection Agency. Export controls should not unduly restrain the free exchange of information and materials among members of the international scientific community.

Promoting Democratic Deliberation

Through democratic deliberation, questions about synthetic biology can be explored and evaluated on an ongoing basis in a manner that welcomes the respectful exchange of opposing views. This principle yields several opportunities for government and non-government actors alike to work together to ensure that synthetic biology advances in ways that respect divergent views and that avoid some of the misunderstanding and confusion, which at times, have hampered other scientific endeavors. To enhance democratic deliberation and thereby ensure that the progress in synthetic biology is widely understood and policy choices are thoughtfully considered, the Commission makes the following recommendations.

Recommendation 14: Scientific, Religious, and Civic Engagement

Scientists, policy makers, and religious, secular, and civil society groups are encouraged to maintain an ongoing exchange regarding their views on synthetic biology and related emerging technologies, sharing their perspectives with the public and with policy makers. Scientists and policy makers in turn should respectfully take into account all perspectives relevant to synthetic biology.

Recommendation 15: Information Accuracy

When discussing synthetic biology, individuals and deliberative forums should strive to employ clear and accurate language. The use of sensationalist buzzwords and phrases such as "creating life" or "playing God" may initially increase attention to the underlying science and its implications for society, but ultimately such words impede ongoing understanding of both the scientific and ethical issues at the core of public debates on these topics. To further promote public education and discourse, a

mechanism should be created, ideally overseen by a private organization, to fact-check the variety of claims relevant to advances in synthetic biology.

This publicly accessible fact-check mechanism is among the most concrete ways by which public perception and acceptance of emerging technologies could be improved. Education also plays a key role in building public support for otherwise unfamiliar technologies. In light of our Nation's dependence on socially responsible scientific innovation for economic progress and individual well-being, the urgency of expanding effective science and ethics education cannot be exaggerated. Dialogue among individuals and public, private, and community groups demonstrates that science and its oversight do not belong exclusively to experts, highly trained professionals, or government officials. Science is a shared resource, affecting and belonging to all citizens.

Recommendation 16: Public Education

Educational activities related to synthetic biology should be expanded and directed to diverse populations of students at all levels, civil society organizations, communities, and other groups. These activities are most effective when encouraged and supported by various sources, not only government, but also private foundations and grassroots scientific and civic organizations. As part of the coordinated approach urged in Recommendation 4, the Executive Office of the President, with input from the scientific community, the public, and relevant private organizations, should identify and widely disseminate strategies to promote overall scientific and ethical literacy, particularly as related to synthetic biology, among all age groups.

Promoting Justice and Fairness

The principle of justice and fairness, at this very early stage of synthetic biology, yields two general recommendations that can be applied to both this technology and other emerging technologies. It directs those in government to consider rules for distribution of risks and benefits in research, and it directs those both in and outside of government to consider processes for just distribution of benefits and risks.

Recommendation 17: Risks in Research

Risks in research should not be unfairly or unnecessarily borne by certain individuals, subgroups, or populations. As part of the coordinated approach urged in Recommendation 4, the Executive Office of the President should lead an interagency evaluation of current requirements and alternative models to identify mechanisms that ensure that the risks of research in synthetic biology, including for human subjects and other affected parties, are not unfairly or unnecessarily distributed. Relevant scientific, academic, and research communities, including those in the private sector, should be consulted. This review should be completed within 18 months and the results made public.

Recommendation 18: Risks and Benefits in Commercial Production and Distribution

Risks to communities and the environment should not be unfairly distributed. Manufacturers and others seeking to use synthetic biology for commercial activities should ensure that risks and potential benefits to communities and the environment are assessed and managed so that the most serious risks, including long-term impacts, are not unfairly or unnecessarily borne by certain individuals, subgroups, or populations. These efforts should also aim to ensure that the important advances that may result from this research reach those individuals and populations who could most benefit from them. As part of the coordinated approach urged in Recommendation 4, the Executive Office of the President should evaluate current statutory mandates or regulatory requirements for distribution of risks and benefits and consider developing guidance materials and voluntary recommendations to assist manufacturers as appropriate.

In summary, the ability to easily manufacture and manipulate DNA in the laboratory has enhanced scientists' productivity and opened new directions for scientific exploration. In the future, scientists may be able to create entirely new organisms and systems previously unknown in the world today. But breakthroughs such as this raise a host of complex and sometimes controversial issues. They can help humanity in many ways, but they invariably carry some risks and often raise public concerns and fears. With these unprecedented achievements comes an obligation to consider carefully both the promise and potential perils that they could realize.

The recommendations detailed in this report provide a publicly accountable basis for ensuring that the field of synthetic biology advances to improve human health and public welfare with processes in place to identify, assess, monitor, and mitigate risks on an ongoing basis as the field matures. Risk assessment should precede field release of the products of synthetic biology. Ongoing assessment and review is required in several areas to avoid unnecessary limits on science and social progress, and to ensure appropriate restrictions to protect individual safety and our shared environment. Ongoing dialogue about concerns regarding the implications of synthetic biology for humans, other species, nature, and the environment should continue as synthetic biology develops from its infancy to a fully mature field of scientific inquiry and innovation.

THE PRESIDENT'S COMMISSION FOR THE STUDY OF BIOETHICAL ISSUES is a presidential advisory body formed by President Barack Obama.

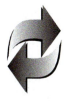

Friends of the Earth et al. → **NO**

The Principles for the Oversight of Synthetic Biology

"**S**ynthetic biology" practitioners begin with computer-assisted biological engineering to design and attempt to construct new biological organisms or biological building blocks, or to redesign existing biological organisms. In building new life forms from scratch using published gene sequence information or by buying inexpensive, made-to-order DNA strands from so-called DNA foundries, synthetic biologists are not just reading and rearranging genetic code, but *writing* it. Synthetic biology is "extreme genetic engineering"—re-engineering and designing genes and creating entire genomes that do not exist in nature as well as designing and building molecules, cell compounds and organelles to desired specifications.

Governments, universities, research institutes and corporations around the world are now racing to develop and commercialize products using synthetic biology. Synthetic biologists have already synthesized working viruses, including the deadly 1918 influenza virus and the poliovirus. In May 2010, the J. Craig Venter Institute announced that its lab had built the first synthetic, self-replicating bacterial cell—that is, researchers inserted an entirely synthetic genome into an existing working cell; the cell accepted the synthetic genome and reproduced. This technical feat is a wake-up call to governments around the world.

Despite industry claims that these technologies are safe, this new technological frontier poses significant health, safety and environmental hazards, as well as profound social, economic and ethical challenges.

The technical ability to synthesize DNA and create synthetic organisms far outpaces our understanding of how these novel products may work. Even engineering supposedly simple organisms could have major ecological and health effects. This unpredictability makes the task of precautionary risk assessment that much more difficult, but also all the more necessary. Research on the effects of these new technologies and synthetic biology-specific regulations must keep pace with the technologies'

development. Commercializing synthetic biology at this stage is premature.

The risks of releasing synthetic organisms into the environment—intentionally or unintentionally—have barely begun to be defined, and the urgently needed ethical, legal and regulatory oversight mechanisms remain undeveloped. Without proper safeguards, we risk letting synthetic organisms and their products out of the laboratory with unknown potential to disrupt ecosystems, threaten human health and undermine social, economic and cultural rights.

This document outlines the following principles necessary for the effective assessment and oversight of the emerging field of synthetic biology:

I. Employ the Precautionary Principle
II. Require mandatory synthetic biology-specific regulations
III. Protect public health and worker safety
IV. Protect the environment
V. Guarantee the right-to-know and democratic participation
VI. Require corporate accountability and manufacturer liability
VII. Protect economic and environmental justice

The Principles

I. Employ the Precautionary Principle

The Precautionary Principle must be applied to synthetic biology because the risks of the technology are inherently unpredictable with potentially far-reaching and irreversible impacts. The Precautionary Principle, integrated into many international conventions and national laws, is aptly described in the Wingspread Consensus Statement on the Precautionary Principle:

> When an activity raises threats of harm to human health or the environment, precautionary measures should be taken even if some cause and effect

relationships are not fully established scientifically. In this context the proponent of an activity, rather than the public, should bear the burden of proof. The process of applying the Precautionary Principle must be open, informed and democratic and must include potentially affected parties. It must also involve an examination of the full range of alternatives, including no action.[iii]

Applying the Precautionary Principle to the field of synthetic biology first necessitates a moratorium on the release and commercial use of synthetic organisms, cells, or genomes until government bodies, with full participation of the public, have:

- Developed a research agenda guided by the public interest.
- Ensured that alternative approaches to synthetic biology applications have fully been considered.
- Conducted full and inclusive assessments of the implications of this technology, including but not limited to devising a comprehensive means of assessing the human health, environmental, and socio-economic impacts of synthetic biology and preventing harms where they are present.
- Developed national and international oversight and security mechanisms equipped to keep pace with the risks as synthetic biology technologies develop.

The Cartagena Protocol on Biosafety provides guidelines for the safe handling, transport and use of any living modified organism.[iv] The 193 nations that are Parties to the UN Convention on Biological Diversity (CBD) agreed at their 10th Conference in 2010 that the release of synthetic biology's products requires precaution. The agreement from the 10th Conference of the Parties reads:

Parties and other Governments [are] to apply the precautionary approach in accordance with the Preamble to the Convention, and the Cartagena Protocol, to the introduction and use of living modified organisms for the production of biofuels as well as to the field release of synthetic life, cell, or genome into the environment, acknowledging the entitlement of Parties, in accordance with domestic legislation, to suspend the release of synthetic life, cell, or genome into the environment.[v]

Additionally, the CBD agreed to study further the risks this technology poses to the environment, biodiversity, livelihoods and human health.

II. Require Mandatory Synthetic Biology-Specific Regulations

Implementing enforceable and prosecutable synthetic biology-specific regulations must be a prior condition for future developments in synthetic biology. Such regulations should complement and strengthen, not replace, any other applicable regulations, such as worker protections, environmental regulations, drug laws and restrictions on pathogens, among others. These regulations should also be considered as a framework for new biotechnology laws as the current regulations around biotechnologies are inadequate and outdated.

Voluntary self-regulation by practitioners is not a substitute for synthetic biology-specific regulations enacted by governments and international treaties. Self-regulation does not allow for oversight or public participation, diminishes transparency and does not provide recourse in the event of worker/public health accidents, environmental disruption or economic harms.

In time, different methods and techniques of synthetic biology may need different forms and levels of oversight. Therefore any new risk assessments, cost-benefit analyses and regulations must flexibly encompass different applications, uses and products. Furthermore, assessments should include full comparative consideration of alternative approaches.

Regulations should specify civil and criminal penalties for violations. Penalties should be imposed for failure to obtain proper licenses, failure to adhere to laboratory standards, unauthorized release of synthetic DNA, RNA, or synthetic organisms, failure to train and equip workers, exposing workers to harm and failure to report adverse incidents to government authorities.

The absence of mandatory synthetic biology-specific regulations necessitates a moratorium on release and commercialization of synthetic organisms, cells or genomes.

III. Protect Public Health and Worker Safety

Adequate and effective synthetic biology oversight requires an immediate emphasis on preventing known and potential human exposures to synthetic organisms that have not been proven safe.

Workers in synthetic biology laboratories will likely be the first to be exposed to any potential hazards. Existing workplace safety procedures and laws must be augmented to take into account the unique risks and challenges to human health posed by organisms created through synthetic biology. Many of the organisms engineered through synthetic biology (e.g., algae) are easily aerosolized and can easily escape confinement or be inhaled. Because these products are imperceptible, workers could unknowingly carry them out of the workplace and into the broader community. Protocols must be in place and strictly adhered to in order to ensure that synthetic organisms and their products are adequately contained.

The public must be informed if such work is being conducted in their community. Workers and the public must be informed of the risks involved with synthetic biology and those working with synthetic organisms must generate clear and reliable means to track, disable and/or destroy strains as a prerequisite to carrying out experiments with them.

Additionally, workers should be allowed to refuse work without fear of retaliation or termination if they report safety concerns regarding the use of synthetic biology products and associated technologies. Workers must have access to qualified safety representatives with whom they can disclose and assess health and environmental safety concerns.

Occupational medical and exposure records must be available to workers and their representatives immediately upon request, and disclosure of such records cannot be withheld as confidential business or trade secret information.

All employees must be notified whenever synthetic biological products are being used within their immediate vicinity or anywhere within their laboratory or workplace.

All containment failures, worker injuries or illnesses, and human exposures must be documented and reported to the proper workplace safety authorities, and details must be available upon request. The public must have prompt access to complete accident reports on government websites, including specific accident locations and the synthetic constructs or organisms involved. The sole exemption should be for personal medical information.

The environmental and health risks of synthetic organisms, their synthetic building blocks and their products must be assessed and disclosed prior to any intended or unintended release or commercial use. Continued systematic disclosure of health and safety information throughout the life cycle of the organism and its products is necessary to improve oversight of government and industry decisions, help people protect themselves, and encourage development of safer alternatives.

The use of synthetic biology to change the human genetic makeup—including the human genome, epigenome and human microbiome—must be prohibited.

The convergence of synthetic biology with other technologies such as gene transfer through viral, nanomaterial or stem cell vectors creates the troubling possibility of altering the human genome. Any alterations to the human genome through synthetic biology—particularly inheritable genetic changes—are too risky and fraught with ethical concerns.

IV: Protect the Environment

Synthetic biology requires the strictest levels of physical, biological and geographic containment as well as independent environmental risk assessment for each proposed activity or product.

Synthetic biology's environmental risks are unknown. In order to identify potential environmental risks and regulatory gaps, governments must require that premarket environmental impact and lifecycle risk assessments are conducted for each distinct synthetic organism, each synthetic construct and each product derived from synthetic organisms and constructs.

The capacity of each synthetic organism to survive in the environment and reproduce must be known before any such organisms leave the laboratory. Unlike most other environmental contaminants that become more diffuse over time, synthetic organisms are designed to reproduce and will evolve. Once released into the environment, these organisms may be impossible to recall or eliminate.

When synthetic organisms are released into the environment, either intentionally or unintentionally, they could find an ecological niche and become a new invasive species that disrupts ecosystems. Moreover, the ability of many microorganisms to take up DNA from living and even dead organisms means that synthetic DNA can be spread in the environment even after the synthetic organism dies.

Confinement strategies for preventing the release of synthetic organisms into the biosphere must include:

1. Means to prevent the whole organism, and its components, from entering and surviving in a receiving environment.
2. Means to prevent gene contamination from the synthetic organism to 'wild' or naturally occurring organisms.

Adequate containment must include:

1. Physical containment to keep the synthetic organism from entering the environment.
2. Geographical containment that only allows growing an organism in a location where it cannot survive in the surrounding environment if it escapes. This also includes locating facilities outside earthquake fault zones, coastal zones where tsunamis

or strong storms could damage the facility, or in flood plains.

3. Biological containment to inhibit the movement of the synthesized organisms, to inhibit the ability of the organism to reproduce outside a contained system, to prevent reproduction once it enters the environment, and to prevent expression of synthesized genetic constructs in other wild-type organisms in the environment.

Some proponents have suggested relying on methods of biological containment originally designed for genetically engineered plants and animals, such as so-called "suicide genes" and other types of self-destruction technologies. These methods are no substitute for physical, geographical and biological containment designed to prevent the release of synthetic organisms. Scientists who have studied "terminator technologies" in seeds have concluded that they are not failsafe. Frequently occurring mutations allow organisms to overcome the intended sterilization, thereby allowing those organisms to remain viable. Specifically, "suicide genes" and other genetic use restriction technologies represent an evolutionary disadvantage; selective pressures will lead organisms to overcome intended biological constraints.[vi] Attempts to develop alternative genetic systems (such as xenobiology[vii], mirror biology[viii] or novel amino acids[ix]) are not well enough understood to claim they provide safety. They should not be tested outside the laboratory.

Importantly, the UN Convention on Biological Diversity has mandated an international moratorium on the use of "terminator technologies," such as "suicide genes," and other genetic use restriction technologies, which has been in place for the past decade. Reliance on an unproven technology that has been deemed unacceptable by 193 nations as a principal method to "contain" synthetic organisms is irresponsible and legally dubious.

Additionally, the intentional release of synthetic organisms into the environment for such things as bioremediation or other applications must be prohibited.

The failure to prioritize (e.g., properly fund) risk relevant environmental impact research[x] necessitates a moratorium on the commercial use of synthetic organisms, cells or genomes and their release into the environment.

V. Guarantee the Right-to-Know and Democratic Participation

Comprehensive public and worker participation should be provided throughout the decision-making processes involving synthetic biology.

Information about human health and environmental effects must be communicated throughout the complete stream of commerce so that all users of products of synthetic biology know the hazards of the organisms and products they use.

Researchers and companies seeking approval for development and commercialization of any products derived from synthetic biology must provide government agencies with the necessary tests to detect synthetic organisms in the case of unintended release or exposure. In addition to requiring synthetic biology researchers to report their activities in detail to the communities in which they work, to their national governments, and publicly on the Internet, researchers must also develop protocols for destroying the organisms when the research is completed and reporting the results to their communities and nations.

All accidental releases into air, water or soil should be reported immediately to the local community and national authorities, and contact information for such reporting must be prominently posted in all laboratories and facilities. Safety data should be available for public inspection on websites and reported to public bodies.

All containers holding synthetic organisms or their synthetic parts should be clearly labeled. Mandatory labeling will help governments track these synthetic organisms. Products, including medicines, vaccines, biofuels and other industrial materials created through synthetic biology should be labeled at all phases—in the lab, while in transport and, if commercialized, on the physical products. Marketing materials and advertisements for these products must state that they are products of synthetic biology.

Closely linked with the right-to-know is our essential right-to-participate in decisions about environmental and societal hazards that affect our lives.

The public must have the legally enforceable right to halt dangerous applications, not just comment after decisions have been made. Governments must provide meaningful involvement for the public and workers throughout the entire decision-making process related to the development of synthetic biology and the products of synthetic biology, including setting the research agenda, the context and the scope of the risk assessment. This includes making sure that communities have access to independent scientific and legal opinions on the proposed projects. Opportunities for participation in decisions on synthetic biology should not be narrowed to only scientific input. Other forms of knowledge including traditional knowledge as well as analysis of cultural, legal, social and economic considerations should also carry weight in decision-making processes.

Public involvement must be open, facilitating equal input from all interested and affected parties around the globe including and especially:

1. Communities that could be impacted—especially poor communities where many of the first commercial facilities using synthetic organisms will be located.[xi]
2. Labor unions and workplace safety groups concerned about exposure.
3. Communities concerned about feedstock procurement, land use and other social, economic and cultural implications (See Principle VII below).

The use of synthetic biology techniques to develop drugs and vaccines is already underway. Data on any health effects from these techniques cannot be considered "confidential business information" by companies and researchers. Additionally, long-term follow-up studies of patients taking synthetic biology-derived medicines or therapies must be mandatory and there must be full disclosure of all the material facts from these studies.

VI. Require Corporate Accountability and Manufacturer Liability for All Products of Synthetic Biology

Those using synthetic biology must be financially and legally accountable for any harm caused to the public, worker health or the environment.

For a product produced through synthetic biology to be placed on and remain in the market, manufacturers must provide all available safety information about the synthetic organism and its products. The information must be sufficient to permit a reasonable evaluation of the safety of the synthetic organism on human health and the environment, including hazard, use and exposure information. This means that if there are no data, the product should not be on the market. Prior to regulatory approval of the products of synthetic biology, developers must demonstrate that they are able to accept the financial and legal liability that could come from manufacture, use and disposal of their products.

Developers of synthetic biology and their funders must establish financial mechanisms, even at the research stage, to assure that adequate funds are available to mitigate and compensate for health, worker or environmental damages. If commercial insurers are unwilling to provide insurance for this purpose, governments should not insure

the developers of synthetic biology. If the risk is too great for private investors, it is too great for the public.

Synthetic biology companies should bear the cost of producing accurate environmental and health safety information. This information must be a precondition for products intended for marketing and be issued before significant quantities of a product are manufactured to assist in protection of workers. Industry should produce data on the earliest phases of the research and development of its products, but full assessments on health and safety should be generated and conducted by governments or independent laboratories at industry expense to ensure the information is publically available and reliable.

Strict standards that prohibit conflicts of interest should be maintained in the oversight of synthetic biology research, including but not limited to prohibiting persons with financial interests in synthetic biology research, development and commercialization from roles in its health and safety oversight.

VII. Protect Economic and Environmental Justice

It is necessary to ensure that the development of synthetic biology does not deepen economic and social injustices.

The impacts that synthetic biology could have on ecosystems and communities in the global South are of special concern. At present, most commercial interest in synthetic biology is focused on enabling a new "biomass-based economy" in which any type of plant matter can be used as feedback for tailored synthetic microbes to transform into high value commercial products—anything from fuels to plastics to industrial chemicals. As major industries shift to biomass-derived feed stocks, larger and larger quantities of plant material will be required. Biomass to feed synthetic microbes will be extracted from or cultivated mostly in the global South, disrupting fragile ecosystems and exacerbating environmental damage from industrial crop production. Further pressure will be placed on land and water resources, already in short supply for food production. There is simply not enough land (or plant matter) for all the uses that are being contemplated. Furthermore, a number of current applications of synthetic biology propose to replace botanical production of natural plant-based commodities (e.g., rubber, plant oils, artemsinin) with vat-based production systems using synthetic microbes or to move production to genetically engineered plants. In time, these substitutions could have devastating economic impacts on farming, fishing and forest communities who depend on natural compounds for their livelihoods. These impacts and the impacts of biomass extraction and associated land grabbing must be considered in any assessment of risk. These assessments must include the full and active participation of the communities that will be impacted.

Corporations have already applied for extremely broadly worded patents on synthetic biology techiniques. If granted, they could give a small number of companies virtual *de facto* monopoly control over entire economic sectors, affecting the rights of small producers, patients (in the case of pharmaceutical patents) and the public at large. Patents on synthetic biology processes, synthetic organisms or products derived from synthetic biology could further the privatization and control of naturally occurring products and processes. Companies and researchers must not be permitted to patent synthetic versions of natural organisms. These patents could open up new avenues for bio-piracy and ways to circumvent access and benefit-sharing agreements. Transparency, public safety and environmental protection must take legal precedence over any patent or intellectual property protections.

Conclusion

Until the above principles are incorporated into international, federal and local law as well as research and industry practices, there must be a moratorium on the release and commercial use of synthetic organisms.

Synthetic biologists predict that new and extreme genetic engineering will usher in dramatic changes in all areas of human life. While some have argued that synthetic biology can be a research tool to better understand biology, it poses significant and unprecedented hazards. The development of synthetic biology without proper oversight and regulation could result in inadequate control over the development of other potentially harmful emerging technologies.

Synthetic biology must, therefore, be accompanied by precautionary mechanisms to safeguard the health of workers and local communities, to preserve the biodiversity of the planet, to ensure public participation, to provide for democratically decided social goals, and to restore public trust in scientific researchers and government regulators. The undersigned organizations call for the governments of the world to incorporate these principles into local, national and international frameworks to provide oversight to this extreme form of biological engineering.

Notes

i. This declaration in no manner limits or binds the signatories from any other relevant actions or statements, including unilateral or joint superseding statements on synthetic biology policy.

Each organization continues to fulfill their respective mission statements in accordance with their own fundamental guiding principles. This joint declaration supplements our organizations' work in this and related areas. This declaration is not intended to be a comprehensive statement of all possible oversight principles or to encompass all subsequent steps needed for their implementation; rather, it is a starting point from which future implementations of oversight policy can build.

ii. See, e.g., RIO DECLARATION ON ENVIRONMENT AND DEVELOPMENT, June 14, 1992, 31 I.L.M. 874, 879 (*"Where there are threats of serious or irreversible damage, lack of full scientific certainty shall not be used as a reason for postponing cost-effective measures to prevent environmental degradation."*); CARTAGENA PROTOCOL ON BIOSAFETY, Jan. 29, 2000, 39 I.L.M. 1027 Art. 10(6) (*"Lack of scientific certainty due to insufficient relevant scientific information and knowledge regarding the extent of the potential adverse effects of a living modified organism on the conservation and sustainable use of biological diversity in the Part of import, taking also into account risks to human health, shall not prevent that party from taking a decision, as appropriate, with regard to the import of the living modified organism in question . . . in order to avoid or minimize such potential adverse effects."*); U.N. FRAMEWORK CONVENTION ON CLIMATE CHANGE, May 9, 1992, 21 I.L.M. 849, (*"The Parties should take precautionary measures to anticipate, prevent or minimize the cause of climate change and mitigate its adverse effects. Where there are threats of serious or irreversible damage, lack of full scientific certainty should not be used as a reason for postponing such measures."*); THE WORLD CHARTER ON NATURE, G.A. Res. 37/7, 11, U.N. Doc. A/RES/37/7 (Oct. 28, 1982) (*"Activities which might have an impact on nature shall be controlled, and the best available technologies that minimize significant risks to nature or other adverse effects shall be used."*); THE LONDON CONVENTION ON THE PREVENTION OF MARINE POLLUTION BY DUMPING WASTES AND OTHER MATTER, 1996 Protocol to the Prevention of Marine Pollution by Dumping of Wastes and Other Matter, Mar. 24, 2006, art. 3, para. 1 (*"Appropriate preventative measures are [to be] taken when there is reason to believe that wastes or other matter introduced into the marine environment are likely to cause harm even when there is no conclusive evidence to provide a causal relation between inputs and their effects."*); AGREEMENT FOR THE IMPLEMENTATION OF THE PROVISIONS OF THE UNITED NATIONS CONVENTION ON THE LAW OF THE SEA OF 10 DECEMBER

1982 RELATING TO THE CONSERVATION AND MANAGEMENT OF STRADDLING FISH STOCKS AND HIGHLY MIGRATORY FISH STOCKS, G. A. 164/37, art. 6, U.N. Doc. A/CONF164/37 ("States shall apply the precautionary approach widely to conservation. . . .").

iii. "The Wingspread Consensus Statement on the Precautionary Principle." Science & Environmental Health Network, 26 Jan. 1998. <http://www.sehn.org/wing.html>.

iv. Text from the Cartagena Protocol to the Convention on Biological Diversity can be viewed here: http://bch.cbd.int/protocol/text/.

v. "COP 10 Decision X/37." *Biofuels and Biodiversity*. UN Convention on Biological Diversity, Oct. 2011. <http://www.cbd.int/decision/cop/?id=12303>.

vi. Steinbrecher, Ricarda A. *V-GURTs (Terminator) as a Biological Containment Tool?* Rep. EcoNexus, June 2005. <http://www.econexus.info/sites/econexus/files/ENx_V-GURTs_brief_2005.pdf>.

vii. Xenobiologists explore the possibility that life might be created without relying on carbon (or water or using the 20 usual amino acids found in life on Earth.

viii. Mirror biology is a biology based on the mirror-image of amino acids. Mirror image molecules were not at first thought to be a problem. That is why the 1960s controversy over the antinausea drug thalidomide was such a surprise—the right-handed version calmed morning sickness in pregnant women, but the left-handed version caused birth defects.

ix. Chemists long have been aware of literally hundreds of amino acids in addition to the normal 20 that make up all protein molecules coded by DNA in biology.

x. For example, Amyris Biotechnologies is currently raising synthetic yeast for the production of biofuels and cosmetics in Brazil. This is to have access to large amounts of cheap sugarcane to feed their yeast.

xi. One study of U.S. and European government funding into synthetic biology research conducted by the Wilson Center's Synthetic Biology Project found that while the U.S. government has spent around $430 million between 2005 and 2010, only 4% of this money went to examine the ethical, legal and social implications of synthetic biology. When researchers searched for projects looking into risk assessment related to potential accidental release of synthetic organisms from a lab or confinement, or risks from intentional release of synthetic organisms they found no such projects. See: "Trends in Synthetic Biology Research Funding in the United States and Europe." *Synthetic Biology Project*. Woodrow Wilson International Center for Scholars, June 2010. Web. <http://www.synbioproject.org/process/assets/files/6420/final_synbio_funding_web2.pdf?>.

FRIENDS OF THE EARTH is a private environmental advocacy organization headquartered in Washington, D.C.

EXPLORING THE ISSUE

Should Scientists Create Artificial Living Things?

Critical Thinking and Reflection

1. If there are significant benefits associated with a new technology, how much risk should be accepted in order to obtain the benefits?
2. How do you understand the idea of "responsible stewardship"?
3. What kinds of activities would satisfy a requirement for "democratic participation" in policy decisions? What sorts of difficulties do you see in carrying out those activities?

Is There Common Ground?

The President's Commission said that it proposed the idea of "prudent vigilance" in order to try to find common ground in the debate about synthetic biology. Opposing sides seemed, in the commission's analysis, to be forming around either a "proactionary" position, according to which those developing the technology should be allowed to experiment with and introduce new products unless there are known risks associated with them (in which case the risks should be ameliorated), or a precautionary position. A strong version of the precautionary approach is often characterized as requiring a moratorium on an endeavor unless the endeavor is known not to have serious risks. Many commentators believe that the strong version can lead to paralysis, given the difficulty of showing that there are no risks. One of the difficulties of examining the precautionary approach is that it has been articulated in a variety of forms, some of which are much more stringent than others.

A call for democratic participation can also be intended to reach for common ground, if it is motivated by the optimistic assumption that crowds can, under the right set of circumstances, work their way through to workable compromises on difficult matters. Of course, crowds may turn out to be no better than experts and advocates at finding common ground. Moreover, a call for democratic participation can also be seen as a battle tactic, rather than an effort to find common ground, insofar as requiring prolonged and difficult public discussion raises further barriers to a technology.

Additional Resources

Omit "New Directions" and "Principles for the Oversight of Synthetic Biology" from the existing list.

The Woodrow Wilson International Center for Scholars offers a variety of resources on synthetic biology at the following website, www.synbioproject.org/.

Bedau's selection is one of a set of essays on synthetic biology that appeared in the *Hastings Center Report* (July–August 2011).

The Boldt and Müller article cited in the Introduction is titled "Newtons of the Leaves of Grass," *Nature Biotechnology* (April 2008).

Jonathan B. Tucker and Raymon A. Zilinskas, "The Promise and Perils of Synthetic Biology," *The New Atlantis,* offers a summary and also a reading list. It is available at www.thenewatlantis.com/publications /the-promise-and-perils-of-synthetic-biology.

Jonathan D. Moreno offers an optimistic view of synthetic biology in "Synthetic Biology Grows Up," *Science Progress* (May 20, 2010), which is available at www.scienceprogress.org/2010/05/synthetic-biology -grows-up.

Internet References . . .

BioBricks Foundation

> http://biobricks.org/

ETC Group

> http://www.etcgroup.org/

The Hastings Center

> http://www.thehastingscenter.org/

The Woodrow Wilson International Center for Scholars: Synthetic Biology Project

> www.synbioproject.org/

Selected, Edited, and with Issue Framing Material by:
Gregory E. Kaebnick, *The Hastings Center*

ISSUE

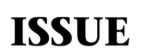

Could Conservation of Wild Species Be Improved through the Use of De-extinction Tools?

YES: Kent H. Redford, William Adams, and Georgina M. Mace, from "Synthetic Biology and Conservation of Nature: Wicked Problems and Wicked Solutions," *Plos Biology* 11 (2013)

NO: Christopher J. Preston, from "De-extinction: A Tale of Two Visions," Center for Humans & Nature (Accessed 2016)

Learning Outcomes

After reading this issue, you will be able to:

- Explain how new biotechnologies can be used to alter the shared environment.
- Discuss the conservation challenge of the current mass extinction.
- Discuss ethical and technical questions that arise in deciding whether to use biotechnologies to create proxies of extinct species.

ISSUE SUMMARY

YES: Kent H. Redford, William Adams, and Georgina M. Mace, who are consultants and researchers working on issues of biodiversity and conservation, propose that synthetic biology, though it is often thought of as providing tool for intervening into nature, can be used as well to protect nature, by aiding in the restoration and protection of species and ecosystems.

NO: Christopher J. Preston, professor of philosophy at University of Montana, counters that biotechnological restoration of a species will cut deeply into environmental values.

Most environmental conservationists believe that a major extinction event has begun on earth—the sixth such event known to have occurred since the beginning of life on earth. The causes of extinctions have been overhunting, pollution, the spread of human-introduced species that threaten existing species, and habitat destruction, but a growing number are expected to be caused by climate change, which is changing species' ranges and leading to rising ocean levels and more acidic ocean water. Most conservationists, dating at least back to Aldo Leopold, accept that humans must manage species in order to save them.

Species management can include, for example, attempting to limit the spread of species that threaten other species (for example, attempting to limit the spread of nonnative insects that threaten tree species in the United States, in reintroducing them where they have gone locally extinct (transporting elk from the Western to the Eastern United States, for example), and sometimes in undertaking expensive and difficult breeding programs (such as with the California condor).

Some conservationists believe that genetic technologies, ranging from crossbreeding programs to highly advanced techniques for genetic engineering and assisted reproduction, may offer new strategies for conserving species. Among the proposals: modifying organisms to tolerate a changed environment (for example, altering coral so that it can withstand warmer and more acidic oceans), modifying organisms to withstand nonnative organisms that attack them (for example, modifying the American chestnut to withstand chestnut blight), and modifying nonnative organisms to reduce the threat they pose to native organisms (for example, modifying nonnative mosquitoes in Hawaii to prevent them from transmitting avian malaria to native Hawaiian birds, which have no immunity to the disease, and modifying nonnative mice and rats on ocean islands to drive them locally into extinction and prevent them from destroying rookeries of ocean birds).

A particularly challenging intervention that some have proposed is the recreation of extinct species. This intervention, which has been dubbed "de-extinction," can sometimes be attempted with crossbreeding, as with a long-standing effort to crossbreeds of cows that are believed to be genetically more closely related to the now-extinct Eurasian aurochs from which they are descended, eventually perhaps producing a line that resembles the aurochs. Sometimes, too, de-extinction can be attempted with cloning techniques: to do this, intact DNA must be recovered from a piece of well-preserved tissue and then inserted into an enucleated egg of a closely related species and brought to term. This strategy has been attempted with the Pyrenean ibex, or bucardo, which was briefly recreated in 2003, although the baby bucardo died after seven minutes due to severe lung deformities. New efforts are reportedly under way both with the bucardo and with the gastric brooding frog. The most ambitious and most difficult de-extinction efforts would involve a mixture of genetic engineering and cloning: if the nuclear DNA of the extinct species can be recreated by genetically modifying the DNA of a closely related species, then it could be used to produce a live animal through cloning. Efforts are under way, with funding from the Long Now Foundation, to recreate the woolly mammoth (creating its genome by modifying an elephant genome) and the passenger pigeon (by modifying the genome of the band-tailed pigeon).

As genetic scientist Beth Shapiro has detailed in her book *How to Clone a Mammoth*, there are many technical hurdles to be overcome to reproduce a mammoth. Genetic engineering on a large scale remains challenging, and cloning has an extremely high failure rate. Identifying the genome of the extinct species is probably an even greater obstacle. And the entire genetic and reproductive process must be successful many times over in order to create a viable population, which must include enough genetic variability to be resistance to disease and environmental threats. Shapiro herself concludes that a mammoth cannot really be cloned, although something somewhat like a mammoth can probably eventually be produced.

Finally, still other challenges must be met if and when the genetic and reproductive challenges are solved: suitable habitat must be available, for example, the threats that first drove the species into extinction must be overcome, and if the species is one that depends on learned behavior, as would be the case for the wooly mammoth and the passenger pigeon, then it must be possible for the newly created animals to learn those behaviors and to reestablish the ecological relationships that initially defined the species. In 2016, a committee formed by the International Union for the Conservation of Nature issued a set of guidelines detailing these challenges and establishing conditions for deciding when de-extinction might be attempted. Many conservationists believe, however, that the challenges are so significant that the recreated species could be at most a proxy for the extinct one-resembling it and perhaps functioning similarly to it in ecosystems, but not perfectly continuing the lost lineage. If these concerns are correct, then the label "de-extinction" is likely misleading.

Another concern among many conservationists is whether de-extinction, and perhaps other technologies for species management, involve a level or kind of human intervention that is inherently at odds with the goals of conservation. This is the concern at the heart of the two readings here. In the first article, a group of authors led by Kent Redford, a conservationist who served at one time with the Wildlife Conservation Society, which runs New York's Bronx Zoo, and is now an independent consultant especially interested in the idea that biotechnologies might be useful for conservation, argues that the threats to species are now so great, and the human impact on nature so great, that there is no turning back from intervention into the natural world. To avoid biotechnological interventions out of a concern about not meddling too deeply in pristine nature would fail to recognize that pristine nature no longer exists, in Redford's view. On the other side of the debate, Christopher J. Preston, professor of philosophy at University of Montana, counters that biotechnological restoration of a species will cut deeply into environmental values.

YES ⬅

Kent H. Redford, William Adams, and Georgina M. Mace

Synthetic Biology and Conservation of Nature: Wicked Problems and Wicked Solutions

Extinction might not be forever if synthetic biologists and others pursue their proposals to use advanced genetic engineering techniques to save endangered species and return extinct ones [1]. This is only the most eye-catching example of a broad engagement that will soon take place between the synthetic biology community and the biodiversity conservation community that may change the relationship between humans and the natural world. Though these communities are strangers to each other now, the work they do and the goals they pursue are in places complementary and in others conflicting but uninformed by each other. A respectful and open discussion between these two communities and society at large is urgent to determine how to proceed on issues that overlap.

Recent international and intergovernmental meetings of the Convention on Biodiversity (CBD) (October 2012) and the International Union for Conservation of Nature (September 2012) have reconfirmed the serious attention the world community is paying to the vital need to conserve the natural world. Commitments made by 94 governments in April 2012 to establish the Intergovernmental Platform on Biodiversity and Ecosystem Services (IPBES) are a tangible response to addressing the ever-increasing threats to global biodiversity, against the approaching beat of a changing climate. These threats have created a set of "wicked problems" [2], that are messy, intractable, subject to multiple interpretations, and for which solutions at present are not evident or inscrutable. Dealing with the causes and consequences of biodiversity loss in a changing environment is one such problem.

Over the past century an array of conservation strategies of increasing sophistication and scope have emerged to address biodiversity loss [3]. The Aichi Biodiversity Strategy, adopted in 2010 by the Conference of the Parties (COP) to the CBD, distills these strategies into a set of 20 targets adopted by the international community. The Strategy is designed to (a) address the underlying causes of biodiversity loss by mainstreaming biodiversity across government and society; (b) reduce the direct pressures on biodiversity and promote sustainable use; (c) improve the status of biodiversity by safeguarding ecosystems, species, and genetic diversity; (d) enhance the benefits to all from biodiversity and ecosystem services; and (e) enhance implementation through participatory planning, knowledge management, and capacity building [4].

The Aichi Targets and Strategic Goals are challenging and will require the full array of tools, techniques and approaches if progress is to be made. Yet, to date both the targets, and the institutional arrangements that support them, are built on an understanding of biodiversity and ideas about conservation strategies developed over the twentieth century, and have barely considered new scientific and engineering prospects such as those found in the emerging field of synthetic biology.

The Presidential Commission for the Study of Bioethical Issues [5] defined synthetic biology as "a scientific discipline that relies on chemically synthesized DNA, along with standardized and automatable processes, to address human needs by the creation of organisms with novel or enhanced characteristics or traits." The field is moving fast [6, 7]. Billions of dollars are being invested globally, and developments of novel applications or improvements of existing ones emerge weekly [8, 9]. Huge claims are routinely made about the potential benefits of synthetic biology: "many of the major global problems, such as famine, disease and energy shortages, have potential solutions in the world of engineered cells" [10]. Lloyds of London's Emerging Risk Group wrote in 2009: "Many believe that Synthetic Biology will be one of the transformative technologies necessary to combat climate change, energy shortages, food security issues and water deficits" [11].

Synthetic biology has the potential to transform many aspects of human economy and society, and the

Redford KH, Adams W, Mace GM (2013) Synthetic Biology and Conservation of Nature: Wicked Problems and Wicked Solutions. PLoS Biol 11(4): e1001530. doi:10.1371/journal.pbio.1001530 environment, not least as a key technology in an emerging "bioeconomy." Citing the impacts of existing biofuel production, some are deeply suspicious of its possible impacts: the ETC Group suggests that "The proposed use of synthetic microbes in the production of the next generation of fuels, medicines and industrial chemicals may massively increase human impact on biodiversity, while accelerating biopiracy and making a mockery of any notion of 'benefit sharing'" [12]. As Marris and Rose [13] observe, when discussing synthetic biology, "utopias and dystopias seem to be the only scenarios possible."

Despite growing general debate, there has been surprisingly limited consideration of the risks or advantages of synthetic organisms to the conservation of biological diversity [14]. In the seven years prior to 2011, some 40 reports (in the English language alone) were published addressing the social, ethical, and legal issues raised by synthetic biology [15]. Ethicists and philosophers have considered the ways synthetic biology may change the relationship between humans and the natural world [16–18], and considerable discussion has taken place about who will be in control of synthetic biology (e.g., [6]). Critics have identified potential dangers of genetically modified organisms on native species, the resilience of natural ecosystems, small-scale producers in developing countries, and public safety [19–22]. Horizon scanning studies have highlighted technologies that involve genetic engineering, such as the transfer of nitrogen-fixing ability to cereals [23].

However, thus far, conservation scientists appear to have paid little attention to synthetic biology as a field of science and technology. Recent surveys in biodiversity science have outlined many of the problems and promises that face the natural world [24–27], yet synthetic biology has gone virtually unnoticed. Noticed or not, change is coming, as the recently completed CBD COP 11 resolved to " . . . consider the potential positive and negative impacts of components, organisms and products resulting from synthetic biology techniques on the conservation and sustainable use of biodiversity"—but only to recommend further study [28].

The limited and timid engagement of conservation science and policy with the development of synthetic biology is unfortunate, because the technology is likely to transform the operating space within which conservation functions, and therefore the prospects for maintaining biodiversity into the future. The shape of this transformation is unclear. There are possibilities that synthetic biology may provide new solutions to established "wicked" problems such as disease affecting wildlife (e.g., [29]) and may alleviate pressure on ecosystems by supplying sustainable food for a future world of 9 billion people. There are also potentially negative impacts on natural and managed

ecosystems and human welfare through the release of novel organisms [19–22]. The potential consequences for biodiversity conservation of even the promise of innovations from synthetic biology are significant. Considering the Aichi Targets (see above), we suggest some plausible consequences of synthetic biology advances for the way that targets are addressed, the side effects of assuming the techniques work, and ultimate impacts on the wild species and habitats for which the targets were devised.

Conservation as a practice has frequently been backwards looking, focusing on reducing loss or on maintaining a status quo, an approach that has clearly not been effective in conserving biodiversity. Potential major shifts in the relationship between humans and nature such as those represented by synthetic biology would be better engaged with early and deeply. Yet of the hundreds of conservation practitioners with whom we have spoken, only a few had even heard of synthetic biology and had any sense of the changes it may bring. In order to expedite the engagement between the two fields, we have organized a meeting entitled "How will synthetic biology and conservation shape the future of nature?" to be held April 9–11, 2013, in Cambridge, United Kingdom (http://www.wcs.org/thefutureofnature). Our hope is that this meeting and this article will ultimately result in a practice of conservation educated about synthetic biology and a practice of synthetic biology educated about the concerns and imperatives of biodiversity conservation.

We do not know what will happen when synthetic biology practice meets conservation practice. There has been some speculation, but data cannot be gathered on what has not yet happened, leaving value-based claims free to proliferate. Yet it is imperative that conservation practitioners engage with synthetic biologists, not only to influence the practice to become "pro-conservation," but also because without such informed engagement it would be too easy for policymakers and politicians to assume that synthetic biology solutions can provide easy fixes to intractable and expensive conservation actions and shift attention and support away from existing efforts such as protected area establishment and strengthening. Biodiversity, ecosystem services, and humans would all suffer from such decisions.

We suggest that conservation needs new thinking and new strategies to cope with the challenges of synthetic biology. We identify here five assertions that we believe highlight key emerging issues that need to be addressed by conservation scientists and practitioners, and institutions such as the CBD and IPBES.

- Extinction may not be forever. There are ongoing attempts to recreate endangered species using the tools of synthetic biology. These include the woolly mammoth, the passenger pigeon, and the thylacine [30]. If successful, would such species be regarded as representatives of the species to which extinct forbears belonged? Or would they be viewed as "invasives from the past" and a threat to existing species? In accounting terms, how would extinction rates in conservation targets deal with recreated species? Currently such experiments are slow and hugely costly, but if such costs fall as some predict (by analogy with the costs and power of computing), such recreations might become routine and affordable. How would choices be made about which species to save? More fundamentally, what conservation value would these forms have if the habitats that once supported them are gone? Might we face the moral hazard whereby confidence in our ability to recreate extinct species undermines our willingness to conserve naturally occurring biodiversity [31]?

- Synthetic life evolves. How will synthetic organisms interact with existing species and how far will such interactions be predictable from current ecological understanding of interspecific interactions? Will they become invasive and damage existing communities, or might they be safe and useful in restoring degraded or polluted ecosystems or address other ecological problems that have been intractable to date? Will the incorporation of synthetic organisms into ecosystems (e.g., through field agriculture, medical application, or accidental release) be seen as adding to the living diversity of the ecosystems in which they are incorporated and, if so, will these be judged as of higher value, or will loss of authenticity mean they are judged degraded [32]? Who will regulate the release of synthetic organisms outside the contained laboratory: will the permissive regulatory environment of "garage biology" be widely endorsed, will national governments try to establish individual regimes, and how will local and international views on the matter be taken into account?

- Our working definition of "natural" is no longer fit for purpose. Much of conservation is based on conserving ecosystems developed through ecological and evolutionary processes over the course of time, sometimes reflecting tight sets of interlinkages that are hard to restore once lost. Will interactions between synthetic and natural organisms arise easily, or might the very different origins lead to largely disruptive impacts on natural communities? What would be the change to public perceptions of what is "natural" and the notion of evolution as a process beyond human construction? Will these technologies challenge the ethical basis for conservation action, as they have done in

other settings [33]? How will we evaluate organisms created using novel nucleic acids as part of their genetic code—products of xenobiology [34]?

- Nature's services can be synthesized. The value of ecosystem to society is increasingly central to arguments about the importance of biodiversity [35]. One of the most common promises of synthetic biology is to engineer organisms that generate services of benefit to people (e.g., carbon sequestration, pollution control). What impact will this have on the relative value attached to natural ecosystems that already deliver these ecosystem services? Might ecosystems containing synthesized elements outcompete existing evolved ecosystems, delivering more services with less biodiversity?

- Synthetic life delivers private benefits. Many forms of life being developed by synthetic biology are being patented. The benefits provided by these organisms will reflect the economic interests of those able to invest in and develop them. This may well favor applications in existing industrial processes and commodity chains (energy, agriculture, aquaculture) and the operations of large business corporations. Impacts on the wider environment will tend to be treated as an externality. Knock-on impacts of price and other economic changes on smaller producers (e.g., smallholder farmers) will affect their decisions about land conversion and management, and hence future patterns of biodiversity loss. How will a balance be struck between private risk and gain versus public benefit and safety?

A serious need exists for wider discussion of the relationship between synthetic biology and biodiversity conservation, and what choices society can and should make. But this discussion is difficult, for two reasons. First, synthetic biology is a technical field little understood by nonexperts. It will be difficult to create conditions for representative groups from society to engage in a well-informed, structured, and balanced discussion. Second, these discussions are hard to frame because it is difficult to identify the right counterfactuals or alternative futures to compare with those underpinned by the new technology. It seems inevitable that synthetic biology will be a major factor in affecting the future. That future world will not be a slightly older version of the world that we currently inhabit. Rather, it will have a significantly altered climate, changed sea levels, novel pests and diseases, nonanalog ecological communities, and a human population with changed priorities. The costs, benefits, and risks of synthetic biology need to be considered against that backdrop, not against a projected version of the present as is the common practice, but rather through mechanisms such as scenario development [36, 37]. This task is complicated by the fact that psychologists have shown how poor people are at thinking about the future—as Gilbert [38] has written, "because predictions about the future are made in the present, they are invariably influenced by the present."

Synthetic biology brings with it a powerful attraction, causing biology to veer toward engineering with its inherent approach of human problem solving. It may prove to be a cure for certain wicked problems. But we suggest that now is the time to consider whether synthetic biology may be a wicked solution, creating problems of its own, some of which may be undesirable or even unacceptable in the area of biodiversity conservation.

But despite these difficulties, the discussion between conservation and synthetic biology must take place. It should not be based on alarmist or triumphalist positions, but on a clear-eyed examination of the norms, oversight, and public education necessary to make decisions about the enormous power of altering life on Earth. Such a careful, respectful, public discussion must examine the continuing role of conservation values. Much of conservation as currently practiced is predicated on the core ideals of wilderness and nature, though others envisage a carefully managed planet with all the biological components in place, albeit carefully tended by conscientious (human) custodians. Synthetic biologists propose to further equip humans to actively and consciously engineer the living world. The transformed world of 2050 will demand new strategies and new approaches in conservation.

References

1. Kumar S (2012) Extinction need not be forever. Nature 492: 9.

2. Rittel HWJ, Webber MM (1973) Dilemmas in a general theory of planning. Policy Sciences 4: 155–169.

3. Adams WM (2004) Against extinction: the story of conservation. London: Earthscan. 311 p.

4. Convention on Biological Diversity. Aichi Biodiversity Targets. Available: http://www.cbd.int/sp/targets/. Accessed December 2012.

5. Presidential Commission for the Study of Bioethical Issues (2010) New directions: the ethics of synthetic biology and emerging technologies. Available: http://bioethics.gov/cms/sites/default/files/PCSBI-Synthetic-Biology-Report-12.16.10.pdf. Accessed December 2012.

6. Carlson RH (2010) Biology is technology. The promise, peril and new business of engineering life. Cambridge, MA: Harvard University Press. 279 p.

7. Church G, Regis E (2012) Regenesis: how synthetic biology will reinvent nature and ourselves. New York, NY: Basic Books. 284 p.

8. Bergin J (2011) Synthetic biology: emerging global markets. BCC Research. Available: http://www.reportsnreports.com/reports/125412-synthetic-biology-emerging-global-markets.html. Accessed December 2012.

9. Pennisi E (2011) DARPA offers $30 million to jump-start cellular factories. Science 333: 147.

10. Collins J (2012) Bits and pieces come to life. Scientists are combining biology and engineering to change the world. Nature 483: S08–S10.

11. Lloyd's Emerging Risks Team Report (2009) Synthetic biology. Influencing development. Available: http://www.lloyds.com/,/media/25352cf96fee4a8fb28f4ab1746f58ac.ashx. Accessed December 2012.

12. ETC Group (2010) Synthetic biology: creating artificial life forms. Briefing and recommendations for CBD delegates to COP 10. Available: http://www.etcgroup.org/sites/www.etcgroup.org/files/publication/pdf_file/ETC_COP10SynbioBriefing081010.pdf. Accessed December 2012.

13. Marris C, Rose N (2012) Let's get real on synthetic biology. New Scientist. 11 June 2012.

14. Dana GV, Kuiken T, Rejeski D, Snow AA (2012) Four steps to avoid a synthetic-biology disaster. Nature 483: 29.

15. Zhang JY, Marris C, Rose N (2011) The transnational governance of synthetic biology. Scientific uncertainty, cross-borderness and the 'art' of governance. BIOS Working Paper no. 4. London School of Economics and Political Science.

16. ECNH (Federal Ethics Committee on Non-Human Biotechnology) (2010) Synthetic biology—ethical considerations. Available: http://www.ekah.admin.ch/fileadmin/ekah-dateien/dokumentation/publikationen/e-Synthetische_Bio_Broschuere.pdf. Accessed December 2012.

17. Gutmann A (2011) The ethics of synthetic biology: guiding principles for emerging technologies. Hastings Center Report 41 no. 4: 17–22.

18. Kaebnick G (2009) Should moral objections to synthetic biology affect public policy? Nat Biotechnol 27(12): 1106–1108.

19. ETC Group (2007) Extreme genetic engineering. An introduction to synthetic biology. Available: http://www.etcgroup.org/upload/publication/602/01/synbioreportweb.pdf. Accessed December 2012.

20. ETC Group (2010) The new biomassters. Synthetic biology and the next assault on biodiversity and livelihoods. Available: http://www.etcgroup.org/content/new-biomassters. Accessed December 2012.

21. Friends of the Earth (2011) Synthetic solutions to the climate crisis: the dangers of synthetic biology for biofuels production. Available: http://www.cbd.int/doc/emerging-issues/foe-synthetic-biology-for-biofuels-2011-013-en.pdf. Accessed December 2012.

22. Hall R (2012) Bio-economy versus biodiversity. Global Forest Coalition. Available: http://globalforestcoalition.org/wp-content/uploads/2012/04/Bioecono-vs-biodiv-report-with-frontage-2.pdf. Accessed December 2012.

23. Sutherland WJ, Aveling R, Bennum L, Chapman E, Clout M, et al. (2012) A horizon scan of global conservation issues for 2012. Trends Ecol Evol 27: 13–18.

24. Biermann F, Abbott K, Andresen S, Backstrand K, Bernstein S, et al. (2012) Navigating the Anthropocene: improving earth system governance. Science 335: 1306–1307.

25. DeFries R, Ellis E, Chapin III FS, Matson P, Turner II BL, et al. (2012) Planetary opportunities: a social contract for global change science to contribute to a sustainable future. Bio Science 62: 603–606.

26. Pereira HM, Leadley PW, Proenca V, Alkemade R, Schartemann JPW, et al. (2010) Scenarios for global biodiversity in the 21st century. Science 330: 1496–1501.

27. Rands MR, Adams WA, Bennum L, Butchart SHM, Clements A, et al. (2010) Biodiversity conservation: challenges beyond 2010. Science 329: 1298–1303.

28. The Conference of the Parties. Advance unedited copy of COP-11 decisions. Available: http://www.cbd.int/cop/cop-11/doc/2012-10-24-advanced-unedited-cop-11-decisions-en.pdf. Accessed December 2012.

29. Fisher MC, Henk DA, Briggs CJ, Brownstein JC, Dadoff LC, et al. (2012) Emerging fungal threats to animal, plant and ecosystem health. Nature 484: 186–194.

30. The Long Now Foundation. Available: http://rare.longnow.org.

31. Norton BG (2010) Synthetic biology: some concerns of a biodiversity advocate. Remarks on synthetic biology to the Presidential Commission on Bioethics. Available: http://bioethics.gov/cms/sites/default/files/Synthetic-Biology.pdf. Accessed December 2012.

32. Dudley N (2011) Authenticity in nature. Making choices about the naturalness of ecosystems. New York: Earthscan. 244 p.

33. Kaebnick GE, editor (2011) The ideal of nature. Debates about biotechnology and the environment. Baltimore, MD: Johns Hopkins University Press, Baltimore. 208 p.

34. Schmidt M (2010) Xenobiology: a new form of life as the ultimate biosafety tool. Bio Essays: 32: 322–331.

35. Mace GM, Norris K, Fitter AH (2011) Biodiversity and ecosystem services: a multilayered relationship. Trends Ecol Evol 27: 19–26. doi:10.1016/j.tree.2011.08.006

36. WCS-Futures Group, bio-era (2007) Futures of the wild. A project of the Wildlife Conservation Society Futures Group. Bronx, N.Y.: Wildlife Conservation Society.

37. Bio-era (2007) Genome synthesis and design futures: implications for the U.S. economy. A Special Bio-era Report. Sponsored by U.S. Department of Energy.

38. Gilbert D (2007) Stumbling on happiness. New York: Random House. 336 p.

KENT H. REDFORD is the principal of Archipelago Consulting, a firm based in Portland, Maine, that addresses issues in conservation.

WILLIAM ADAMS is a professor of geography at the University of Cambridge.

GEORGINA M. MACE is the head of the Centre for Biodiversity and Environment Research at University College London.

Christopher Preston

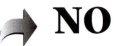 **NO**

De-extinction: A Tale of Two Visions

Consider two different narratives for thinking about extinction reversal for species such as the Passenger Pigeon or Woolly Mammoth. Think of it first as simply a remarkable technological achievement, a chance to show just how far genomic technologies can take us. Applaud the audacity of deciphering and recreating the full DNA sequence of a lost species; the chemically encoded character of pigeon-hood or mammoth-dom decisively cracked and the genome painstakingly rebuilt through human ingenuity. The narrative intoxicates. De-extinction allows us to prove our chops at things that only gods used to do, as Stuart Brand might observe. For this reason some have called it "resurrection ecology." Anthropogenic extinctions have, till now, felt like a blot on our soul. The ability to recreate a life form would seem to give the raw excitement of the technological endeavor a healthy shot of moral legitimacy. The website *Revive and Restore* suggests it would be a "suitable and extraordinary twist to the story of the Passenger Pigeon." Thanks to our skills, we could rewrite a melancholic tale of loss and despair as a much more satisfying story of technological prowess and moral restitution.

Think now of de-extinction in a different light. Think of it as another step down a path of increasing human manipulation of the earth and its systems, a step in which humans, for the first time, manage to reverse what used to be a fundamental Darwinian truth about speciation and evolution. Not content with merely transforming ecological systems to fulfill an endlessly growing reservoir of needs and desires, humanity now concentrates its attention on transforming, restoring, and creating the essence of life itself. An explosion of knowledge at the nanoscale makes reading, adjusting, and even rebuilding life forms possible through incredibly precise interventions into the chemistry of life. Nature, and the respiring, photosynthesizing, and mutating forms contained therein, no longer originates in biochemical processes operating independently of us but becomes part of the realm of human endeavor. The biosphere would here take its most decisive step into the technosphere. Welcome, one might say, to the Anthropocene.

These two differing visions capture just a tiny sliver of what is divisive about de-extinction. One vision contains an uplifting account of human potential and possibility, the other offers a cautionary tale about exceeding boundaries and crossing moral lines in the sand. Each vision has legitimate complaints to make about the other. In one case, the complaint might be, hubris causes humans to erroneously view themselves as virtually omnipotent. In the other, humanity sees itself as shackled by an unnecessary and debilitating image entirely of its own making. The truth is clearly more ambiguous than this bifurcation suggests. We are at the same time both powerful and constrained. We are both part of nature and separate from it. We are both killers and creators.

Surrounding these two competing visions are the numerous scientific and ethical questions that have tended to form the heart of the de-extinction debate. Would the revived Passenger Pigeon really be a Passenger Pigeon or would it be some kind of inauthentic hybrid? Would the restored creature be able to find a suitable ecology in which to live and breed? Would it outcompete existing species for forage or destabilize ecosystems? Would it suffer pain in the process of being subject to our experiments with life? Would the ability to reverse extinction distract us from more important conservation priorities? These are all good questions that require the attention of ecologists, animal welfarists, and other interested communities.

But backing away from the scientific and ethical questions that tend to occupy the foreground, we can see that the two visions capture two different approaches towards moral questions. The first looks entirely within humanity for guidance. It focuses upon our ingenuity, our mistakes, and our potential to make good. It is an account that asks us to secure a worthy destiny for ourselves. It casts us as fallible but redeemable through our ingenuity. We can make good on our mistakes and make amends for even our gravest of errors. It asks us to fulfill our potential and to excel.

The second seems less obsessed with humanity in its own right and finds morality located somewhere outside of us, or at least in the in-between. It suggests the need for a certain type of relationship between humans and the environing world. It recognizes limits. It proposes that there is such a thing as "right relation" and some searchable answers to the lasting mystery of how to act with regards to the life and land that surrounds us. It asks us to question just how far our knowledge and the meddling it permits should be extended.

Distinguishing these two approaches does not itself answer the moral conundrum about de-extinction. Nor are the two approaches entirely exclusive of each other. One of them, however, travels a path that seems to me more dangerous than the other; the vision focusing on human ingenuity runs the risk of cutting us adrift. If we look only inside of us for guidance on how to interact with the surrounding world we find no foil against which to evaluate our choices, no resistance that might set boundaries or limits, and no honest acknowledgment of an exteriority upon which we might gaze in awe. The focus is too much on us.

If, alternatively, we look outside and ask questions about right relationship to what exists independently of us then, at the very least, we are compelled to score our actions in relation to something separate from us. If we take this path, we insist that the biosphere is not something contained entirely within the technosphere but remains something of its own kind with its own integrity. Figuring out how to place ourselves in proper relation to it becomes the heart of the moral quest, just as placing ourselves in proper relation to other people is our objective when we think of morality between humans. We see ourselves as necessarily bound into an essential and ongoing dialogue with something. This sort of dialogue lies close to the core of morality.

The ethics of de-extinction is obviously complex. As we inspect the many different pieces that coalesce to make it such a puzzle, we might do well to think of these pieces not exclusively as questions about human possibilities and risks but as questions about how to place ourselves in relation to something that necessarily exceeds us. The moral quest remains a search for a proper place in the biosphere. For it is on this earth that we exist and must continue to do so, alongside a wondrous plenitude of species, both living and dead.

CHRISTOPHER PRESTON, Professor, Writer—University of Montana, teaches and writes in environmental philosophy at the University of Montana, Missoula. Raised in England and now living in Montana, he has particular interest in the idea of "sense of place."

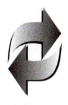

EXPLORING THE ISSUE

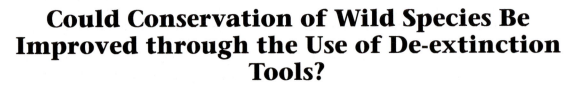

Could Conservation of Wild Species Be Improved through the Use of De-extinction Tools?

Critical Thinking and Reflection

1. Redford and his coauthors describe conservation as "backward-looking." What do they mean by this? Do you think that Preston sets out a backward-looking vision, and do you see that as a problem? Is the prospect of "reviving and restoring" a species forward-looking or backward-looking?
2. Preston describes two visions of de-extinction and two approaches to moral questions. Compare the position articulated by Redford and his coauthors to the visions and approaches articulated by Preston.
3. Redford et al. contrast a management-oriented approach to nature with the traditional conservationist orientation. Do you think Preston is wholly opposed to managing nature? Are there kinds of management he might accept, and do you think that his acceptance of them would be a step toward reaching a compromise of some sort with Redford et al.?
4. What do you think these authors think "nature" means? Would they say that humans are part of nature?
5. Would other ways of using genetic technologies for conservation purposes—for example, to alter threatened species in order to help them survive or to sequence their genomes so that we understand them better and can help in other, more traditional ways—be more acceptable to Preston?

Is There Common Ground?

As arresting as the prospect of de-extinction is, its actual impact is likely to be fairly modest. There are relatively few species that can really be said to be amenable to de-extinction, and both the technical challenges and the costs involved in performing it may also end up being limiting factors. Most conservationists are likely to agree that protecting extant species remains the most important conservationist biodiversity goal.

De-extinction is contested more because it is seen as potentially leading to many other more significant kinds of biotechnological interventions. The declaration in 2010 by scientists at the J. Craig Venter Institute that they had succeeded in creating the synthesizing a version of a microbe known as Mycoplasma mycoides offered a prospect of entirely "synthetic," or artificial, life forms. More recently, the discovery of strategies for constructing so-called "gene drives" has introduced the possibility that extant populations of wild organisms, perhaps entire species, could be modified, replaced with new versions, or deliberately driven into extinction. There could be very good reasons for using gene drives; for example, it's possible that gene drives could be used to modify mosquitoes so that they could no longer serve as vectors for plasmodium, the microbe that causes malaria. Such a drive appears to have enormous benefits for public health and for human well-being, particularly in low-income countries. It also sharpens a question that conservationists may have about de-extinction. One of the benefits of de-extinction might turn out to be simply that it's exciting, that seeing a wooly mammoth would be fascinating and maybe worth a lot of money. If that came to be an acceptable rationale for de-extinction, then finding limits to other, more significant biotechnologies could prove very challenging.

Additional Resources

Beth Shapiro's book How to Clone a Mammoth: The Science of De-extinction (Princeton University Press, 2016) is a balanced and very accessible book that details the many technical steps necessary to achieve de-extinction and makes a limited case for a limited form of de-extinction. She argues that creating proxy species may be appropriate to achieve broader ecological goals.

How Will Synthetic Biology and Conservation Shape the Future of Conservation? (published in 2013 by The Wildlife Conservation Society and The Nature Conservancy and available at http://e.wcs.org/pdf/Synthetic_Biology_and_Conservation_Framing_Paper.pdf) is a framing paper prepared for a meeting of conservationists and scientists doing work in synthetic biology. It gives a high-level overview of conservation and synthetic biology and describes some ways in which synthetic biology might be useful to conservation.

The prominent genetic scientist George Church teamed with the science writer Ed Regis to write Regenesis: How Synthetic Biology Will Reinvent Nature and Ourselves (Basic Books, 2014). The book describes de-extinction and some other, even more challenging developments and makes a case for unrestrained technological intervention into nature.

Internet References . . .

De-extinction: Bringing Extinct Species Back to Life

http://www.nationalgeographic.com/deextinction/

How Far Should We Go to Bring Back Lost Species?

http://www.humansandnature.org/how-far-should-we-go-to-bring-back-lost-species

Revive & Restore: Genetic Rescue for Endangered and Extinct Species

http://reviverestore.org

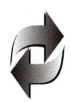

Unit 6

UNIT

Access to Health Care

*I*n its modern infancy, biomedical ethics was almost exclusively concerned with issues relating to individual doctor–patient relationships. Questions of resource allocation and public policy occurred, but they arose mostly within the context of decisions about whether a patient could pay for certain kinds of care. In the past several decades, as medical care costs have skyrocketed, the issues concerning equitable distribution of scarce resources have become paramount. As medical care became more costly, it became less accessible to the uninsured and to the underinsured (people who have some employment-based health insurance but not enough to cover their own illnesses or those of their families). In this new world of market-driven health care, some old problems of resource allocation and public policy take on new urgency. Can government step in to help organize effective insurance markets, which might require mandates both to insurance providers and insurance purchasers? How much trust do we put in unrestricted markets? Could we even allow things like human organs to be bought and sold in market exchanges? This unit takes up these issues with readings that explore trade-offs, in several different contexts, between individual liberty and community standards.

Selected, Edited, and with Issue Framing Material by:
Gregory E. Kaebnick, *The Hastings Center*

ISSUE

Does Government Overreach by Mandating Health Insurance?

YES: **James Stacey Taylor**, from "The Carelessness of Affordable Care," *Hastings Center Report* (2012)

NO: **Timothy Stoltzfus Jost**, from "A Mutual Aid Society?" *Hastings Center Report* (2012)

Learning Outcomes
After reading this issue, you will be able to:
• Identify core issues in recent health-care reform initiatives.
• Discuss moral and policy arguments for and against mandating that individuals purchase health insurance.
• Discuss the tension in a liberal democracy between individual liberty and community cohesion.

ISSUE SUMMARY

YES: Philosopher James Stacey Taylor argues that the Affordable Care Act passed into law during President Obama' first term is unduly paternalistic, failing to pass muster even on the simple utilitarian grounds that could most easily support policies to require citizens to buy insurance.

NO: Timothy Stoltzfus Jost, a legal scholar, holds that the ACA is intended to create a national community of community aid, relying on the power of Congress to impose taxes.

On March 23, 2010, President Obama signed into law the Patient Protection and Affordable Care Act (often cited as ACA), a major change in the way health care is financed and delivered in the United States. The United States has long been the only industrialized country without a national health-care system, despite the efforts over the past 50 years of Republican and Democratic presidents to introduce change. The ACA is intended to address two major health-care problems: lack of access and high costs.

Most of the people who have health insurance today obtain it through their employers. It was not always the case, however. Employer-based insurance was introduced in World War II as an incentive to recruit and retain workers because wartime regulations prevented them from offering higher wages.

Even though there is no national health-care system, government programs have long played a major role. Medicare, a federal program, was enacted in 1965 to cover people over the age of 65 and those with end-stage kidney disease. Medicaid, introduced at the same time, is a joint federal–state program that covers people below the poverty line. There are other government-sponsored programs—TRICARE (formerly CHAMPUS) for uniformed service members, retirees, and their families; federal employees' insurance; and the Children's Health Insurance Program (CHIP) for poor children. These government-sponsored programs are administered by private insurance companies.

Even with these programs aimed at special populations, around 50 million people lack health insurance in the United States. According to the Commonwealth Fund, a private foundation that addresses health reform, data from the U.S. Census Bureau shows that provisions of the ACA that have already gone into effect have lowered the number of young adults who lack insurance. Because of the weak job market, however, the overall number of uninsured still increased by about 5 million between 2007 and 2009. Many employers also dropped or limited coverage or raised employee contributions.

Most of the adults without health insurance are in working families but have low incomes. Twenty-seven percent of people whose families have incomes under $25,000 were without health insurance in 2010, according to the Commonwealth Fund, and nearly 22 percent of those in families with incomes between $25,000 and $50,000 were uninsured. About 80 percent of the uninsured are U.S. citizens.

Hospitals with emergency departments are required by law to treat patients whether they have insurance or not. "Treatment," however, is limited to stabilizing the patient, not providing follow-up care. And hospitals can still bill for the care, at a rate that is often higher than the one negotiated with health insurance plans.

The ACA sought to address the lack of access by expanding Medicaid to cover nearly all of the nonelderly lowest-income adults. To spread this cost over the greatest number, almost every American (with a few exemptions) is required either to have health insurance or to pay a fine. An individual can choose to enroll in an employer-based plan as long as it meets certain standards. Insurance is available through state-based insurance marketplaces called exchanges, with subsidies for low-income people. People younger than 30 are able to satisfy the mandate by buying low-cost, high-deductible plans. In 2006, Massachusetts expanded access through a similar plan with an individual mandate provision.

The public has been deeply divided about the ACA. The idea of government running health care—as suggested by the name "Obamacare," which critics quickly gave to the ACA—raises alarms about the extent of government control over citizens' lives. In fact, the ACA does not run health care; patients receive coverage mostly through private insurers and receive care from doctors and hospitals affiliated with their plan. The ACA organizes markets for health insurance plans and sets some of the terms for health insurance plans. The requirement that individuals either obtain health insurance or pay a fine, however—a requirement known as the ACA's "individual mandate"—is undeniably an intrusion on individual liberty, however, and it is one of the most controversial aspects of the health reform law. The ACA was challenged by several states, but in June 2012, the U.S. Supreme Court ruled that the mandate was constitutional. The Court's opinion concluded that the mandate would be unconstitutional if it were considered a "penalty" but that it could be considered a tax and as such fell within the federal government's power to levy taxes.

Since the ACA went into effect, the percentage of the U.S. population under 65 that lack health insurance has fallen, as of October 2016, to 11.9 percent, although that leaves 24 million people without coverage. There are several reasons people may still not have insurance: undocumented immigrants are excluded from coverage, nineteen states (taking advantage of a portion of the Supreme Court's 2012 decision) have opted not to use the ACA's mechanisms to expand Medicaid eligibility, many of the uninsured either don't know about the health insurance marketplaces or have found enrolling too difficult, and many of the uninsured still believe that the plans available in the marketplace are still not affordable for them. The ACA's ability to attract insurers and keep insurance costs down has been mixed. Health plan costs were initially lower than expected, but significant increases occurred in 2015 and 2016.

Other lawsuits against the ACA have been working their way slowly through the courts, and in the 2016 U.S. presidential election, the Republican nominee, Donald J. Trump, promised to repeal the ACA, while the Democratic nominee, Hillary Clinton, was committed to keeping it but amending it.

The following selections discuss the merits of individual mandates. Philosopher James Stacey Taylor sets out a libertarian position. Taylor argues that the ACA will eventually fail to provide affordable care and that, partly because it fails economically, its intrusion on individual liberty is morally unacceptable. Legal scholar Timothy Stoltzfus Jost argues that the core idea of the ACA is that a cohesive, morally good community endorses a principle of "mutual aid"—a good community will take care of its sick. The United States has sometimes tended to endorse a more atomistic view of human relationships. The ACA attempts to remedy that situation.

YES ↵

James Stacey Taylor

The Carelessness of Affordable Care

The Affordable Care Act (ACA) has been touted as a long-overdue remedy for what is perceived to be the chronic problem of large numbers of Americans living without adequate health insurance. While much of the discussion of the ACA has focused on its legality, it should also be assessed on the basis of its economic implications and its moral acceptability. On its face, the ACA appears to do well on both counts. Given that the uninsured often secure their health care from expensive emergency room treatment (from which they cannot be excluded and whose cost is often borne by third parties), expanding insurance to cover them (and hence to give them access to less expensive treatments) appears to make economic sense. Similarly, it might appear that providing access to insurance for people who otherwise could not afford it, or who would be denied it as a result of having medical conditions that they are not responsible for, would be morally laudable. But these appearances deceive: The ACA is neither economically sound nor morally acceptable. To paraphrase Oscar Wilde, to fail on one of these criteria may be misfortune; to fail on both looks like carelessness.

The ACA has three major provisions. First, it requires insurers in the individual and group markets to "guarantee issue"—to cover all who apply for insurance, regardless of health status. It also requires insurers to cover preexisting conditions and to set their premium levels independently of the health status of the insured. Second, using the threat of the loss of federal funding to secure compliance, it requires states to expand their Medicaid programs to cover all their citizens whose income is at or below 138 percent of the poverty level. Finally, using the threat of a financial penalty to secure compliance, the ACA includes an "individual mandate" requiring everyone who can afford health insurance to buy it, whether through employment, a public program, or directly purchased by individuals.

The obvious moral objection to the ACA is that it appears to be unjustifiably paternalistic. While this is certainly a legitimate concern, the requirement of the individual mandate is likely to be motivated more by economic

necessity than by paternalistic benevolence. If the ACA required insurers to cover the preexisting conditions of those they insured and to set premiums without regard to health status without also requiring them to guarantee the issue of insurance to all applicants, then insurers would simply refuse to issue insurance to those whose health care would probably cost more than the premiums would garner. To ensure that people with preexisting conditions or whose health status is likely to be costly can secure health insurance, insurers must be required to issue it to all applicants. The natural result of requiring insurers to guarantee issue is to raise the price of health-care insurance, for now the premiums must reflect the increased costs of the persons insured. These price increases would lead to the adverse selection of persons seeking health-care insurance, for healthy persons would now be less likely to choose to purchase it. The cost—and hence the price—of health-care insurance would thus rise further, since the insured population would now, on average, be less healthy. As insurers are now required to cover preexisting conditions and to guarantee issue, no one need carry health insurance until they needed it.

Moreover, given these requirements imposed on insurers, since government action would artificially raise the price of health-care insurance to higher than market-based levels, it would be economically rational for people to avoid purchasing it until they actually need health care. Insurers' expenditures would inevitably exceed their income from premiums. To avoid bringing about the collapse of the health insurance industry, then, the government must further coercively interfere with it by requiring that all persons who can afford to buy insurance do so. The individual mandate, then, might be motivated less by a concern for the well-being of uninsured Americans than by the need to coerce the healthy to subsidize the health care of their unhealthy fellow citizens.

Before turning to the moral criticisms of the ACA, let us outline its economic drawbacks. The first of these is simply that its imposition will require a small army of lawyers and bureaucrats. Unless the costs of these can be composed of the economic equivalent of phlogiston, the imposition of the ACA will automatically raise the cost of health care. The second economic drawback of the ACA is also obvious. In requiring healthy people to subsidize the health-care costs of the unhealthy, it leads to the moral hazard of people having no financial incentive to avoid unhealthy behavior. The absence of this financial incentive would drive health-care costs still higher.

The final economic drawback of the ACA is that requiring insurers to guarantee issue would lead to the expansion of elective rather than remedial health care. The combination of guaranteed issue and the individual mandate further removes health-care insurance from the market realm and places it more firmly within the political arena. This will lead to an increase in the cost—and hence the price—of health care by opening the door to increased lobbying by interest groups who favor required coverage of certain medical procedures. Under a market system, health-care providers would have to secure business from people who both desired the procedures they offered and were willing and able to pay the market price for them (or obtain insurance that pays for them). If the government determines what coverage insurers must provide, then health-care providers will now have an interest in lobbying to have insurers required to cover the procedures that they offer.

The ACA thus gives health-care providers who specialize in nonessential procedures incentive to lobby for coverage. Of course, insurers might be motivated to lobby against expanded coverage. However, given the individual mandate, the costs of the additional procedures will be more widely distributed. As such, people would have less reason to balk at increases in the price of coverage. Moreover, since people could not exit the insurance market, insurers would be more weakly motivated to lobby against requirements to cover new procedures, for the increasing price of insurance would not lead people to reject their services.

The greater the government involvement in health-care insurance, then, the greater the motivation of health-care providers to lobby for expanded coverage, while the presence of an individual mandate undermines insurers' motivations to lobby against such expansion. Since these two factors are both associated with the ACA, it is to be expected that, with time, insurers will be required to cover increasing numbers of nonessential procedures. Moreover, as the cost of nonessential procedures will not be directly borne by those who undergo them, more people would be motivated to undergo them. The resulting increase in these procedures will lead to an increase in both the cost and the price of health-care insurance.

For these three reasons—increasing bureaucracy, moral hazard, and increased coverage of elective procedures—the ACA will increase both the cost and the price of health-care insurance. This is not merely economic speculation: it is supported by empirical evidence. According to the Kaiser Family Foundation and the American Health Insurance Plans Center for Policy Research, there were in 2009 five "guaranteed issue" states in America, and four of them—Massachusetts, Vermont, New Jersey, and New York—had the highest annual health insurance premiums in the country. The other, Maine, was ranked ninth.

These economic drawbacks lead to the first of the moral objections to the ACA, which is that by increasing both the overall cost and the price of health insurance, the ACA will make people worse off. As a utilitarian objection, however, this moves too quickly. The ACA will have different effects on different subsections of the population. If the decrease in well-being to one part of the population is less than the benefit to another part, then utilitarians should support the ACA.

And, in fact, there are reasons to believe that the benefit to some would be greater than the cost to others. The uninsured include persons who are impoverished. Owing to the diminishing marginal utility of money, the transfer of wealth (in the form of paid health insurance premiums) to the impoverished uninsured should be (at least prima facie) supported by utilitarians. The utilitarian argument would be further strengthened by the apparently high number of uninsured people in the United States.

But the appearance is misleading. It is widely believed that in 2009, there were 47 million uninsured Americans—roughly 16 percent of the population. But these data are mistaken. Roughly 6 million of these 47 million actually have insurance through either Medicaid or the State Children's Health Insurance Program (SCHIP) but report that they are uninsured because they do not have private insurance. A further four million are eligible for Medicaid or SCHIP but have not yet registered. These persons are de facto insured, since neither of these social programs can refuse persons insurance based on preexisting conditions, and they would be enrolled were they to go to an emergency room. Of the remaining 37 million, 20 million were uninsured for less than four months—but owing to the methodology of the Census Bureau they would be counted as uninsured for the whole of a given year if they were uninsured at any point during it. Of the remaining seventeen million people (or roughly 6 percent of the population), five million were childless adults between the ages of 18 and 34—the people who are likely to have least need of insurance. In sum, only about 12 million people—or roughly 4 percent of the population—were uninsured for an extended period and in need of aid. (These data are from the Bureau of Labor Statistics and the Census Bureau.)

These data considerably weaken the utilitarian case for the ACA, for it makes it much less likely that the benefit to some is greater than the cost to others. Moreover, it is highly likely that a portion of the 4 percent of persons who lacked health insurance for an extended period were uninsured because they had expensive health problems. These people would, from a utilitarian point of view, be those that either should receive palliative treatment only, or perhaps even not receive treatment at all, given the opportunity costs of their treatment. This further reduces the number of persons to whom a utilitarian would support the redistribution of wealth.

Finally, and on a separate note, it is not clear that a utilitarian would support the ACA even if she would support the transfer of wealth to the small subsection of the population that are both uninsured and the likely recipients of health care under a utilitarian system. It is overwhelmingly likely that the members of this subsection would be made better off (at least if well-being is judged subjectively) if this wealth was transferred to them in the form of cash rather than health insurance. They could use the money to buy whatever they believed would give them most pleasure, or best satisfy their preferences—which might not be health insurance.

There is, then, good reason to believe that even a utilitarian who favors the redistribution of wealth would hold the ACA to be immoral. Of course, that a utilitarian would be likely to reject the ACA need not persuade one of its immorality, for one might reject utilitarianism itself on the grounds that, as a theory, it fails directly to respect the autonomy of persons. But if one is concerned with the moral value of personal autonomy, then one should be even more strongly opposed to the ACA. As noted, the individual mandate appears to be paternalistic. One who is concerned with autonomy's moral value would have prima facie reason to object to the ACA. But this objection is based on the most charitable interpretation of the rationale behind the individual mandate. The mandate is likely motivated not by paternalism but by the recognition that healthy people who are disinclined to buy insurance must be forced back into the health-care market to subsidize the costs of the unhealthy. And while paternalistically coercing persons for their own good is clearly objectionable to one who values autonomy, coercing them for the good of others is worse.

The ACA does not, however, merely fail to respect the autonomy of those who are forced to purchase health-care insurance; it also fails to respect the autonomy of those whom they are forced to subsidize. One can fail to respect another person's autonomy in one of two ways. One might act so as to compromise her autonomy by, for example, manipulating her or subjecting her to coercion (such as by forcing her to buy health insurance). Alternatively, one might fail to respect a person's autonomy by holding that it is not *worthy* of respect, even if one does not actually act so as to compromise it. It is in this latter sense that the ACA fails to respect the autonomy of those whose health care it is intended to subsidize. Recall that part of the utilitarian objection to the ACA was that it redistributes wealth from the healthy to the unhealthy in the form of health-care insurance, rather than as cash. Implicit in this health-care-based approach to redistribution is the view that the recipients of the plunder (to use Claude Frédéric Bastiat's apt term) *should* use it to buy health insurance. This is why they are given insurance rather than cash. Inherent in the ACA, then, is the belief that those to whom the plunder is redistributed cannot be trusted to make their own decisions concerning their use of it—in other words, that their autonomy is not worthy of respect. The ACA, then, respects the autonomy of no one.

Of course, one might respond to these arguments that it is simply the nature of the political process to subject some groups to coercion for the public good, and so the ACA is no worse than any other (well-meaning?) act of legislation. But there are two rejoinders. First, pleading that a violation is routine is no defense of the act. Second, even if coercing some subset of the population for the public good is morally acceptable (and this is highly contestable), the ACA is still morally problematic, for even a utilitarian who would endorse such coercion is likely to find it morally objectionable.

In short, the serious economic drawbacks of the ACA mean that it will probably make those subject to it worse off overall, and so it is morally objectionable from a utilitarian view. It is also morally objectionable from the view of people who value autonomy because it respects neither the autonomy of those coerced into buying health insurance nor those to whom the plunder thus extracted is provided. To reprise Wilde, the passing of the ACA is thus careless indeed.

Acknowledgments

The author thanks Antony Davies for exceptionally helpful conversations on the economics of the ACA, and for providing me with the data concerning the number of Americans who are uninsured.

JAMES STACEY TAYLOR is a professor of philosophy at The College of New Jersey.

Timothy Stoltzfus Jost

NO

A Mutual Aid Society?

In her classic 1993 article, "The Struggle for the Soul of Health Insurance," Deborah Stone contrasted the principle of mutual aid—"the essence of community" in the face of sickness—and the principle of actuarial fairness, under which "each person should pay for his own risk." Stone claimed that "in most societies sickness is widely accepted as a condition that should trigger mutual aid," while in the United States, a competitive insurance industry fosters in people "a sense of their difference, rather than their commonalities, and their responsibility for themselves only, rather than their interdependence," leading to the fragmentation of "communities into ever-smaller, more homogeneous groups" and "the destruction of mutual aid" [1].

Except within families, and perhaps in small communities like the Amish, Hutterites, or religious orders, mutual aid as a means of sharing the cost of sickness rarely happens out of simple altruism. However, the health care financing systems of virtually all developed nations are, as Stone claims, based on the principle of "solidarity," or mutual aid. But although this mutual aid is fundamentally based on a societal commitment to community in the face of sickness, in the end it is implemented through the coercive authority of the state. Either members of society are required by law to purchase insurance, as in the Netherlands and Switzerland, or to participate in a "sickness fund," as in Germany or Israel, or they are required to pay taxes that finance a public insurance system, as in the United Kingdom or Canada. Anyone who, without a legal excuse, refuses to purchase insurance, join a sickness fund, or pay taxes will be penalized in some way by the state.

The United States has, as Stone observes, long been an outlier in its approach to financing care for sickness. Over the past half century, we have developed mutual aid-based programs to care for some—Medicare for the elderly and disabled, and Medicaid for poor elderly, disabled and blind persons, pregnant women, and dependent children and their families. We have also required hospitals that participate in Medicare to provide emergency care regardless of the patient's ability to pay and hospitals that receive charitable tax exemptions to provide care free or at reduced cost to indigents.

But most Americans have had to pay the "actuarially fair" cost of their care, either as individuals or as employee groups. Mutual aid has existed only on a limited scale, in the sense that discrimination based on health status has, since 1996, been limited within employee groups. Individuals who purchase insurance on their own have had to pay premiums based on their projected health-care costs, have faced preexisting condition exclusions and lifetime and annual coverage limits, or have been denied coverage altogether because of their health status. Employment-based groups have been "experience rated." Small groups with older employees or employees with serious health problems have found insurance unaffordable. Households that cannot afford health insurance and that fail to qualify for Medicaid (either because their income is over the often draconian eligibility limits set by states or because they do not fall within one of the categories of poor persons eligible for Medicaid) remain uninsured. Thus, over 50 million Americans are uninsured—16.3 percent of the population. The consequences of this situation in terms of mortality, morbidity, and financial insecurity have been devastating.

The Affordable Care Act (ACA) is the most comprehensive attempt to date to remedy this situation. The ACA brings to bear the coercive power of the federal government to bring about several major changes. First, it compels health insurers in the individual and small group markets to abandon actuarial fairness and convert to a mutual aid-based approach to underwriting—henceforth, insurers in these markets must cover all applicants regardless of health status, ignore health status in setting premiums, and cover preexisting conditions. Second, all households that can afford health insurance, either through their jobs, a public program, or with their own resources, must become insured or pay a penalty. Third, the states must expand their Medicaid programs to cover all of their citizens with incomes at or below 138 percent of the poverty level or risk losing federal funding.

Within minutes of President Obama signing the ACA, a lawsuit was filed by a group of states and private parties challenging its constitutionality. The plaintiffs argued that Congress lacks the authority under the Constitution to coerce individuals to purchase health insurance. They also contended that Congress cannot coerce the states to expand their Medicaid programs to cover poor households regardless of the reason they are poor. While the plaintiffs did not argue in so many words that the U.S. Constitution endorses actuarial fairness, they did contend that Congress is limited in its authority to institute a national community based on the principle of mutual aid for covering the cost of sickness.

After a fitful two-year course up through the lower courts, these questions reached the Supreme Court. In a decision written by Chief Justice Roberts, a closely divided Court both rejected and accepted the authority of Congress to establish a mutual aid-based health-care financing system in the United States, but largely rejected the idea that the principle of actuarial fairness is enshrined in the Constitution.

The requirement that insurers abandon health status-based underwriting was not squarely before the Court. A long line of precedent has established that the constitutional authority of Congress to regulate interstate commerce empowers it to regulate insurance. Nonetheless, the ACA underwriting reforms were distinctly visible in the background of the ACA litigation: if Congress could not compel healthy individuals to participate in a mutual aid-based insurance community, could insurers realistically be required to abandon the principle of actuarial fairness? As Justice Kennedy (who ultimately voted to nullify the entire ACA) asked at oral argument, "Is it within the proper exercise of this Court's function to impose" the financial risk that insurers would incur if they were forced to abandon the principle of actuarial fairness without a mandate that healthy persons purchase health insurance? The four justices who joined the joint dissent concluded that the insurance reforms could not go forward if the individual mandate was stricken from the ACA.

The primary question raised by the litigation was whether Congress had authority under the Constitution to coerce uninsured individuals to join the community of the insured—to engage in mutual aid. In particular, does the authority of Congress to regulate interstate commerce extend to requiring healthy individuals who would prefer to remain uninsured to purchase health insurance—can Congress mandate health insurance coverage? Proponents of the mandate asserted that Congress was in fact regulating commerce in imposing the mandate; indeed,

that it was regulating both the market for health care and the market for health insurance. Without the mandate, individuals could refuse to contribute toward the cost of insuring the entire community while freeloading on the existing scheme of mutual aid that requires hospitals to offer emergency care regardless of ability to pay. Congress had the power, ACA proponents argued, to require individuals to purchase insurance because everyone eventually uses health care, and the cost of providing that health care to the uninsured—estimated at $43 billion a year—would otherwise be passed on to others. The federal government also argued that the mandate was necessary to implement the insurance reforms. Insurers could not be expected to embrace the mutual aid principle if insurance purchasers still based their participation in the market on the principle of actuarial fairness.

Chief Justice Roberts, writing for himself but supported by four justices in a joint dissent, concluded that Congress has no authority under the Constitution to compel individuals to join a health insurance mutual aid community. The power of Congress to regulate commerce does not extend to requiring individuals to engage in commerce.

But this does not mean that Congress is powerless to create a national community of mutual aid. It can do this, but must do it under its power to tax. Congress can, that is, impose a tax on those who do not join the mutual aid community. The only question was whether Congress had in fact done so. Is the exaction imposed on those who can afford health insurance but refuse to purchase it a penalty or a tax? Roberts concluded it was a tax and thus permissible. Congress often imposes taxes or offers tax preferences to influence behavior, and that's what it was doing in this case.

Does it make a difference that the exaction that Americans who refuse to join the health insurance mutual aid community face is a tax rather than a penalty? The amount of the payment will remain the same. But people may experience it differently, which raises a question whether it will make a practical difference. If individuals conclude that they simply face an economic choice—either to buy insurance or to pay a tax, whichever is financially more advantageous—rather than a legal requirement, enforced by a penalty, that they buy insurance, then they may be less likely to feel a social obligation to purchase insurance. Normatively, a mandate enforced by a penalty would seem to communicate a strong endorsement of the principle of mutual aid. The ACA, in fact, seems to embrace this: "An applicable individual shall for each month beginning after 2013 ensure that the individual, and any dependent of the individual who is an applicable individual, is covered under minimum essential coverage for such month." But the Court seemed to endorse a weaker version—join the mutual aid community or pay a tax for refusing to participate—in effect insisting on actuarial fairness.

The Supreme Court's decision also addressed a second question about coercion: can the federal government redefine the mutual aid community embraced by the federal-state cooperative Medicaid program to consist not only of the "worthy poor" categories originally included, but all persons with incomes below 138 percent of the poverty level, making continued state participation in the program contingent on a state's accepting this broader definition of the mutual aid community? The states argued that the federal government was coercing them, as independent sovereigns, to expand the Medicaid mutual aid community against their will, and that this exceeded the constitutional authority of Congress. Since Medicaid is one of the largest expenditures in state budgets and their largest source of federal funds, Congress could not threaten them with the loss of all Medicaid funding as a condition of expanding their Medicaid programs.

The Court sided with the states on this claim by a seven-to-two majority. Chief Justice Roberts proclaimed that the Medicaid expansion was a "shift in kind, not merely of degree" in the Medicaid program, and that Congress could only offer it as an option, not require states' participation. Given the terms on which the option is offered to the states, however, the difference in terms of coercion between an option and a mandate may be a difference in degree, not in kind.

For 2014, 2015, and 2016, the federal government picks up 100 percent of the cost of the expansion, with the federal share gradually declining to 90 percent by 2020. This contrasts with the traditional federal matching rate of 50 percent to 83 percent. No other federal funding is available to cover citizens with incomes below 100 percent of the federal poverty rate who do not qualify for traditional Medicaid—which is to say, childless adults. This population will continue to rely on uncompensated care, burdening hospitals and the medical safety net. Managed care companies, drug companies, and other providers of health-care drugs and services who were expecting a large increase in Medicaid managed care revenues will miss out on a major expansion of their markets in states that refuse to participate and will inform state policy-makers of this fact. The residents of states that refuse to expand their Medicaid programs will still pay federal taxes to expand programs in other states. Although a number of governors are defiantly proclaiming that they will refuse to expand Medicaid, on sober second thought many will reconsider—if not in time for January 1, 2014, then at some point in the future.

In the end, the mutual aid principle would seem to have triumphed in the Court. But the triumph may be short-lived. More lawsuits are reportedly brewing. Republican states continue to resist implementation. And most importantly, the 2012 presidential, congressional, and state house elections may bring to power officials deeply committed to the principle of actuarial fairness and opposed to an expansion of mutual aid. The struggle for the soul of health insurance in the United States may be far from over.

Reference

1. D. Stone, "The Struggle for the Soul of Health Insurance," *Journal of Health Politics, Policy and Law,* **18** (1993):287–317, at 289–290.

TIMOTHY STOLTZFUS JOST is a professor of law at the Washington and Lee University School of Law.

EXPLORING THE ISSUE

Does Government Overreach by Mandating Health Insurance?

Critical Thinking and Reflection

1. Explain Jost's idea, drawn from Deborah Stone, that health insurance can reflect a principle of mutual aid.
2. Communitarians argue that an individual's identify, life prospects, and personal successes are dependent on the individual's relationship to the community, whereas libertarians hold that the individual's identity, life prospects, and personal successes are the responsibility of that individual. Where do you fall on this debate? Do you see a spectrum of possible views? How does it relate to the debate about health care? How does it relate to the debate about the individual mandate?
3. These readings make competing claims about how the individual mandate can affect the cost of health-care insurance. Explain these claims and evaluate them.
4. Do you agree with Taylor that the ACA also fails to respect the autonomy of those whose health care it subsidizes?
5. Jost holds that a societal commitment to community can be brought about coercively; do you agree that is possible?

Is There Common Ground?

The divisive political debate since 2009 over the Patient Protection and Affordable Care Act would seem to leave little hope of finding common ground on this issue. During the 2012 presidential election, both candidates held that the law illustrated the gap between the competing visions or philosophies endorsed by Republicans and Democrats. Nonetheless, maybe turning to the underlying values offers some hope of discovering some common ground beneath the political infighting.

The philosopher Paul Menzel is one commentator on health-care reform who has made this kind of case. Menzel points out, for example, that conservatives in most of the rest of the world have health-care reform efforts that aim to achieve broader access to health care because that goal promotes conservative goals such as personal responsibility, individual opportunity, and the strong and stable social foundation that allows for prosperity. The problem, then, is to identify the particular reform strategies that both liberals and conservatives can recognize as advancing their underlying values.

Additional Resources

For an older but still helpful overview of the contrasting positions on the mandate, see Sara Rosenbaum and Jonathan Gruber, "Buying Health Care, the Individual Mandate, and the Constitution," *The New England Journal of Medicine* (July 29, 2010), and Glen Whitman, "Hazards of the Individual Health Care Mandate," *Cato Policy Report* (September/October 2007); http://www.cato.org/pubs/policy_report/v29n5/cpr29n5-1.html.

The readings here are part of a larger set of essays found in the September–October 2012 issue of the *Hastings Center Report*. Another, earlier writing from the *Report* is Paul Menzel and Donald W. Light, "A Conservative Case for Universal Access to Health Care," *Hastings Center Report* (July–August 2006).

Internet References . . .

Alliance for Health Reform

> http://www.allhealth.org

Health Reform GPS

> http://www.healthreformgps.org/

Kaiser Family Foundation, Health Reform

> http://kff.org/health-reform/

ObamaCare Facts

> http://obamacarefacts.com

The Robert Wood Johnson Foundation

> http://www.rwjf.org

Selected, Edited, and with Issue Framing Material by:
Gregory E. Kaebnick, *The Hastings Center*

ISSUE

Is There an Ethical Duty to Provide Health Care to Undocumented Immigrants?

YES: **Rajeev Raghavan and Ricardo Nuila**, from "Survivors—Dialysis, Immigration, and U.S. Law," *The New England Journal of Medicine* (2011)

NO: **David W. Stratas**, from *"Toussaint v. Attorney General of Canada"* (2011)

Learning Outcomes

After reading this issue, you will be able to:

- Explain the societal challenge of extending health insurance to undocumented immigrants.
- Discuss arguments for and against extending health insurance to undocumented immigrants.

ISSUE SUMMARY

YES: Rajeev Raghavan and Ricardo Nuila, physicians who work with end-stage renal disease patients, argue that standardized coverage for dialysis treatments would alleviate the burden on taxpayers where the most undocumented residents live and would improve these patients' health, allowing them to return to work.

NO: David Stratas, a justice with the Federal Court of Appeals of Ontario, Canada, explains why Canada was justified in not providing health care benefits to an undocumented immigrant who lived in Toronto.

In October 2009, Grady Memorial Hospital in Atlanta, a "safety-net" public hospital, announced it was closing its free dialysis center because it was losing too much money. Fifty patients, many of them undocumented immigrants who had no insurance coverage, had until January 2010 to find alternative dialysis providers in the United States or in their home countries. Without regular dialysis treatment for their kidney disease, they would die. Yet, other dialysis providers would not accept the patients without payment. In December 2009, a federal judge dismissed a lawsuit challenging the center closing, and it closed as planned. Grady paid for 3 months' treatment for the 13 patients who agreed to be repatriated. And it contracted with a large for-profit provider to cover the other patients' treatment until September 2010.

At different points in American history, immigrants have been welcomed as cheap, unskilled labor; at others, immigrants have been excluded as potential revolutionaries or threats to social order. An immigrant's health status was considered crucial in the massive waves of immigration from Eastern and Southern Europe in the nineteenth and early twentieth centuries. Public health officials examined immigrants at Ellis Island in New York harbor and marked with chalk the coats of those suspected of having a "loathsome or dangerous contagious disease." They might be sent to a hospital on site or sent back home. In fact, immigration officials were really worried about accepting people whose conditions were likely to make them "public charges." In 1924, legal immigration was sharply curtailed.

Even so, immigration to the United States increased dramatically in the 1990s and thereafter (but has recently

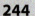

slowed somewhat), as waves of people from Mexico, other Latin American countries, and Asia, as well as other countries, came seeking work. Again health status is an issue, but this time the questions are not about people seeking legal entry (although they still have to answer medical questions) but about people who have crossed the border without the required permission. Are these undocumented immigrants entitled to health care? And if so, who should pay if they are uninsured?

In 2005, there were an estimated 36 million foreign-born residents in the United States, about 35 percent of them naturalized citizens, 33 percent documented immigrants, and 31 percent (about 12 million) undocumented immigrants. Many of these families include children. In 1995, the Personal Responsibility and Work Opportunity Reconciliation Act made recent immigrants ineligible for Medicaid and other public benefits for 5 years. Although one goal of the Affordable Care Act is to increase access to health insurance to the 45 million Americans without it, the act specifically excludes undocumented immigrants from all its programs aimed at this goal. This ban also applied to the State Children's Health Insurance Program (SCHIP) of 1997.

Undocumented immigrants are likely to be poor, work at low-wage jobs without health insurance, and avoid going to doctors until an emergency because they fear being deported. Under the Emergency Medical Treatment and Active Labor Act (EMTALA), they are entitled to emergency treatment but not follow-up care. There is no evidence that undocumented immigrants use emergency rooms more than any other group of uninsured people. In fact, most people who come to emergency rooms for treatment have insurance.

While undocumented immigrants are moving into states that have previously not been known for foreign-born residents, certain areas of the country and even certain hospitals are more likely to treat them for emergency conditions. A major financial problem arises when the patient cannot safely be discharged, requires further rehabilitation or chronic treatment, or lacks family to provide needed care.

The YES and NO selections address this dilemma. Neither selection advocates a drastic solution such as deportation but each brings a different perspective. Physicians Rajeev Raghavan and Ricardo Nuila believe that a better and cheaper solution to the needs of undocumented dialysis patients would be to provide standardized coverage so that patients would not come to treatment as a last resort. David W. Stratas argues that a country is justified in setting eligibility requirements for financially burdensome benefits, and it may then exclude from those benefits individuals who have not taken appropriate measures to become eligible for them.

YES

Rajeev Raghavan and Ricardo Nuila

Survivors—Dialysis, Immigration, and U.S. Law

Santiago is in the ER again. He sits in a special row of 20 patients, all of whom are waiting for one result: the potassium. Is it high enough today? Two days ago he was here, and it was only 6 meq per liter. We discharged him. Right now his chest hurts, and he is short of breath. Nothing new, and Santiago knows that if he's to be dialyzed today, these symptoms don't matter. Only the potassium matters.

One of us is the nephrologist on service, and the other is the hospitalist taking admissions. We both trained here as medical students and have continued to work in the county hospital system as faculty members. Some of these patients remember us as residents. Now they recognize us as the gatekeepers, the people deciding which patients go home and which sit in the chair. We know them, too. There's Juan, who is 67 years old and lives 50 miles away in Hempstead. His children take turns bringing him in. There's Maria; she's 38, a mother of three. She began dialysis 5 years ago, initially just once a month; now it's twice every week. Hugo is back. He was admitted for line sepsis last month and spent 2 weeks in-house receiving antibiotics and a new catheter. He was referred for an arteriovenous fistula 6 months ago, but the waiting list is more than a year long. Hugo was brought to the United States at the age of 5; he works in an upscale restaurant and speaks perfect English. Some of the patients appear miserable, but most are like Santiago—they are just waiting patiently for a doctor to quantify their malaise.

Santiago emigrated from Mexico at the age of 20. He had no papers and no job, but he had a family to support, so he hired a smuggler to help him cross the border. He worked in construction from his first day here and helped to build Houston's highways, until one day he became inexplicably ill. He presented to our county hospital, where on his first encounter with a doctor, he was found to have a serum creatinine concentration of 15 mg per

deciliter. An ultrasound and laboratory tests confirmed the diagnosis: irreversible kidney failure. A tunneled hemodialysis catheter was inserted into his right internal jugular vein, and the demands of his new life were explained: you are to come to the emergency room every time you feel sick. And every fourth day for 5 years now, Santiago has come to our ER.

More than 11 million undocumented residents live in the United States, and 6000 of them have end-stage renal disease (ESRD).[1] This number seems small in the context of the 400,000-plus Americans currently undergoing dialysis,[2] but the direct and indirect costs are not small. The annual cost of hemodialysis is approximately $72,000 per patient.[2] Through the End Stage Renal Disease program, passed by Congress in 1973, all U.S. citizens with advanced kidney failure qualify for Medicare or Medicaid to defray these high costs.[1] The Consolidated Omnibus Budget Reconciliation Act (COBRA) passed in 1986 explicitly prohibits the use of federal funds for covering undocumented residents for nonemergency services such as dialysis.[3] Some states such as California and Massachusetts use state-allocated Medicaid or county taxes to pay for thrice-weekly hemodialysis for undocumented residents. Most states—including ours, Texas—do not. Here, undocumented residents with ESRD depend on public safety-net hospitals for emergency dialysis. That is to say, even though we know when these patients become ill, we must wait until their lives are at risk before we provide dialysis.

Nephrology guidelines recommend initiating dialysis when the estimated glomerular filtration rate (GFR) falls below 15 ml per minute in patients with diabetes or 10 ml per minute in patients without diabetes. Because of a lack of resources, we often delay initiation of dialysis in undocumented residents until the GFR is much lower or a patient requires emergency treatment. Our inpatient dialysis unit has 12 chairs, and priority is given to admitted patients. The line in the ER begins to swell by 6 a.m. Over the years, we've had some small victories—a special row of chairs, blood for laboratory tests drawn at triage, EKGs performed in assembly-line fashion—which have helped us maximize the provision of hemodialysis. Still, our capacity is grossly insufficient to meet the demands of the more than 180 undocumented residents (and counting) who depend on emergency dialysis in our city.[3]

Emergency dialysis is good for nobody. It places patients' lives at risk, and it results in more ER visits, more hospitalizations, and more blood transfusions than does scheduled dialysis. In total, these excesses result in costs of more than $200,000 per emergency-dialysis patient annually.[4] Furthermore, the community loses these patients' labor, and they lose out on wages, because of their irregular dialysis schedules and poor health. These effects are apparent in our population of patients, the majority of whom immigrated to the United States to work. In our experience, very few patients immigrate to this country because of their illness. Most are like Santiago: they are survivors.

This issue lies at the intersection of debates over the soaring cost of health care and the need for immigration reform. Do we have an ethical duty to provide the same standard of care for all sick patients within our borders? Or would mandating the provision of health care (and of maintenance-dialysis treatments) create an incentive for illegal immigration and worsen the current situation?

There is no easy solution. But with this particular disease, there are cheaper, more compassionate alternatives: dialyzing at home using peritoneal dialysis, kidney transplantation, or funding of maintenance hemodialysis. Resources in our city have allowed for 100 undocumented residents to receive thrice-weekly hemodialysis treatments in a county-funded clinic.[3] Patients undergoing dialysis in this clinic are healthier and happier than those who must receive emergency treatment, and many of them have returned to work.[3] Like the undocumented residents cared for in other centers, our patients are young, with an average age of 43 years.[3] These patients are excellent candidates for transplantation, and many have potential donors. However, the out-of-pocket costs for transplantation and immunosuppressive medications make this option untenable, despite the potential savings for taxpayers.[5]

In order for any of these options to work, dialysis coverage for this patient population must be standardized throughout the country. Standardization would alleviate the burden that is unfairly placed on taxpayers in areas where the most undocumented residents live, such as California and Texas.[3] In states like ours, standardization of care would improve these patients' health and allow them to return to work.

Santiago would love to work, but he can't work like this—not with his body so weak. On the days he qualifies for dialysis, he arrives here by bus at 5 a.m. and leaves in the evening, exhausted. When he doesn't qualify, he comes back the very next day. Today he waits. It's July in Houston—the heat index is 110°F—and Santiago is wearing his blue hoodie. He's cold. By any moral or medical standard, he should already be upstairs, but he "looks stable," and so we wait for the potassium. There are mouths to feed and bills to pay, but though Santiago would like nothing more than to work, his body tells him he can't, and so he rests. And in 2 days, he will begin the process again.

References

1. Campbell GA, Sanoff S, Rosner MH. Care of the undocumented immigrant in the United States with ESRD. Am J Kidney Dis 2010;55:181–91.
2. USRDS. 2008 Annual data report: atlas of chronic kidney disease and end-stage renal disease in the United States. Bethesda, MD: National Institutes of Health, National Institute of Diabetes and Digestive and Kidney Diseases; 2008.
3. Raghavan R, Sheikh-Hamad D. Descriptive analysis of undocumented residents with ESRD in a public hospital system. Dial Transplant 2011;2:78–81.
4. Sheikh-Hamad D, Paiuk E, Wright AJ, Kleinmann C, Khosla U, Shandera WX. Care for immigrants with end-stage renal disease in Houston: a comparison of two practices. Tex Med 2007;103:54–8.
5. Goldberg MJ, Simmerling M, Frader JE. Why nondocumented residents should have access to kidney transplantation: arguments for lifting the federal ban on reimbursement. Transplantation 2007;83:17–20.

RAJEEV RAGHAVAN is a staff member of the Department of Medicine, Division of Nephrology, Baylor College of Medicine, Houston, Texas.

RICARDO NUILA is a staff member of the Department of Medicine, Department of Family and Community Medicine, Baylor College of Medicine, Houston, Texas.

David W. Stratas   ⮕ **NO**

Toussaint v. Attorney General of Canada

Reasons for Judgment

[1] The applicant is a citizen of Grenada. In 1999, she entered Canada as a visitor. She never left. She has stayed in Canada, contrary to Canada's immigration laws.

[2] For her first seven years in Canada, the appellant worked and earned enough to sustain herself. However, in 2006, her health began to deteriorate. She could no longer work.

[3] Since 2006, the appellant has received some medical care without having to pay for it, but much more medical care is required. Her medical condition has become most serious.

[4] In September 2008, still in Canada contrary to Canada's immigration laws, the appellant took steps to try to regularize her status in Canada. She applied to Citizenship and Immigration Canada for permanent residence status. A few months later, she applied to Citizenship and Immigration Canada for a temporary residence permit so she could become eligible for health coverage under the Ontario Health Insurance Program. In both applications, she asked for a waiver of the fees. The waivers were refused, the fees remained unpaid, and so the applications were never considered.

[5] In May 2009, the appellant applied to Citizenship and Immigration Canada for medical coverage under its Interim Federal Health Program. As we shall see, this Program is actually embodied in one of Canada's immigration laws, Order in Council OIC 1957-11/848. Under this Order in Council, Citizenship and Immigration Canada covers the cost of emergency medical care for indigent persons that it has legally admitted to Canada.

[6] A Director with Citizenship and Immigration Canada found that the appellant was ineligible to receive medical coverage and rejected her application.

[7] The appellant brought an application for judicial review to the Federal Court, submitting that she was eligible for medical coverage. In the alternative, she submitted that her exclusion from medical coverage infringed her rights under sections 7 and 15 of the Charter. She requested the Federal Court to "read" the Order in Council as including her—in effect, to make this law compliant with sections 7 and 15 of the Charter by extending its terms to provide her with medical coverage.

[8] If the Federal Court accepted the appellant's request, the curiosity of some might be piqued: even though the appellant has disregarded Canada's immigration laws for the better part of a decade, she would be able to take one of Canada's immigration laws (the Order in Council), get a court to include her by extending the scope of that law, and then benefit from that extension while remaining in Canada contrary to Canada's immigration laws.

[9] But the Federal Court (*per* Justice Zinn) did not accept the appellant's request to extend the scope of the Order in Council. It rejected her submissions and dismissed the application for judicial review: 2010 FC 810 (main decision) and 2010 FC 926 (decision on motion for reconsideration).

[10] The appellant appeals to this Court, making submissions substantially similar to those that were made in the Federal Court.

[11] I also reject the appellant's submissions and would dismiss the appeal.

. . .

E. Assessment of the Federal Court's decision that the appellant was ineligible to receive medical coverage under the Order in Council

(1) Introduction and overview

[24] In my view, the Federal Court's bottom line conclusion is correct: the appellant was ineligible to receive medical coverage under the Order in Council.

. . .

[32] The Order in Council does not define "immigrant." However, the term "immigrant" was defined in *The Immigration Act*, S.C. 1952, c. 42, subsection 2(*i*) as "a person who seeks admission to Canada for permanent residence."

. . .

[35] The appellant does not qualify . . . . She was not admitted into Canada as an applicant for permanent residence. . . . The appellant was simply a visitor who decided to remain in Canada, contrary to Canada's immigration law.

(4) Section 15 of the Charter

(a) General principles

[89] When assessing the merits of a subsection 15(1) claim, we must apply a two-part test: (1) whether the law creates a distinction that is based on an enumerated or analogous ground and (2) whether the distinction creates a disadvantage by perpetuating prejudice or stereotyping. . . .

[90] The first step tells us that not all distinctions, in and of themselves, are contrary to s. 15(1) of the Charter. . . . Subsection 15(1) only covers distinctions made on the basis of the grounds enumerated in subsection 15(1), or grounds analogous to them.

[91] The second step tells us that the focus under subsection 15(1) is not differential treatment, but rather discrimination. Therefore, in order to succeed, a section 15 claimant must show that the impact of the law is discriminatory. . . .

[92] Discrimination has been described as follows:

...a distinction, whether intentional or not but based on grounds relating to personal characteristics of the individual or group, which has the effect of imposing burdens, obligations, or disadvantages on such individual or group not imposed upon others, or which withholds or limits access to opportunities, benefits, and advantages available to other members of society. Distinctions based on personal characteristics attributed to an individual solely on the basis of association with a group will rarely escape the charge of discrimination, while those based on an individual's merits and capacities will rarely be so classed. (*Andrews, supra,* at pages 174–175.)

(b) Application of the principles to this case

[93] The appellant submits that her exclusion from the medical coverage afforded by the Order in Council infringed subsection 15(1) of the Charter because that exclusion was based on an enumerated and analogous ground, and was discriminatory.

[94] The Federal Court rejected the appellant's subsection 15(1) submission, primarily on the basis (at paragraphs 79-83) that the appellant had failed to establish that her exclusion from coverage under the Order in Council was based on an enumerated or analogous ground.

[95] I find no error in the Federal Court's rejection of the appellant's section 15 submissions. In my view, there are four main reasons why the appellant's section 15 submissions must fail.

- I -

[96] In my view, the appellant has failed to demonstrate that the Order in Council makes a distinction based on any enumerated or analogous ground that is relevant to her situation. On this point, I substantially agree with the Federal Court reasons.

[97] In this Court, the appellant suggests that the Order in Council creates a "primary distinction" enhanced by a "secondary intersecting ground."

[98] The primary distinction is said to be between foreign nationals possessing certain immigration status who are covered under the Order in Council, and other foreign nationals who possess another immigration status who are not covered. As we have seen, however, coverage is potentially available under paragraph (b) to all persons regardless of immigration status. For example, the appellant herself might have been covered by the Order in Council upon her arrival in Canada. Upon entry, she was legally admitted as a visitor. Had she been in desperate need of emergency medical attention at that time and could not otherwise afford it, and if the immigration authorities felt obligated to assist, she would have been covered by the Order in Council.

[99] Further, I do not accept that "immigration status" qualifies as an analogous ground under section 15 of the Charter. . . . "Immigration status" is not a "[characteristic] that we cannot change." It is not "immutable or changeable only at unacceptable cost to personal identity." Finally "immigration status"—in this case, presence in Canada illegally—is a characteristic that the government has a "legitimate interest in expecting [the person] to change." Indeed, the government has a real, valid and justified interest in expecting those present in Canada to have a legal right to be in Canada. . . .

[100] The "secondary intersecting ground" is said by the appellant to be "a distinction between undocumented migrants with disabilities, who are adversely affected by the policy, and those without disabilities, who are similarly disqualified from coverage, but who do not have serious disabilities or related healthcare needs, therefore experiencing a differential effect." . . . As the appellant has failed to establish her primary distinction, immigration status, and since there are other obstacles to her section 15 claim, discussed below, I need not consider this further.

[101] Therefore, in my view, the appellant has failed to demonstrate that the Order in Council makes a distinction based on any enumerated or analogous ground that is relevant to her situation.

. . .

- II -

[103] The appellant has failed to establish that the Order in Council relies upon, perpetuates or promotes prejudice or stereotyping.

[104] The appellant has been denied coverage because she did not enter as an applicant for permanent residence, is not a person under immigration jurisdiction, and is not a person for whom the immigration authorities feel responsible. In imposing these eligibility criteria, the Order in Council does not suggest that the appellant and others like her are less capable or less worthy of recognition or value as human beings. The Order in Council does not single out, stigmatize or expose the appellant and others like her to prejudice and stereotyping, nor does it perpetuate any pre-existing prejudice and stereotyping. Indeed, the Order in Council, with its eligibility criteria, denies medical coverage to the vast majority of us, and not just the appellant and others like her. The Order in Council treats the appellant—a non-citizen who has remained in Canada contrary to Canadian immigration law—in the same way as all Canadian citizens, rich or poor, healthy or sick.

- III -

[105] In my view, the facts and the holding of the Supreme Court in *Auton* . . . are directly on point and confirm that the Order in Council does not infringe section 15 of the Charter. In *Auton*, the claimants sought an order that British Columbia's medicare program should be extended to cover a particular treatment for autism. The denial of coverage was said to be discriminatory under section 15 of the Charter. The Supreme Court refused to order British Columbia to extend its medicare program to cover the treatment.

[106] At paragraph 41, the Supreme Court held that "[i]t is not open to Parliament...to enact a law whose policy objectives and provisions single out a disadvantaged group for inferior treatment." I note that the Order in Council does not do this. The Supreme Court then added (at paragraph 41):

On the other hand, a legislative choice not to accord a particular benefit absent demonstration of discriminatory purpose, policy or effect...does not give rise to s. 15(1) review. This Court has repeatedly held that the legislature is under no obligation to create a particular benefit. It is free to target the social programs it wishes to fund as a matter of public policy, provided the benefit itself is not conferred in a discriminatory manner: *Granovsky v. Canada (Minister of Employment and Immigration)*, [2000] 1 S.C.R. 703, 2000 SCC 28 at para. 61; *Nova Scotia (Attorney General)*

v. Walsh, [2002] 4 S.C.R. 325, 2002 SCC 83, at para. 55; *Hodge, supra,* at para. 16.

[107] On the issue whether the benefit was conferred in a discriminatory manner, the Supreme Court stated (at paragraph 42):

Where stereotyping of persons belonging to a group is at issue, assessing whether a statutory definition that excludes a group is discriminatory, as opposed to being the legitimate exercise of legislative power in defining a benefit, involves consideration of the purpose of the legislative scheme which confers the benefit and the overall needs it seeks to meet. If a benefit program excludes a particular group in a way that undercuts the overall purpose of the program, then it is likely to be discriminatory: it amounts to an arbitrary exclusion of a particular group. If, on the other hand, the exclusion is consistent with the overarching purpose and scheme of the legislation, it is unlikely to be discriminatory. Thus, the question is whether the excluded benefit is one that falls within the general scheme of benefits and needs which the legislative scheme is intended to address.

[108] The exclusion of the appellant from the coverage provided by the Order in Council does not undercut its overall purpose. On the other hand, the exclusion of the appellant from the coverage provided by the Order in Council is consistent with its purpose. The Order in Council is designed to provide emergency care to legal entrants into Canada who are under immigration jurisdiction or for whom immigration authorities feel responsible. Extending these benefits to all foreign nationals in Canada, even those in Canada illegally, stretches the program well beyond its intended purpose. Excluding persons such as the appellant keeps the program within its purpose. In the words of *Auton* (at paragraph 43), the appellant's exclusion from the Order in Council "cannot, without more, be viewed as an adverse distinction based on an enumerated ground"; rather, "it is an anticipated feature" of the Order in Council.

[109] Since the Order in Council does not confer benefits in a discriminatory manner, the general rule expressed by the Supreme Court in paragraph 41 of *Auton* prevails. The government was "under no obligation to create a particular benefit" in the Order in Council and was left "free to target the social programs it [wished] to fund as a matter of public policy."

- IV -

[110] Finally, I query whether the Order in Council, said by the appellant to be discriminatory, is the operative cause of the disadvantage the appellant is encountering.

The observations I made in paragraphs 67-73 also apply to the appellant's section 15 claim.

[111] Therefore, for all of the foregoing reasons, I conclude that the Order in Council does not infringe the appellant's rights under section 15 of the Charter.

G. Justification and remedy

[112] On the issue of justification under section 1 of the Charter—whether the Order in Council is a reasonable limit prescribed by law in a free and democratic society—the Federal Court held (at paragraph 94) that if the Order in Council were extended to prove medical coverage to persons illegally in Canada, such as the appellant, Canada would become a "health care safe haven." . . .

[113] In any analysis of justification under section 1 of the Charter in this case, the interests of the state in defending its immigration laws would deserve weight. If the appellant were to prevail in this case and receive medical coverage under the Order in Council without complying with Canada's immigration laws, others could be expected to come to Canada and do the same. Soon, as the Federal Court warned, Canada could become a health care safe haven, its immigration laws undermined. Many, desperate to reach that safe haven, might fall into the grasp of human smugglers, embarking upon a voyage of destitution and danger, with some never making it to our shores. In the end, the Order in Council—originally envisaged as a humanitarian program to assist a limited class of persons falling within its terms—might have to be scrapped.

[114] In this case, it is not necessary to comment on justification under section 1 any further. Nor is it necessary to comment on what constitutional remedy might be awarded under subsection 24(1) of the Charter. The appellant's constitutional challenge fails for want of proof of rights breach. The Order in Council does not infringe sections 7 and 15 of the Charter.

H. Concluding comments

[115] Just before the release of these reasons, this Court released its judgment in *Toussaint v. Canada (Citizenship and Immigration)*, 2011 FCA 146. It held that the Minister must consider the appellant's request for a waiver of fees for her application for permanent residence in Canada.

[116] On the evidence in this record, . . . a decision by the Minister to waive the fees and accept the appellant's application will not entitle her to medical coverage under the Order in Council. However, depending upon the terms of legislation in Ontario, she may be entitled to health coverage or assistance from Ontario, now or at some point in the future. That will be for others to decide.

DAVID W. STRATAS is a justice with the Federal Court of Appeals of Ontario in Canada.

EXPLORING THE ISSUE

Is There an Ethical Duty to Provide Health Care to Undocumented Immigrants?

Critical Thinking and Reflection

1. There are two contrasting ways to frame the question of whether health insurance should be extended to undocumented immigrants: We might ask whether they have a right to it, or we might ask whether our society is the kind of society that accepts an obligation to address their needs. Which would you find more persuasive? How do Raghavan and Nuila argue for extending insurance?
2. What kind of response to the problem of undocumented workers does Stratas propose? Do you think Stratas is addressing the problem more honestly, or sidestepping the problem?

Is There Common Ground?

Extending health insurance to undocumented immigrants remains controversial. Although the Affordable Care Act (ACA) excludes undocumented immigrants from the state-run health-care exchanges through which, starting in 2014, citizens without employer-provided insurance should be able to buy health insurance, the ACA does include increased funding for constructing and staffing Federally Qualified Health Centers, which provide primary care for medically underserved populations, including seasonal and migrant workers.

In August 2010, Grady Memorial Hospital and several Atlanta dialysis providers reached an agreement to provide dialysis for 38 end-stage renal disease patients, most of them undocumented immigrants. The hospital agreed to help pay for continuing dialysis for most of the immigrants, while the rest would be distributed among the local providers as charity cases. There is no plan for managing the care of newly diagnosed patients, except for emergency room care when they become desperately ill.

Additional Resources

A selection of resources are available at a website developed by The Hastings Center, "Undocumented Patients: Undocumented Immigrants & Access to Health Care," www.undocumentedpatients.org/.

For further reading, see Stephen Zukerman, Timothy A. Waldman, and Emily Lawton, "Undocumented Immigrants, Left Out of Health Reform, Likely to Continue to Grow as Share of the Uninsured," *Health Affairs* (pp. 1997–2007, October 2011). Also, Susan Okie, "Immigrants and Health Care—At the Intersection of Two Broken Systems," *The New England Journal of Medicine* (pp. 525–529, August 9, 2007).

Elizabeth R. Chesler argues that denying undocumented immigrants' access to Medicaid under the 1996 Personal Responsibility and Work Opportunity Reconciliation Act violates their right to equal protection (www.bu.edu/law/central/jd/organizations/journals/pilj/vol17no2/documents/17-2CheslerNote.pdf).

"Immigrants in the U.S. Health Care System: Five Myths That Misinform the American Public" (2007), by Meredith L. King, is available on the website of the Center for American Progress (www.americanprogress.org/projects/healthprogress/articles.html). Among the beliefs she cites as erroneous is "Restricting immigrants' access to the health care system will not affect American citizens."

For a different view, see James R. Edwards Jr., "The Medicaid Costs of Legalizing Illegal Aliens," a July 2010 memorandum from the Center for Immigration Studies, an organization opposed to expanding immigration.

The National Conference of State Legislatures has an immigration policy project that provides updates on activities in state legislatures. The most recent report covers the period from January 1, 2011 to December 7, 2011; www.ncsl.org/?tabid=19897.

The Kaiser Commission on Medicaid and the Uninsured has data on immigrants' health care coverage and access; www.kff.org/medicaid/upload/Connecting-Eligible-Immigrant-Families-to-Health-Coverage-and-Care-Key-Lessons-from-Outreach-and-Enrollment-Workers-pdf.pdf

Internet References . . .

California Immigrant Policy Center

http://www.caimmigrant.org/healthcare.html

Human Rights Watch

http://www.hrw.org/topic/migration

Undocumented Patients

www.undocumentedpatients.org/

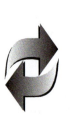

Selected, Edited, and with Issue Framing Material by:
Gregory E. Kaebnick, *The Hastings Center*

ISSUE

Should New Drugs Be Given to Patients Outside Clinical Trials?

YES: Emil J. Freireich, from "Should Terminally Ill Patients Have the Right to Take Drugs That Pass Phase I Testing?" *British Medical Journal* (2007)

NO: George J. Annas, from "Cancer and the Constitution—Choice at Life's End," *The New England Journal of Medicine* (2007)

Learning Outcomes

After reading this issue, you will be able to:

- Discuss the ethical and policy issues that arise in the development and marketing of new drugs.
- Explore critically the individual right to make one's own risk–benefit decisions and society's reasons for limiting that right.

ISSUE SUMMARY

YES: Physician Emil J. Freireich believes that patients with advanced cancer and limited life expectancy should have the same privilege as all individuals in a free society.

NO: Law professor George J. Annas argues that there is no constitutional right to demand experimental interventions, and that fully open access would undermine the FDA's ability to protect the public from unsafe drugs.

At the beginning of the twentieth century, any American could manufacture a medication and sell it to the public. The era of "patent medicines" led at best to harmless but useless "cure-alls," and at worst, to illness and death. Alarmed by this practice, in 1906 the U.S. Congress enacted the Food and Drug Act, prohibiting the sale of misbranded, mislabeled, and adulterated foods and drugs in interstate commerce. In 1938, more than 100 people died as a result of taking elixir sulfanilamide, a powder that had been made into a liquid form by adding diethylene glycol, a poison used in antifreeze. In response, Congress created the Food and Drug Administration (FDA) to prevent future tragedies.

Under the current rules, drug manufacturers must submit "investigational new drug" applications to the agency and provide evidence of their safety and effectiveness before they can bring new drugs to the market. In general, drug trials involve stages of testing and data are collected from small, carefully selected groups, analyzed, and then tested in wider populations. Phase I includes a small number of patients and is designed to determine levels of toxicity (bad reactions). This process is costly and can take considerable time.

Over the years, the FDA has been criticized on grounds that it allows unsafe drugs to be marketed to the public, and in recent years several drugs have been taken off the market. It has also been criticized for its slow review process because of which promising new drugs are unavailable to people who desperately need them. In the 1980s and 1990s, HIV/AIDS activists in particular lobbied for faster access to drugs, and the FDA responded with a plan to allow access to some experimental drugs for patients with serious diseases and no other therapeutic options.

But for many people facing death, the FDA does not go far enough. They want to be able to take drugs that are in early stages of development and without being enrolled in a clinical trial, for which they may not be eligible. The Abigail Alliance, founded in 2001 by Frank Burroughs, is one of the most prominent advocates of this position. Mr. Burroughs' daughter Abigail died that year from cancer of the head and neck. He had tried unsuccessfully to obtain two drugs that were then in clinical trials, although not for her type of cancer. (One of the drugs has since been approved for that indication.) Abigail was not eligible for the clinical trials because as Mr. Burroughs said, "She had the right cells in the wrong place."

In 2003, the Alliance sued the FDA in federal district court, claiming that the agency's failure to permit the sale of investigational new drugs to terminally ill patients violated the patients' rights to privacy and due process under the Fifth Amendment of the U.S. Constitution. The three-judge panel on the first court to hear the case agreed that there was a constitutional right to such access, but 15 months later this decision was reversed by the District of Columbia Circuit Court of Appeals. In January 2008, the U.S. Supreme Court declined to hear the case.

The YES and NO selections take different views of the basic issue. Physician Emil J. Freireich asserts that dying individuals for whom all approved medications have failed should have the right to take drugs still in the investigational stage. Law professor George J. Annas believes that access to unproven drugs has to be limited to protect the public.

YES ↵

Emil J. Freireich

Should Terminally Ill Patients Have the Right to Take Drugs That Pass Phase I Testing?

Around half a million people will die from cancer-related causes in the United States this year. In the US, as in much of the Western world, patients know their diagnosis and are often given a hopeless prognosis. For most, the option of participating in phase I and phase II clinical trials of new drugs that offer some promise helps them remain optimistic. Clearly, they should have the right to take drugs that have passed phase I testing.

The problem is that most cancer patients cannot participate in phase II trials because they are either ineligible or they are unable to fulfil the financial and social requirements for participating in such trials, such as staying in the centres conducting these trials, sometimes for many weeks or months. The problem is clearly not one of safety because these drugs have completed phase I clinical trials and there is sufficient information about them to justify a phase II trial to determine efficacy.

Phase II trials are designed to give the highest probability of a positive outcome. Thus, they have patient eligibility requirements which assure that only the healthiest patients at the earliest point in their disease are entered. These decisions are not based on any reasonable evidence that patients who are ineligible would not benefit, but are strictly designed to fulfil the regulatory requirements established by bodies such as the Food and Drug Administration (FDA) and the regulatory components of industry and academia that govern these clinical trials.

Compassionate Prescribing

In the modern electronic era, most of the patients with hopeless cancer diagnoses have access through the media and the internet to information about promising new drugs that are in phase II clinical trials. These patients would like very much to receive these drugs to offer them some hope, but for the reasons mentioned above are unable to participate in those trials. So why not offer these drugs to these patients on a compassionate basis?

The first reason given is usually the safety concerns. Without knowledge about how renal function, cardiac function, age, etc. affect the action of the phase I drug, side effects might occur that could be harmful to the patient or, perhaps more importantly, the continued development of the drug. I think this objection is relatively minor since it simply states the benefit:risk ratio problem—that is, these patients are prepared to volunteer to expose themselves to increased risk because of their hopeless prognosis and because of the promise of the new drug.

The second objection is that it will interfere with the development of the drug. However, in the past, the FDA and the National Cancer Institute have allowed compassionate use of drugs and have found that it actually accelerates development. This is because when patients are offered compassionate use of an experimental drug, their doctors have to collect information as systematically as in the research protocol and submit it to the sponsor. Information is therefore available about use of the drug outside trial conditions. For example, if patients with impaired renal function not only tolerate the drug but respond, it will assist in drug development to have that knowledge collected systematically.

Drug Industry Profits

Another objection is that the drug industry might use this device to profit from investigation of a phase I drug. I believe this is a trivial objection because the usual strategy for compassionate use is that the drug is provided at cost. The last, and perhaps the most serious, objection is that expanded access would interfere with the clinical trial process. This certainly should not be the case. The clinical trial process is governed by the regulatory bodies in government, in industry, and in academic institutions.

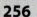

The unfortunate consequence of this is that physician scientists, who have the most experience, the most training, the most knowledge, the most productivity, and the most creativity, are completely excluded from this process. Because of the relationship between the regulatory organisations of government, industry, and academia, the academic physician scientist can only implement protocols that have been developed by the drug developer with direction from the regulatory agencies. Expanded access would bring the doctors back into the drug development process and, rather than damage the clinical trial system, would greatly expand its effectiveness and value.

In summary, patients with advanced cancer and limited life expectancy should have the same privilege as all individuals in a free society—that is, to decide their own benefit:risk ratio. It is tragic that regulatory bodies have created a circumstance where people have to live in an aura of hopelessness even though they have the will, the resources, and the ability to expose themselves to the risk of participating in investigational studies and to enjoy the potential for benefit. The solution is legislation or judicial action to permit expanded access to experimental treatments for patients with limited life expectancy.

EMIL J. FREIREICH is a professor of special medical education at the MD Anderson Cancer Center, Houston, Texas.

George J. Annas 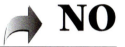 **NO**

Cancer and the Constitution— Choice at Life's End

J.M. Coetzee's violent, anti-apartheid *Age of Iron,* a novel the *Wall Street Journal* termed "a fierce pageant of modern South Africa," is written as a letter by a retired classics professor, Mrs. Curren, to her daughter, who lives in the United States. Mrs. Curren is dying of cancer, and her daughter advises her to come to the United States for treatment. She replies, "I can't afford to die in America. . . . No one can, except Americans."[1] Dying of cancer has been considered a "hard death" for at least a century, unproven and even quack remedies have been common, and price has been a secondary consideration. Efforts sponsored by the federal government to find cures for cancer date from the establishment of the National Cancer Institute (NCI) in 1937. Cancer research was intensified after President Richard Nixon's declaration of a "war on cancer" and passage of the National Cancer Act of 1971.[2] Most recently, calls for more cancer research have followed the announcement by Elizabeth Edwards, wife of presidential candidate John Edwards, that her cancer is no longer considered curable.

Frustration with the methods and slow progress of mainstream medical research has helped fuel a resistance movement that distrusts both conventional medicine and government and that has called for the recognition of a right for terminally ill patients with cancer to have access to any drugs they want to take. Prominent examples include the popularity of Krebiozen in the 1950s and of laetrile in the 1970s. As an NCI spokesperson put it more than 20 years ago, when thousands of people were calling the NCI hotline pleading for access to interleukin-2, "What the callers are saying is, 'Our mother, our brother, our sister is dying at this very moment. We have nothing to lose.'"[2] Today, families search the Internet for clinical trials, and even untested chemicals such as dichloroacetate, that seem to offer them some hope. In addition, basing advocacy on their personal experiences with cancer, many families have focused their frustrations on the Food and Drug Administration (FDA), which they see as a government agency denying them access to treatments they need.

In May 2006 these families won an apparent major victory when the Court of Appeals for the District of Columbia, in the case of *Abigail Alliance v. Von Eschenbach* (hereafter referred to as *Abigail Alliance*),[3] agreed with their argument that patients with cancer have a constitutional right of access to investigational cancer drugs. In reaction, the FDA began the process of rewriting its own regulations to make it easier for terminally ill patients not enrolled in clinical trials to have access to investigational drugs.[4] In November 2006, the full bench of the Court of Appeals vacated the May 2006 opinion, and the case was reheard in March 2007.[5] The decision of the full bench, expected by the fall, will hinge on the answer to a central question: Do terminally ill adult patients with cancer for whom there are no effective treatments have a constitutional right of access to investigational drugs their physicians think might be beneficial?

The Constitutional Controversy

The Abigail Alliance for Better Access to Developmental Drugs (hereafter called the Abigail Alliance) sued the FDA to prevent it from enforcing its policy of prohibiting the sale of drugs that had not been proved safe and effective to competent adult patients who are terminally ill and have no alternative treatment options. The Abigail Alliance is named after Abigail Burroughs, whose squamous-cell carcinoma of the head and neck was diagnosed when she was only 19 years old. Two years later, in 2001, she died. Before her death she had tried unsuccessfully to obtain investigational drugs on a compassionate use basis from ImClone and AstraZeneca and was accepted for a clinical trial only shortly before her death. Her father founded the Abigail Alliance in her memory.[6]

The district court dismissed the Abigail Alliance lawsuit. The appeals court, in a two-to-one opinion written by Judge Judith Rogers, who was joined by Judge Douglas Ginsburg, reversed the decision. It concluded that competent, terminally ill adult patients have a constitutional "right to access to potentially life-saving post-Phase I investigational new drugs, upon a doctor's advice, even where that medicine carries risks for the patient," and remanded the case to the district court to determine whether the FDA's current policy violated that right.[3]

The Right to Life

The appeals court found that the relevant constitutional right was determined by the due-process clause of the Fifth Amendment: "no person shall be . . . deprived of life, liberty, or property without due process of law." In the court's words, the narrow question presented by *Abigail Alliance* is whether the due-process clause "protects the right of terminally ill patients to make an informed decision that may prolong life, specifically by use of potentially life-saving new drugs that the FDA has yet to approve for commercial marketing but that the FDA has determined, after Phase I clinical human trials, are safe enough for further testing on a substantial number of human beings."[3]

The court answered yes, finding that this right has deep legal roots in the right to self-defense, and that "Barring a terminally ill patient from the use of a potentially life-saving treatment impinges on this right of self-preservation."[3] In a footnote, the court restated this proposition: "The fundamental right to take action, even risky action, free from government interference, in order to save one's own life undergirds the court's decision."[3] The court relied primarily on the *Cruzan* case,[7] in which the Supreme Court recognized the right of a competent adult to refuse life-sustaining treatment, including a feeding tube:

> The logical corollary is that an individual must also be free to decide for herself whether to assume any known or unknown risks of taking a medication that might prolong her life. Like the right claimed in *Cruzan,* the right claimed by the [Abigail] Alliance to be free of FDA imposition does not involve treatment by the government or a government subsidy. Rather, much as the guardians of the comatose [sic] patient in Cruzan did, the Alliance seeks to have the government step aside by changing its policy so the individual right of self-determination is not violated.[3]

The appeals court concluded that the Supreme Court's 1979 unanimous decision on laetrile,[8] in which the Court concluded that Congress had made no exceptions

in the FDA law for terminally ill cancer patients, was not relevant because laetrile had never been studied in a phase 1 trial and because the Court did not address the question of whether terminally ill cancer patients have a constitutional right to take whatever drugs their physicians prescribe.

The Dissent

Judge Thomas Griffith, the dissenting judge, argued that the suggested constitutional right simply does not exist. He noted, for example, that the self-defense cases relied on are examples of "abstract concepts of personal autonomy," and cannot be used to craft new rights. As to the nation's history and traditions, he concluded that the FDA's drug-regulatory efforts have been reasonable responses "to new risks as they are presented."[3] Accepting his argument leaves the majority resting squarely on *Cruzan* and the laetrile case. As to *Cruzan,* the dissent argued that "A tradition of protecting individual *freedom* from life-saving, but forced, medical treatment does not evidence a constitutional tradition of providing affirmative *access* to a potentially harmful, even fatal, commercial good."[3] As to the laetrile case, the judge noted simply that the Court had agreed with the FDA that, "For the terminally ill, as for anyone else, a drug is unsafe if its potential for inflicting death or physical injury is not offset by the possibility of therapeutic benefit."[3,8]

Finally, the dissenting judge argued that if the new constitutional right were accepted, it was too vague to be applied only to terminally ill patients seeking drugs that had been tested in phase 1 trials. Specifically, the judge asked, must the right also apply to patients with "serious medical conditions," to patients who "cannot afford potentially life-saving treatment," or to patients whose physicians believe "marijuana for medicinal purposes . . . is potentially life saving?"[3] In other words, there is no principled reason to restrict the constitutional right the majority created to either terminally ill patients or to post–phase 1 drugs.

Discussion

The facts as illustrated by stories of patients dying of cancer while trying unsuccessfully to enroll in clinical trials are compelling, and our current system of ad hoc exceptions is deeply flawed. The central constitutional issue, however, rests primarily on determining whether this case is or is not like the right-to-refuse-treatment case of Nancy Cruzan, a woman in a permanent vegetative state whose family wanted tube feeding discontinued because they believed that discontinuation was what she would have wanted. I do not think *Abigail Alliance* is like *Cruzan*. Rather, it is substantially identical to cases involving physician-assisted suicide, in which a terminally ill patient claims a constitutional right of access to physician-prescribed drugs to commit suicide.

The Supreme Court has decided, unanimously, that no right to physician-prescribed drugs for suicide exists.[9,10] There is no historical tradition of support for this right. And although the right seems to be narrowly defined, it is unclear to whom it should apply—why only to terminally ill patients? Don't patients in chronic pain have even a stronger interest in suicide? Why is the physician necessary, and why are physician-prescribed drugs the only acceptable method of suicide? None of these questions can be answered by examining the Constitution.[11]

Similarly, in *Abigail Alliance,* the new constitutional right proposed has no tradition in the United States, and it cannot be narrowly applied. For example, why should a constitutional right apply only to people who have a particular medical status? And why should a physician be involved at all? If patients have a right to autonomy, why isn't the requirement of a government-licensed physician's recommendation at least as burdensome as the requirement of the FDA's approval of the investigational drug? And why would the Constitution apply only to investigational drugs for which phase 1 trials have been completed? Why not include access to investigational medical devices, like the artificial heart, or even to Schedule I controlled substances, like marijuana or lysergic acid diethylamide (LSD)? If it is a constitutional right, these should be available too, at least unless the state can demonstrate a "compelling interest" in regulating them.

My prediction is that after rehearing this case en banc, the full Circuit Court will reject the position of the Abigail Alliance for the same reasons that the Supreme Court rejected the "right" of terminally ill patients to have access to physician-prescribed drugs they could use to end their lives.[9,11] To decide otherwise would entirely undermine the legitimacy of the FDA. Patients in the United States have always had a right to refuse any medical treatment, but we have never had a right to demand mistreatment, inappropriate treatment, or even investigational or experimental interventions. This will not, however, be the end of the matter. After the physician-assisted–suicide cases, the fight appropriately shifted to the states, although so far only one, Oregon, has provided its physicians with immunity for prescribing life-ending drugs to their competent, terminally ill patients.[12] In the Abigail Alliance case, the

debate will continue in the forum in which it began—the FDA—and in Congress.

Congress

Congressional action also had its birth with the story of one patient with cancer and was also heavily influenced by another individual patient involved in a controversy over removal of a feeding tube. "Terri's Law" was enacted in Florida in 2003 to try to prevent the removal of a feeding tube from Terri Schiavo; the case was substantially similar to *Cruzan*. Terri's case gained national attention 2 years later.[13] In the midst of it, in March 2005, the *Wall Street Journal* asserted, in an editorial titled "How About a 'Kianna's Law'?," "If Terri Schiavo deserves emergency federal intervention to save her life, people like Kianna Karnes deserve it even more."[14] At the time, Kianna Karnes was a 44-year-old mother of four who was dying of kidney cancer. Her only hope of survival, according to the editorial, was to gain access to one of two experimental drugs in clinical trials, but neither of the two companies running the trials (Bayer and Pfizer) would make the drugs available to her on a compassionate-use basis. This was because, according to the *Wall Street Journal*, the FDA "makes it all but impossible" for the manufacturers "to provide [drugs] to terminal patients on a 'compassionate use' basis."[14]

Almost immediately after the editorial was published, both drug manufacturers contacted Kianna's physicians to discuss releasing the drugs to her. But within 2 days after publication, she was dead. The *Wall Street Journal* editorialized, "Isn't it a national scandal that cancer sufferers should have to be written about in the *Wall Street Journal* to be offered legal access to emerging therapies once they've run out of other options?"[15] It noted that Mrs. Karnes' father, John Rowe—himself a survivor of leukemia—was working with the Abigail Alliance on a "Kianna's Law." That law, formally titled the "Access, Compassion, Care, and Ethics for Seriously Ill Patients Act" or the "ACCESS Act," was introduced in November 2005 and is an attempt to make it much easier for seriously ill patients to gain access to experimental drugs.[16,17]

The act begins with a series of congressional findings, including that "Seriously ill patients have a right to access available investigational drugs, biological products, and devices." The act permits the sponsor to apply for approval to make an investigational drug, biologic product, or device available on the basis of data from a completed phase 1 trial, "preliminary evidence that the product may be effective against a serious or life-threatening condition or disease," and an assurance that the clinical trial will continue.[17] The patient, who must have exhausted all approved treatments, must provide written informed consent and must also sign "a written waiver of the right to sue the manufacturer or sponsor of the drug, biological product, or device, or the physicians who prescribed the product or the institution where it was administered, for an adverse event caused by the product, which shall be binding in every State and Federal court."[17]

Although Congress is the proper forum to address this issue, this initial attempt has some of the same problems as the *Abigail Alliance* decision: the patients to whom it applies are ambiguously classified, and clinical research seems to be equated with clinical care. Also troubling is that the patients (and would-be subjects) are asked to assume all of the risks of the uncontrolled experiments, and current rules of research—which protect subjects by prohibiting mandatory waivers of rights—are jettisoned, with the requirement of such waivers becoming the price of obtaining the investigational agent from an otherwise reluctant drug company.

FDA Proposal

In direct response to *Abigail Alliance*, the FDA proposed amending its rules to encourage more drug companies to offer their investigational drugs through compassionate-use programs.[4] These programs first came into prominence during the early days of infection with the human immunodeficiency virus (HIV) and AIDS, when there were no effective treatments and AIDS activists insisted that they have early access to investigational drugs because, in the words of their inaccurate slogan, "A Research Trial Is Treatment Too."[18] Because the FDA could not stand the political pressure generated by the activists, the compassionate-use program was developed as a kind of political safety valve to provide enough exceptions to save their basic research rules. In early December 2006, the FDA continued this political-safety-valve approach by issuing new proposed regulations with a title that could have been taken directly from the AIDS Coalition to Unleash Power (ACT-UP): "Expanded Access to Investigational Drugs for Treatment Use."[19]

The FDA's expanded-access proposal applies to "seriously ill patients when there is no comparable or satisfactory alternative therapy to diagnose, monitor, or treat the patient's disease or condition."[4] Manufacturers are required to file an "expanded access submission," and the product must be administered or dispensed by a licensed physician who will be considered an "investigator," with all the reporting requirements that role entails.[3]

Whether or not the proposal is adopted, it will do little to increase access, since the major bottleneck in the compassionate-use program has never been the FDA. The manufacturers have no incentives to make their investigational products available outside clinical trials. This is because direct access to investigational drugs by individuals may make it more difficult to recruit research subjects, and thus to conduct the clinical trials necessary for drug approval, and could also subject the drug manufacturer to liability for serious adverse reactions. Even without a lawsuit, a serious reaction to a drug outside a trial could adversely affect the trial itself.[4,16,20] The drug companies are right to worry that the approaches of the judiciary, Congress, and the FDA will probably make clinical trials more difficult to conduct, because few seriously ill patients who have exhausted conventional treatments would rather be randomly assigned to an investigational drug than have a guarantee that they will receive the investigational drug their physician recommends for them. This could result in significant delays in the approval and overall availability of drugs that demonstrate effectiveness—a result no one favors. Even if patients with cancer are willing buyers, drug manufacturers are not willing sellers.

Physicians and Patients

The cover story for all the proposed changes is patients' choice. But without scientific evidence of the risks and benefits of a drug, choice cannot be informed, and for seriously ill patients, fear of death will predictably overcome fear of unknown risks. This is understandable. As psychiatrist Jay Katz, the leading scholar on informed consent, has noted, when medical science seems impotent to fight nature, "all kinds of senseless interventions are tried in an unconscious effort to cure the incurable magically through a 'wonder drug,' a novel surgical procedure, or a penetrating psychological interpretation."[21] Another *Wall Street Journal* article, entitled "Saying No to Penelope,"[22] illustrates the impossibility of limiting access to unproven cancer drugs to competent adults. The article tells the story of 4-year-old Penelope, who is dying from neuroblastoma that has proved resistant to all conventional treatments. Her parents seek "anything [that] has a prayer of saving her." In her father's words, "The chance of anything bringing her back from the abyss now is very low. But the only thing I know for sure is if we don't treat her, she will die." With Penelope hospitalized and in pain, her parents continue "searching Penelope's big brown eyes for clues as to how long she wants to continue to battle for life."

It is suggested that the requirement of a physician's recommendation can safeguard against "magical thinking" and help make informed consent real.[23] But as Katz has noted, although physicians (and, he could have added, drug companies) often justify such last-ditch interventions as simply being responsive to patient needs, the interventions "may turn out to be a projection of their own needs onto patients."[21]

Government and the Market

Another recurrent theme is the belief that government regulation is evil, a central tenet of the laetrile litigation of the 1970s. The court hearing *Abigail Alliance* was correct to note that laetrile never underwent a phase 1 trial, but every indication was that the drug, also known as vitamin B_{17}, was harmless, albeit also ineffective against cancer. Laetrile became a legal cause celebre in 1972, when California physician John A. Richardson was prosecuted for promoting laetrile. Richardson was a member of the John Birch Society, which quickly formed the Committee for Freedom of Choice in Cancer Therapy, with more than 100 committees nationwide.[24] It took another 7 years before the FDA prevailed in its case against laetrile before the Supreme Court.[8] The basic arguments against FDA regulation remain the same today: the FDA follows a "paternalistic public policy that prevents individuals from exercising their own judgment about risks and benefits. If the FDA must err, it should be on the side of patients' freedom to choose."[25]

Public Policy

The FDA will prevail again today, not only because there is no constitutional right of access to unapproved drugs but also because even if there were, the state has the same compelling interest in approving drugs as it has in licensing physicians. From a public policy view, the *Abigail Alliance* court, the Congress, and the FDA all seem to be suffering from the "therapeutic illusion" in which research, designed to test a hypothesis for society, is confused with treatment, administered in the best interests of individual patients.[21,26,27] Of course there is a continuum, and it is perfectly understandable that many patients with cancer, told that there is nothing conventional medicine can do for them, will want access to whatever is available in or outside the context of clinical trials. But this is a problem for patients, physicians, the FDA, and drug manufacturers. First, because terminally ill patients can be harmed and exploited, there are better and worse ways to die.[21,26] Second, it is only through research, not "treatment," that cancer may become a chronic illness that is treated with a complex array of drugs, given either together or in a progression.[28,29] The right to choose in medicine is a central right of patients, but the choices can and should be

limited to reasonable medical alternatives, which themselves are based on evidence.

This is, I believe, good public policy. But it is also much easier said than done.[30] Death is feared and even dreaded in our culture, and few Americans are able to die at home, at peace, with our loved ones in attendance, without seeking the "latest new treatment." There always seems to be something new to try, and there is almost always anecdotal evidence that it could help. This is one reason that even extremely high prices do not affect demand for cancer drugs, even ones that add little or no survival time.[31,32] When does caring for the patient demand primary attention to palliation rather than to long-shot, high-risk, investigational interventions? Coetzee's Mrs. Curren, who rejected new medical treatment for her cancer and insisted on dying at home, told her physician, whom she saw as "withdrawing" from her after giving her a terminal prognosis—"His allegiance to the living, not the dying"—"I have no illusions about my condition, doctor. It is not [experimental] care I need, just help with the pain."[1]

References

No potential conflict of interest relevant to this article was reported.

From the Department of Health Law, Bioethics, and Human Rights, Boston University School of Public Health, Boston.

1. Coetzee JM. Age of iron. London: Seeker & Warburg, 1990.
2. Patterson JT. The dread disease: cancer and modern American culture. Cambridge, MA: Harvard University Press, 1987.
3. Abigail Alliance v. Von Eschenbach, 445 F.3d 470 (DC Cir 2006). Vacated 469 F.3d 129 (DC Cir 2006).
4. Proposed rules for charging for investigational drugs and expanded access to investigational drugs for treatment use. Rockville, MD: Food and Drug Administration, 2006. (Accessed July 6, 2007, at http://www.fda.gov/cder/regulatory/applications /IND_PR.htm.)
5. Abigail Alliance v. Von Eschenbach, 429 F.3d 129 (DC Cir 2006).
6. Jacobson PD, Parmet WE. A new era of unapproved drugs: the case of Abigail Alliance v Von Eschenbach. JAMA 2007;297:205–8.
7. Cruzan v. Director, Missouri Dept. of Health, 497 U.S. 261 (1990).
8. United States v. Rutherford, 442 U.S. 544 (1979).
9. Washington v. Glucksberg, 521 U.S. 702 (1997).
10. Vacco v. Quill, 521 U.S. 793 (1997).
11. Annas GJ. The bell tolls for a constitutional right to assisted suicide. N Engl J Med 1997;337:1098–103.

12. Gonzales v. Oregon, 546 U.S. 243 (2006).
13. Annas GJ. "I want to live": medicine betrayed by ideology in the political debate over Terri Schiavo. Stetson Law Rev 2005;35:49–80.
14. How about a "Kianna's Law"? Wall Street Journal. March 24, 2005:A14.
15. Kianna's legacy. Wall Street Journal. March 29, 2005:Al4.
16. Groopman J. The right to a trial: should dying patients have access to experimental drugs? The New Yorker. December 18, 2006:40–7.
17. ACCESS Act (Access, Compassion, Care, and Ethics for Seriously Ill Patients), S. 1956, 109th Cong (2005).
18. Annas GJ. Faith (healing), hope and charity at the FDA: the politics of AIDS drug trials. Villanova Law Rev 1989;34:771–97.
19. FDA proposes rules overhaul to expand availability of experimental drugs: the agency also clarifies permissible charges to patients. Rockville, MD: Food and Drug Administration, December 11, 2006. (Accessed July 6, 2007, at http://www.fda.gov/bbs/topics/NEWS/2006/NEW01520.html.)
20. Prud'homme A. The cell game: Sam Waksal's fast money and false promises—and the fate of ImClone's cancer drug. New York: Harper Business, 2004.
21. Katz J. The silent world of doctor and patient. New Haven, CT: Yale University Press, 1984:151.
22. Anand G. Saying no to Penelope: father seeks experimental cancer drug, but a biotech firm says risk is too high. Wall Street Journal. May 1, 2007:A1.
23. Robertson J. Controversial medical treatment and the right to health care. Hastings Cent Rep 2006;36:15–20.
24. Culbert ML. Vitamin B17: Forbidden weapon against cancer. New Rochelle, NY: Arlington House, 1974.
25. Miller HI. Paternalism costs lives. Wall Street Journal. March 2, 2006:A15.
26. Annas GJ. The changing landscape of human experimentation: Nuremberg, Helsinki, and beyond. Health Matrix J Law Med 1992;2:119–40.
27. Appelbaum PS, Lidz CW. Re-evaluating the therapeutic misconception: response to Miller and Joffe. Kennedy Inst Ethics J 2006;16:367–73.
28. Nathan D. The cancer treatment revolution: how smart drugs and other therapies are renewing our hope and changing the face of medicine. New York: John Wiley, 2007.
29. Brugarolas J. Renal-cell carcinoma—molecular pathways and therapies. N Engl J Med 2007;356:185–6.
30. Callahan D. False hopes: why America's quest for perfect health is a recipe for failure. New York: Simon and Schuster, 1998.
31. Berenson A. Hope, at $4,200 a dose: why a cancer drug's cost doesn't hurt demand. New York Times. October 1, 2006:BU1.
32. Anand G. From Wall Street, a warning about cancer drug prices. Wall Street Journal. March 15, 2007:A1.

GEORGE J. ANNAS is the Edward R. Utley Professor of Health Law and chairman of the Health Law Department at the Boston University School of Public Health in Boston, Massachusetts. He is also the cofounder of Global Lawyers & Physicians and the Patients' Rights Project.

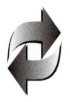

EXPLORING THE ISSUE

Should New Drugs Be Given to Patients Outside Clinical Trials?

Critical Thinking and Reflection

1. What other kinds of risk–benefit decisions does society allow individuals to make for themselves? What are some examples of risk–benefit decisions that society attempts to impose on individuals?
2. How do the examples above compare to the proposed right to make decisions about experimental drugs? How far does the right to make one's own decisions about risks extend, in your view—are there risks one could not claim a right to accept?
3. In recent years, some libertarians have called for eliminating the FDA altogether. In your view, on the basis of the YES and NO selections, would that improve or worsen access to drugs?

Is There Common Ground?

In August 2008, another case involving access to experimental treatment reached the courts. While the appeals court in the Abigail Alliance case determined that there was no constitutional right to experimental drugs, Judge William J. Martini of the United States District Court in Newark ruled that 16-year-old Jacob Gunvalson, suffering from a rare and fatal form of Duchenne muscular dystrophy, should be allowed to use an experimental drug for that condition. Jacob did not meet the criteria for a clinical trial organized by the manufacturer. Jacob's mother claimed that drug company officials had led her to believe that her son would be allowed to take part in a clinical trial, but then refused to accept him. In December 2008, the U.S. Court of Appeals reversed Judge Martini's decision and ruled that PTC therapeutics did not have to provide the experimental drug to Jacob Gunvalson.

The Access, Compassion, Care, and Ethics for Seriously Ill Patients Act, known as the Compassionate Access Act, were introduced in the Senate in 2008 and in the House in 2010. The act would require the Secretary of Health and Human Services to permit a still-experimental drug or device to be made available to sick people under certain circumstances. The law has not been passed.

An alternative approach is simply to speed the review of drugs. In 2012, the Food and Drug Administration announced that it had developed several different mechanisms to accelerate the approval of drugs and make them available to patients faster.

Additional Resources

Additional information about the Abigail Alliance's activities can be found at www.Abigail-Alliance.org. The Alliance supports the Compassionate Access Act of 2010 (H.R. 4732), introduced in March 2010, to create a new conditional approval process for drugs, biologics, and devices for seriously ill patients.

Jerome Groopman addresses the issue and its background in "The Right to a Trial: Should Dying Patients Have Access to Experimental Drugs?" *The New Yorker* (December 18, 2006). This article is available online at www.newyorker.com/archives.

See also Susan Okie, "Access before Approval—A Right to Take Experimental Drugs?" *The New England Journal of Medicine* (August 3, 2006); and Peter D. Jacobson and Wendy E. Parmet, "A New Era of Unapproved Drugs: The Case of Abigail Alliance v. Von Eschenbach," *Journal of the American Medical Association* (January 10, 2007). These articles express concerns about unregulated access to experimental drugs.

For opposing views, see Roger Pilon, "New Right to Life," *Wall Street Journal* (August 13, 2007); and A. Puckett, "The Proper Focus for FDA Regulations: Why the Fundamental Right to Self-Preservation Should Allow Terminally Ill Patients with No Treatment Options to Attempt to Save Their Lives," *SMU Law Review* (Spring 2007).

The FDA's accelerated review policies are described in "Fast Track, Accelerated Approval and Priority Review: Accelerating Availability of New Drugs for Patients with Serious Diseases," www.fda .gov/forconsumers/byaudience/forpatientadvocates /speedingaccesstoimportantnewtherapies/ucm128291.htm.

Internet References . . .

American Cancer Society: Compassionate Drug Use

http://www.cancer.org/treatment/treatmentsandside effects/clinicaltrials/compassionate-drug-use

Patient Advocate Foundation, Questions and Answers about Investigational Drugs

http://www.patientadvocate.org/resources .php?p=102

U.S. Food and Drug Administration, Learn about Other Treatment Options

http://www.fda.gov/ForPatients/Other/default.htm

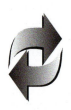

Selected, Edited, and with Issue Framing Material by:
Gregory E. Kaebnick, *The Hastings Center*

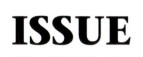

Should Vaccination for HPV Be Mandated for Teenage Girls?

YES: R. Alta Charo, from "Politics, Parents, and Prophylaxis—Mandating HPV Vaccination in the United States," *New England Journal of Medicine* (2007)

NO: Gail Javitt, Deena Berkowitz, and Lawrence O. Gostin, from "Assessing Mandatory HPV Vaccination: Who Should Call the Shots?" *The Journal of Law, Medicine and Ethics* (2008)

Learning Outcomes

After reading this issue, you will be able to:

- Identify and discuss the ethical issues raised by public health policies that attempt to influence or compel individuals' behavior.
- Explain the public health problem posed by the human papillomavirus (HPV) and how the HPV vaccine can be used to address it.

ISSUE SUMMARY

YES: Law professor R. Alta Charo argues that vaccination against the human papillomavirus, which causes most cases of cervical cancer, should be mandatory except in cases of medical, religious, or philosophical objection.

NO: Law professors Gail Javitt and Lawrence O. Gostin and physician Deena Berkowitz believe that, given the limited data and experience, and the fact that HPV does not pose imminent and significant risk to others, mandating HPV vaccine is premature.

Human papillomavirus (HPV) is the most common sexually transmitted infection in the United States, with about 6.2 million individuals newly infected every year. Over a quarter (26.8 percent) of females aged 14–24 have an HPV infection, and among the age group 20–24, almost half (44.8 percent) are infected. There is no treatment, but the vast majority (90 percent) of the women clear the virus within 2 years.

HPV is the cause of nearly all cases of cancer of the cervix (the narrow end of the uterus, or womb), which the National Institutes of Health lists as the third most common cancer among women globally. Each year around the world, a little less than half a million new cases of cervical cancer are diagnosed, and up to 300,000 deaths from this disease are reported. Most of these cases are among young women in their child-bearing and child-rearing years. More than 80 percent of the cases occur in developing countries, and this percentage is rising. In the United States, the incidence of cervical cancer is low, but still significant; about 11,000 new cases occur every year, and about 4,000 women die of the disease. The risk of death in the United States is much lower because of the widespread use of the Papanicolaou (Pap) test, which detects cervical cancer at an early and usually treatable stage.

But for those whose infection does not go away, the consequences are serious, especially if the infection comes from the high-risk strain of HPV. The high-risk strain is present in nearly all (99 percent) of cervical cancers. If a young woman is infected with the lower-risk variation, the association with cervical cancer is relatively low.

Clearly, cervical cancer related to HPV infection in the developing world is a major public health problem. But what about the United States? The chances of becoming infected with HPV are quite high, but the chances of this infection leading to cervical cancer are relatively low.

This issue was moved from the theoretical to the real world in June 2006 when the Food and Drug Administration (FDA), which must approve the safety and effectiveness of a medication or vaccine before it is introduced to the general public, licensed a prophylactic (preventive) vaccine against four strains of HPV. The vaccine protects against 70 percent of cervical cancers linked to HPV, but not against all cancer-causing types of HPV. The vaccine was approved for females aged 9–26. Commonly known as Gardasil, its trade name, the vaccine is manufactured and marketed by Merck. In October 2009, the FDA approved a second HPV vaccine, Cervarix, which targets a different HPV strain and is manufactured by GlaxoSmithKline.

The Advisory Committee on Immunization Practices of the Centers for Disease Control and Prevention (CDC) recommends routine vaccination of 11- and 12-year-old girls with three doses of the vaccine as well as vaccination of 13- to 26-year-olds who had no opportunity to receive the vaccine when they were younger. The three-dose vaccination costs about $375, making it one of the most costly vaccines available.

The CDC's recommendations were just that—recommendations. The controversy began when Merck officials lobbied state legislatures to require the vaccine as a condition of school entry for girls entering the sixth grade. By executive order from the governor, in 2007 Texas became the first state to mandate this use of the vaccine, but the state legislature passed legislation to override the executive order and the governor did not veto it. As a result of the controversy, Merck withdrew its lobbying campaign.

The following selections explore this controversy from different perspectives. Law professor R. Alta Charo argues that states are justified in promoting HPV vaccination and even in making it mandatory unless parents object. Gail Javitt and Lawrence O. Gostin, law professors, and Deena Berkowitz, a physician, based their objections on the lack of long-term data on safety and effectiveness and on the lack of imminent risk to others posed by HPV. They believe that mandates would undermine trust in the vaccine and contribute to the widespread fear of vaccination in general.

YES

R. Alta Charo

Politics, Parents, and Prophylaxis—Mandating HPV Vaccination in the United States

Cancer prevention has fallen victim to the culture wars. Throughout the United States, state legislatures are scrambling to respond to the availability of Merck's human papillomavirus (HPV) vaccine, Gardasil, and to the likely introduction of GlaxoSmithKline's not-yet-approved HPV vaccine, Cervarix, which have been shown to be effective in preventing infection with HPV strains that cause about 70% of cases of cervical cancer. At the Centers for Disease Control and Prevention (CDC), the Advisory Committee on Immunization Practices (ACIP) has voted unanimously to recommend that girls 11 and 12 years of age receive the vaccine, and the CDC has added Gardasil to its Vaccines for Children Program, which provides free immunizations to impoverished or underserved children.

Yet despite this federal imprimatur, access to these vaccines has already become more a political than a public health question. Though the more important focus might be on the high cost of the vaccines—a cost that poses a genuine obstacle to patients, physicians, and insurers—concern has focused instead on a purported interference in family life and sexual mores. This concern has resulted in a variety of political efforts to forestall the creation of a mandated vaccination program. In Florida and Georgia, for example, efforts to increase adoption of the vaccine have been stalled by legislative maneuvering. The Democratic governor of New Mexico has announced that he will veto a bill that mandates vaccinations. And the Republican governor of Texas came under fire (and under legal attack from his own attorney general) when he issued an executive order to the same effect, mandating that all girls entering the sixth grade receive the vaccine; the policy was attacked as an intrusion on parental discretion and an invitation to teenage promiscuity. But all these measures included a parental right to opt out, whether on religious or secular grounds. The opposition seemed more about acknowledging the realities of teenage sexuality than about the privacy and autonomy of the nuclear family.

For more than a century, it has been settled law that states may require people to be vaccinated, and both federal and state court decisions have consistently upheld vaccination mandates for children, even to the extent of denying unvaccinated children access to the public schools. State requirements vary as to the range of communicable diseases but are often based on ACIP recommendations. School-based immunization requirements represent a key impetus for widespread vaccination of children and adolescents[1] and are enforceable even when they allegedly conflict with personal or religious beliefs.[2] In practice, however, these requirements usually feature exceptions that include individual medical, religious, and philosophical objections.

HPV-vaccination mandates, which are aimed more at protecting the vaccinee than at achieving herd immunity, have been attacked as an unwarranted intrusion on individual and parental rights. The constitutionality of vaccination mandates is premised on the reasonableness of the risk–benefit balance, the degree of intrusion on personal autonomy, and, most crucial, the presence of a public health necessity. On the one hand, to the extent that required HPV vaccination is an example of state paternalism rather than community protection, mandatory programs lose some of their justification. On the other hand, the parental option to refuse vaccination without interfering in the child's right to attend school alters this balance. Here the mandates act less as state imperatives and more as subtle tools to encourage vaccination. Whereas an opt-in program requires an affirmative effort by a parent, and thus misses many children whose parents forget to opt in, an opt-out approach increases vaccination rates among children whose parents have no real objection to the program while perfectly preserving parental autonomy.

From *The New England Journal of Medicine*, vol. 356, no. 19, May 10, 2007, pp. 1905–1907. Copyright © 2007 by Massachusetts Medical Society.

Opposition to HPV vaccination represents another chapter in the history of resistance to vaccination and, on some levels, reflects a growing trend toward parental refusal of a variety of vaccines based on the (erroneous) perception that many vaccines are more risky than the diseases they prevent. In most cases, pediatricians have largely restricted themselves to educating and counseling objecting families, since it is rare that the risks posed by going unvaccinated are so substantial that refusal is tantamount to medical neglect. In the case of HPV vaccine, parents' beliefs that their children will remain abstinent (and therefore uninfected) until marriage render it even more difficult to make the case for mandating a medical form of prevention. Even with an opt-out program, critics may argue that the availability of a simple and safe alternative—that is, abstinence—undermines the argument for a state initiative that encourages vaccination through mandates coupled with an option for parental refusal.

But experience shows that abstinence-only approaches to sex education do not delay the age of sexual initiation, nor do they decrease the number of sexual encounters.[3] According to the CDC, though only 13% of American girls are sexually experienced by 15 years of age, by 17 the proportion grows to 43%, and by 19 to 70%.[4] School-based programs are crucial for reaching those at highest risk of contracting sexually transmitted diseases, and despite the relatively low rate of sexual activity before age 15, the programs need to begin with children as young as 12 years: the rates at which adolescents drop out of school begin to increase at 13 years of age,[1] and younger dropouts have been shown to be especially likely to engage in earlier or riskier sexual activity.

Another fear among those who oppose mandatory HPV vaccination is that it will have a disinhibiting effect and thus encourage sexual activity among teens who might otherwise have remained abstinent. This outcome, however, seems quite unlikely. The threat of pregnancy or even AIDS is far more immediate than the threat of cancer, but sex education and distribution of condoms have not been shown to increase sexual activity. Indeed, according to a study conducted by researchers at the University of Pennsylvania, it is the comprehensive sex-education approaches that include contraceptive training that "delay initiation of sexual intercourse, reduce frequency of sex, reduce frequency of unprotected sex, and reduce the number of sexual partners."[5] Opposition to the HPV-vaccination mandates, then, would seem to be based more on an inchoate concern: that to recognize the reality of teenage sexual activity is implicitly to endorse it.

Public health officials may have legitimate questions about the merits of HPV vaccine mandates, in light of the financial and logistic burdens these may impose on families and schools, and also may be uncertain about adverse-event rates in mass-scale programs. But given that the moral objections to requiring HPV vaccination are largely emotional, this source of resistance to mandates is difficult to justify. Since, without exception, the proposed laws permit parents to refuse to have their daughters vaccinated, the only valid objection is that parents must actively manifest such refusal. Such a slight burden on parents can hardly justify backing away from the most effective means of protecting a generation of women, and in particular, poor and disadvantaged women, from the scourge of cervical cancer. To lighten that burden even further, the governor of Virginia has proposed that refusals need not even be put in writing. Perhaps it is time for parents who object to HPV vaccinations to take a lesson from their children and heed the words of Nancy Reagan: Just say no.

References

1. Adolescent vaccination: bridging from a strong childhood foundation to a healthy adulthood. Bethesda, MD: National Foundation for Infectious Diseases, 2005....
2. Hodges J, Gostin L. School vaccination requirements: historical, social, and legal perspectives. Ky Law J 2001–2002;90:831–90.
3. Trenholm C, Devaney B, Fortson K, Quay L, Wheeler J, Clark M. Impacts of four Title V, Section 510 abstinence education programs: final report. Princeton, NJ: Mathematica Policy Research, April 2007....
4. Dailard C. Legislating against arousal: the growing divide between federal policy and teenage sexual behavior. Guttmacher Policy Rev 2006;9:12–6.
5. Bleakley A, Hennessy M, Fishbein M. Public opinion on sex education in US schools. Arch Pediatr Adolesc Med 2006;160:1151–6.

R. Alta Charo is the Warren P. Knowles professor of law and bioethics at the University of Wisconsin at Madison.

Gail Javitt, Deena Berkowitz, and Lawrence O. Gostin   ➡ **NO**

Assessing Mandatory HPV Vaccination: Who Should Call the Shots?

Why Mandating HPV Is Premature

The approval of a vaccine against cancer-causing HPV strains is a significant public health advance. Particularly in developing countries, which lack the health care resources for routine cervical cancer screening, preventing HPV infection has the potential to save millions of lives. In the face of such a dramatic advance, opposing government-mandated HPV vaccination may seem foolhardy, if not heretical. Yet strong legal, ethical, and policy arguments underlie our position that state-mandated HPV vaccination of minor females is premature.

A. Long-Term Safety and Effectiveness of the Vaccine Is Unknown

Although the aim of clinical trials is to generate safety and effectiveness data that can be extrapolated to the general population, it is widely understood that such trials cannot reveal all possible adverse events related to a product. For this reason, post-market adverse event reporting is required for all manufacturers of FDA-approved products, and post-market surveillance (also called "phase IV studies") may be required in certain circumstances. There have been numerous examples in recent years in which unforeseen adverse reactions following product approval led manufacturers to withdraw their product from the market. . . .

In the case of HPV vaccine, short-term clinical trials in thousands of young women did not reveal serious adverse effects. However, the adverse events reported since the vaccine's approval are, at the very least, a sobering reminder that rare adverse events may surface as the vaccine is administered to millions of girls and young women. Concerns have also been raised that other carcinogenic HPV types not contained in the vaccines will replace HPV types 16 and 18 in the pathological niche.

The duration of HPV vaccine-induced immunity is unclear. The average follow-up period for Gardasil during clinical trials was 15 months after the third dose of the vaccine. Determining long-term efficacy is complicated by the fact that even during naturally occurring HPV infection, HPV antibodies are not detected in many women. Thus, long-term, follow-up post-licensure studies cannot rely solely upon serologic measurement of HPV-induced antibody titers. . . .

The current ACIP recommendation is based on assumptions about duration of immunity and age of sexual debut, among other factors. As the vaccine is used for a longer time period, it may turn out that a different vaccine schedule is more effective. In addition, the effect on co-administration of other vaccines with regard to safety is unknown, as is the vaccines' efficacy with varying dose intervals. Some have also raised concerns about a negative impact of vaccination on cervical cancer screening programs, which are highly effective at reducing cervical cancer mortality. These unknowns must be studied as the vaccine is introduced in the broader population.

At present, therefore, questions remain about the vaccine's safety and the duration of its immunity, which call into question the wisdom of mandated vaccination. Girls receiving the vaccine face some risk of potential adverse events as well as risk that the vaccine will not be completely protective. These risks must be weighed against the state's interest in protecting the public from the harms associated with HPV. As discussed in the next section, the state's interest in protecting the public health does not support mandating HPV vaccination.

B. Historical Justifications for Mandated Vaccination Are Not Met

HPV is different in several respects from the vaccines that first led to state-mandated vaccination. Compulsory vaccination laws originated in the early 1800s and were driven by fears of the centuries-old scourge of smallpox and the advent of the vaccine developed by Edward Jenner in 1796. By the 1900s, the vast majority of states had enacted compulsory smallpox vaccination laws.[1] While such laws were not initially tied to school attendance, the coincidental rise of smallpox outbreaks, growth in the number of public schools, and compulsory school attendance laws provided a rationale for compulsory vaccination to prevent the spread of smallpox among school children as well as a means to enforce the requirement by barring unvaccinated children from school.[2] In 1827, Boston became the first city to require all children entering public school to provide evidence of vaccination.[3] Similar laws were enacted by several states during the latter half of the 19th century.[4]

The theory of herd immunity, in which the protective effect of vaccines extends beyond the vaccinated individual to others in the population, is the driving force behind mass immunization programs. Herd immunity theory proposes that, in diseases passed from person to person, it is difficult to maintain a chain of infection when large numbers of a population are immune. With the increase in number of immune individuals present in a population, the lower the likelihood that a susceptible person will come into contact with an infected individual. There is no threshold value above which herd immunity exists, but as vaccination rates increase, indirect protection also increases until the infection is eliminated. . . .

The smallpox laws of the 19th century, which were almost without exception upheld by the courts, helped lay the foundation for modern immunization statutes. Many modern-era laws were enacted in response to the transmission of measles in schools in the 1960s and 1970s. In 1977, the federal government launched the Childhood Immunization Initiative, which stressed the importance of strict enforcement of school immunization laws.[5] Currently, all states mandate vaccination as a condition for school entry, and in deciding whether to mandate vaccines, are guided by ACIP recommendations. At present, ACIP recommends vaccination for diphtheria, tetanus, and acellular pertussis (DTaP), Hepatitis B, polio, measles, mumps, and rubella (MMR), varicella (chicken pox), influenza, rotavirus, haemophilus Influenza B (HiB), pneumococcus, Hepatitis A, meningococcus, and, most recently HPV. State mandates differ; for example, whereas all states require DTaP, polio, and measles in order to enter kindergarten, most do not require Hepatitis A.[6]

HPV is different from the vaccines that have previously been mandated by the states. With the exception of tetanus, all of these vaccines fit comfortably within the "public health necessity" principle articulated in *Jacobson* [v. *Massachusetts* (1905)], in that the diseases they prevent are highly contagious and are associated with significant morbidity and mortality occurring shortly after exposure. And, while tetanus is not contagious, exposure

to *Clostridium tetani* is both virtually unavoidable (particularly by children, given their propensity to both play in the dirt and get scratches), life threatening, and fully preventable only through vaccination. Thus, the public health necessity argument plausibly extends to tetanus, albeit for different reasons.

Jacobson's "reasonable relationship" principle is also clearly met by vaccine mandates for the other ACIP recommended vaccines. School-aged children are most at risk while in school because they are more likely to be in close proximity to each other in that setting. All children who attend school are equally at risk of both transmitting and contracting the diseases. Thus, a clear relationship exists between conditioning school attendance on vaccination and the avoidance of the spread of infectious disease within the school environment. Tetanus, a non-contagious disease, is somewhat different, but school-based vaccination can nevertheless be justified in that children will foreseeably be exposed within the school environment (e.g., on the playground) and, if exposed, face a high risk of mortality.

HPV vaccination, in contrast, does not satisfy these two principles. HPV infection presents no public health necessity, as that term was used in the context of *Jacobson*. While non-sexual transmission routes are theoretically possible, they have not been demonstrated. Like other sexually transmitted diseases which primarily affect adults, it is not immediately life threatening; as such, cervical cancer, if developed, will not manifest for years if not decades. Many women will never be exposed to the cancer-causing strains of HPV; indeed the prevalence of these strains in the U.S. is quite low. Furthermore, many who are exposed will not go on to develop cervical cancer. Thus, conditioning school attendance on HPV vaccination serves only to coerce compliance in the absence of a public health emergency.[7]

The relationship between the government's objective of preventing cervical cancer in women and the means used to achieve it—that is, vaccination of all girls as a condition of school attendance—lacks sufficient rationality. First, given that HPV is transmitted through sexual activity, exposure to HPV is not directly related to school attendance.[8] Second, not all children who attend school are at equal risk of exposure to or transmission of the virus. Those who abstain from sexual conduct are not at risk for transmitting or contracting HPV. Moreover, because HPV screening tests are available, the risk to those who choose to engage in sexual activity is significantly minimized. Because it is questionable how many school-aged children are actually at risk—and for those who are at risk, the risk is not linked to school attendance—there is not a sufficiently rational reason to tie mandatory vaccination to school attendance.

To be sure, the public health objective that proponents of mandatory HPV vaccination seek to achieve is compelling. Vaccinating girls before sexual debut provides an opportunity to provide protection against an adult onset disease. This opportunity is lost once sexual activity begins and exposure to HPV occurs. However, that HPV vaccination may be both medically justified and a prudent public health measure is an insufficient basis for the state to compel children to receive the vaccine as a condition of school attendance.

C. In the Absence of Historical Justification, the Government Risks Public Backlash by Mandating HPV Vaccination

Childhood vaccination rates in the United States are very high; more than half of the states report meeting the Department of Health and Human Services (HHS) Healthy People 2010 initiative's goal of ≥95 percent vaccination coverage for childhood vaccination.[9] However, from its inception, state mandated vaccination has been accompanied by a small but vocal anti-vaccination movement. Opposition has historically been "fueled by general distrust of government, a rugged sense of individualism, and concerns about the efficacy and safety of vaccines."[10] In recent years, vaccination programs also have been a "victim of their tremendous success,"[11] as dreaded diseases such as measles and polio have largely disappeared in the United States, taking with them the fear that motivated past generations. Some have noted with alarm the rise in the number of parents opting out of vaccination and of resurgence in anti-vaccination rhetoric making scientifically unsupported allegations that vaccination causes adverse events such as autism.[12]

The rash of state legislation to mandate HPV has led to significant public concern that the government is overreaching its police powers authority. As one conservative columnist has written, "[F]or the government to mandate the expensive vaccine for children would be for Big Brother to reach past the parents and into the home."[13] While some dismiss sentiments such as this one as simply motivated by right wing moral politics, trivializing these concerns is both inappropriate and unwise as a policy matter. Because sexual behavior is involved in transmission, not all children are equally at risk. Thus, it is a reasonable exercise of a parent's judgment to consider his or her child's specific risk and weigh that against the risk of vaccination.

To remove parental autonomy in this case is not warranted and also risks parental rejection of the vaccine

because it is perceived as coercive. In contrast, educating the public about the value of the vaccine may be highly effective without risking public backlash. According to one poll, 61 percent of parents with daughters under 18 prefer vaccination, 72 percent would support the inclusion of information about the vaccine in school health classes, and just 45 percent agreed that the vaccine should be included as part of the vaccination routine for all children and adolescents.[14]

Additionally, Merck's aggressive role in lobbying for the passage of state laws mandating HPV has led to some skepticism about whether profit rather than public health has driven the push for state mandates.[15] Even one proponent of state-mandated HPV vaccination acknowledges that Merck "overplayed its hand" by pushing hard for legislation mandating the vaccine.[16] In the face of such criticisms, the company thus ceased its lobbying efforts but indicated it would continue to educate health officials and legislators about the vaccine.[17]

Some argue that liberal opt-out provisions will take care of the coercion and distrust issues. Whether this is true will depend in part on the reasons for which a parent may opt out and the ease of opting out. For example, a parent may not have a religious objection to vaccination in general, but nevertheless may not feel her 11-year-old daughter is at sufficient risk for HPV to warrant vaccination. This sentiment may or may not be captured in a "religious or philosophical" opt-out provision.

Even if opt-out provisions do reduce public distrust issues for HPV, however, liberal opt outs for one vaccine may have a negative impact on other vaccine programs. Currently, with the exception of those who opt out of all vaccines on religious or philosophical grounds, parents must accept all mandated vaccines because no vaccine-by-vaccine selection process exists, which leads to a high rate of vaccine coverage. Switching to an "a la carte" approach, in which parents can consider the risks and benefits of vaccines on a vaccine-by-vaccine basis, would set a dangerous precedent and may lead them to opt out of other vaccines, causing a rise in the transmission of these diseases. In contrast, an "opt in" approach to HPV vaccine would not require a change in the existing paradigm and would still likely lead to a high coverage rate.

Conclusion

Based on the current scientific evidence, vaccinating girls against HPV before they are sexually active appears to provide significant protection against cervical cancer. The vaccine thus represents a significant public health advance. Nevertheless, mandating HPV vaccination at the present time would be premature and ill-advised. The vaccine is relatively new, and long-term safety and effectiveness in the general population is unknown. Vaccination outcomes of those voluntarily vaccinated should be followed for several years before mandates are imposed. Additionally, the HPV vaccine does not represent a public health necessity of the type that has justified previous vaccine mandates. State mandates could therefore lead to a public backlash that will undermine both HPV vaccination efforts and existing vaccination programs. Finally, the economic consequences of mandating HPV are significant and could have a negative impact on financial support for other vaccines as well as other public health programs. These consequences should be considered before HPV is mandated.

The success of childhood vaccination programs makes them a tempting target for the addition of new vaccines that, while beneficial to public health, exceed the original justifications for the development of such programs and impose new financial burdens on both the government, private physicians, and, ultimately, the public. HPV will not be the last disease that state legislatures will attempt to prevent through mandatory vaccination. Thus, legislatures and public health advocates should consider carefully the consequences of altering the current paradigm for mandatory childhood vaccination and should not mandate HPV vaccination in the absence of a new paradigm to justify such an expansion.

Note

The views expressed in this article are those of the author and do not reflect those of the Genetics and Public Policy Center or its staff.

References

1. J. G. Hodge and L. O. Gostin, "School Vaccination Requirements: Historical, Social, and Legal Perspectives," *Kentucky Law Journal* 90, no. 4 (2001–2002): 831–890.
2. J. Duffy, "School Vaccination: The Precursor to School Medical Inspection," *Journal of the History of Medicine and Allied Sciences* 33, no. 3 (1978): 344–355.
3. See Hodge and Gostin, *supra* note 1.
4. *Id.*
5. A. R. Hinman et al., "Childhood Immunization: Laws that Work," *Journal of Law, Medicine & Ethics* 30, no. 3 (2002): 122–127; K. M. Malone and A. R. Hinman, "Vaccination Mandates: The Public Health Imperative and Individual Rights," in R. A.

Goodman et al., *Law in Public Health Practice* (New York: Oxford University Press, 2006).
6. Centers for Disease Control and Prevention, *Childcare and School Immunization Requirements, 2005–2006,* August 2006, *available at* <http://www.immunize.org/laws/2005-06_izrequirements.pdf> (last visited March 5, 2008).
7. B. Lo, "HPV Vaccine and Adolescents' Sexual Activity: It Would Be a Shame If Unresolved Ethical Dilemmas Hampered This Breakthrough," *BMJ* 332, no. 7550 (2006): 1106–1107.
8. R. K. Zimmerman, "Ethical Analysis of HPV Vaccine Policy Options," *Vaccine* 24, no. 22 (2006): 4812–4820.
9. C. Stanwyck et al., "Vaccination Coverage Among Children Entering School—United States, 2005–06 School Year," *JAMA* 296, no. 21 (2006): 2544–2547.
10. See Hodge and Gostin, *supra* note 1.
11. S. P. Calandrillo, "Vanishing Vaccinations: Why Are So Many Americans Opting Out of Vaccinating Their Children?" *University of Michigan Journal of Legal Reform* 37 (2004): 353–440.
12. *Id.*
13. B. Hart, "My Daughter Won't Get HPV Vaccine," *Chicago Sun Times,* February 25, 2007, at B6.
14. J. Cummings, "Seventy Percent of U.S. Adults Support Use of the Human Papillomavirus (HPV) Vaccine: Majority of Parents of Girls under 18 Would Want Daughters to Receive It," *Wall Street Journal Online* 5, no. 13 (2006). . . .
15. J. Marbella, "Sense of Rush Infects Plan to Require HPV Shots," *Baltimore Sun,* January 30, 2007. . . .
16. S. Reimer, "Readers Worry About HPV Vaccine: Doctors Say It's Safe," *Baltimore Sun,* April 3, 2007.
17. A. Pollack and S. Saul, "Lobbying for Vaccine to Be Halted," *New York Times,* February 21, 2007. . . .

GAIL JAVITT is the law and policy director at the Genetics and Public Policy Center in Washington, DC. She is also a research scientist at the Berman Institute of Bioethics at Johns Hopkins University in Baltimore, Maryland.

DEENA BERKOWITZ is an assistant professor of pediatrics at Georgetown University School of Medicine and Health Sciences in Washington, DC.

LAWRENCE O. GOSTIN is a professor of law at Georgetown University, a professor of public health at the Johns Hopkins University, and the director of the Center for Law and the Public's Health at Johns Hopkins and George Town universities.

EXPLORING THE ISSUE

Should Vaccination for HPV Be Mandated for Teenage Girls?

Critical Thinking and Reflection

1. How great must a vaccine's public benefit be in order to justify that the vaccine be mandated? How would you apply your thinking to other public health measures, such as campaigns to promote healthy eating or limit the consumption of sugary drinks?
2. Is an opt-out approach sufficient to ensure that individual liberty is respected? Would there be different ways of making the opt-out known and available to patients that you would find either acceptable or unacceptable?

Is There Common Ground?

As of July 2012, according to the National Conference of State Legislatures, at least 41 states and the District of Columbia have introduced legislation to require the vaccine or to fund or educate the public about the vaccine, and at least 21 states have enacted legislation.

In October 2009, Gardasil also was licensed for use in males aged 9–26 years. It works better in younger males, however, and the CDC now recommends routine vaccination of boys aged 11 or 12 years with three doses of Gardasil. On August 1, 2008, Gardasil became one of the required vaccinations for young immigrant females. A 1996 immigration law requires applicants for a green card (legal entry into the United States) have all the vaccinations recommended (not required) by the CDC. This action has been criticized by immigration advocates and even members of the original CDC panel that recommended the use of the vaccine, as well as Merck representatives. Even though only one dose is required, this adds about $120 to an already expensive list of requirements.

The trend in public policy toward greater use of HPV vaccines is occurring against a backdrop of widespread public resistance toward vaccines in general. In October 2008, the CDC announced that one in four girls aged 13–17 have been vaccinated with Gardasil since its introduction. This is a lower percentage than vaccine advocates had anticipated.

Additional Resources

J. L. Schwartz, A. L. Caplan, R. R. Faden, and J. Sugarman review the "unexpectedly early" activity in state legislatures from an ethical perspective ("Lessons from the Failure of Human Papillomavirus Vaccine State Requirements," *Clinical Pharmacological Therapy* [December 2007]).

R. I. Field and A. L. Caplan see the controversy as one between autonomy (in this case freedom from government intrusion) and beneficence, utilitarianism, and justice, all of which lend support to intervention. They would support a mandate based on utilitarianism if certain conditions are met and if "herd immunity" (protecting the community by vaccinating the few) is a realistic objective ("A Proposed Ethical Framework for Vaccine Mandates: Competing Values and the Case of HPV," *Kennedy Institute of Ethical Journal* [June 2008]).

For a complete list of state legislation from the National Conference of State Legislatures, go to www.ncsl.org/programs/health/HPVVaccine.htm.

For additional commentary on the HPV vaccine, see these articles in the May 10, 2007, issue of *The New England Journal of Medicine*: George F. Sawaya and Karen Smith-McCune, "HPV Vaccination—More Answers, More Questions"; Lindsey R. Baden, Gregory D. Curfman, Stephen Morrissey, and Jeffry M. Drazen, "Human Papillomavirus Vaccine—Opportunity and Challenge"; Jan M. Agosti and Sue J. Goldie, "Introducing HPV Vaccine in Developing Countries—Key Challenges and Issues." The scientific report that inspired these commentaries, also in this issue, is "Quadrivalent Vaccine against Human Papillomavirus to Prevent High-Grade Cervical Lesions," by The FUTURE II Study Group.

Internet References . . .

Centers for Disease Control and Prevention: HPV Vaccine for Preteens and Teens

http://www.cdc.gov/vaccines/who/teens/vaccines/hpv.html

MedlinePlus: HPV

http://www.nlm.nih.gov/medlineplus/hpv.html

ProCon.org: Vaccines Pros and Cons

http://vaccines.procon.org/

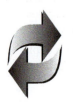

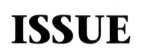

Selected, Edited, and with Issue Framing Material by:
Gregory E. Kaebnick, *The Hastings Center*

ISSUE

Should There Be a Market in Human Organs?

YES: Sally Satel, from "Kidney for Sale: Let's Legally Reward the Donor," *Globe and Mail* (2010)

NO: The Institute of Medicine Committee on Increasing Rates of Organ Donation, from *Organ Donation: Opportunities for Action*, National Academies Press (2006)

Learning Outcomes

After reading this issue, you will be able to:

- Discuss the use of markets to allocate vital scarce resources, and explain the kinds of ethical claims offered for and against using markets to solve allocation problems.
- Discuss the concept of commodification and the relevance of that concept to topics such as organ transplantation.

ISSUE SUMMARY

YES: Psychiatrist Sally Satel contends that a regulated and legal system of rewarding organ donors will not only save lives but also stop the illegal trafficking that offers no protections for poor people around the world.

NO: The Institute of Medicine Committee on Increasing Rates of Organ Donation argues that a free market in organs is problematic because in live organ donation, both buyers and sellers may not have complete or accurate information, and selling organs of dead people raises concerns about commodification of human bodies.

Human organ transplantation, unachievable at mid-twentieth century and still experimental a few decades ago, has now become routine. Dr. Joseph E. Murray of Brigham and Women's Hospital in Boston performed the first successful kidney transplant in 1954. By the 1980s, livers, hearts, pancreases, lungs, and heart–lungs had also been successfully transplanted. Surgical techniques, as well as methods for preserving and transporting organs, had improved over the years. But the most significant advance came from a single drug, cyclosporine, discovered by Jean Borel in the mid-1970s and approved by the Food and Drug Administration in 1983. Cyclosporine suppresses the immune system so that the organ recipient's body does not reject the transplanted organ. However, the drug does not suppress the body's ability to fight infection from other sources.

This achievement has its darker side in that there is a shortage of transplantable organs and many seriously ill people wait for months to receive one. Some die before one becomes available. In 2009 almost 7,000 people on waiting lists died while waiting to receive an organ. According to the United Network of Organ Sharing (UNOS), the national agency responsible for allocating organs, on October 11, 2010, 108,952 people were waiting for organs. Over 86,000 of these patients were waiting for kidney transplants, and over 16,000 for liver transplants. Heart transplants were the next highest category, with over 3,000 patients on the waiting list.

By contrast, the UNOS data show that in 2009 only 28,463 transplants were performed, with kidney-alone transplants leading the list at 16,829. Of the total transplants, 21,854 came from deceased donors, and 6,609 from living donors. Living donors are almost always relatives of the recipient, although there have been several highly publicized cases in which the donor was not related. Like any surgery, transplantation presents risks to the donor but these are usually not grave. A person can live with one kidney, although should that kidney fail, the donor would require regular dialysis (cleansing the blood of toxic substances through a machine) or a transplant.

The shortage of transplantable organs in the United States is attributed to many factors: the reluctance of families to approve donation after death, even if the donor has indicated the desire to do so; the reluctance of medical personnel to approach families at a time of crisis; religious objections; and mistrust of the medical system. Despite many educational programs and publicity about donation, Americans seem unwilling either to move to a system of required request (mandated in a few states) or to presume that potential donors would agree to having their organs used for transplantation, unless they had explicitly consented in advance.

The shortage of organs is even more acute in other parts of the world, where cultural or religious objections to removing organs from the deceased remain strong. Organ transplantation is one area in which "technology transfer"—the export of the science and training for the procedure—has been particularly strong. Organ transplant centers have grown rapidly in areas of the world that lack even basic public health measures. However, although some countries have the technology for transplantation, they do not have enough organs to meet the demand.

In the United States, the National Organ Transplant Act (Public Law 98-507), passed in 1984, made it illegal to buy and sell organs. Violators are subject to fines and imprisonment. Congress passed this law because it was concerned that traffic in organs might lead to inequitable access to donor organs with the wealthy having an unfair advantage. (Even with the ban, the wealthy have an advantage in being able to pay for the transplant and the necessary post-transplant supportive services, and thus are more likely to be accepted for a waiting list.)

Although many countries and international medical organizations officially ban the sale of organs as well, the practice goes on. The YES and NO selections present opposing views on whether the ban should be reexamined or more aggressively implemented. Sally Satel, a psychiatrist and recipient of a kidney donated by a friend, maintains that the ban on selling organs is unfair and should be replaced by a legal system of rewarding donors with in-kind rewards, such as lifetime health insurance. The Institute of Medicine's Committee on Transplantable Organs argues that selling organs of either living or dead people raises serious questions about the commodification of human bodies.

YES ↵

Sally Satel

Kidney for Sale: Let's Legally Reward the Donor

World Kidney Day [held every March] is part of a global health campaign meant to alert us to the impact of kidney disease. Sadly, there is little to celebrate.

According to the International Society of Nephrology, kidney disease affects more than 500 million people worldwide, or 10 per cent of the adult population. With more people developing high blood pressure and diabetes (key risks for kidney disease), the picture will only worsen.

There are nearly two million new cases of the most serious form of kidney disease—renal failure—each year. Unless patients with renal failure receive a kidney transplant or undergo dialysis—an expensive, lifelong procedure that cleanses the blood of toxins—death is guaranteed within a few weeks.

[In 2008], Australian nephrologist Gavin Carney held a press conference in Canberra to urge that people be allowed to sell their kidneys. "The current system isn't working," The Sydney Morning Herald quoted him as saying. "We've tried everything to drum up support" for organ donation, but "people just don't seem willing to give their organs away for free."

Dr. Carney wants to keep patients from purchasing kidneys on the black market and in overseas organ bazaars. As an American recipient of a kidney who was once desperate enough to consider doing that myself (fortunately, a friend ended up donating to me), I agree wholeheartedly that we should offer well-informed individuals a reward if they are willing to save a stranger's life.

If not, we will continue to face a dual tragedy: on one side, the thousands of patients who die each year for want of a kidney; on the other, a human-rights disaster in which corrupt brokers deceive indigent donors about the nature of surgery, cheat them out of payment and ignore their postsurgical needs.

The World Health Organization estimates that 5 per cent to 10 per cent of all transplants performed annually— perhaps 63,000 in all—take place in the clinical netherworlds of China, Pakistan, Egypt, Colombia and Eastern Europe.

Unfortunately, much of the world transplant establishment—including the WHO, the international Transplantation Society, and the World Medical Association—advocates only a partial remedy. They focus on ending organ trafficking but ignore the time-tested truth that trying to stamp out illicit markets either drives them further underground or causes corruption to reappear elsewhere.

For example, after China, India and Pakistan began cracking down on illicit organ markets, many patients turned to the Philippines. Last spring, after the Philippines banned the sale of kidneys to foreigners, a headline in The Jerusalem Post read: "Kidney transplant candidates in limbo after Philippines closes gates." (Israel has one of the lowest donation rates in the world, so the government pays for transplant surgery performed outside the country.) Similarly, patients from Qatar who travelled to Manila are "looking for alternative solutions," according to the Qatari daily The Peninsula.

True, more countries must develop efficient systems for posthumous donation, a very important source of organs. But even in Spain, which is famously successful at retrieving organs from the newly deceased, people die while waiting for a kidney.

The truth is that trafficking will stop only when the need for organs disappears.

Opponents allege that a legal system of exchange will inevitably replicate the sins of the black market. This is utterly backward. The remedy to this corrupt and unregulated system of exchange is a regulated and transparent regime devoted to donor protection.

My colleagues and I suggest a system in which compensation is provided by a third party (government, a charity or insurance) with public oversight. Because bidding and private buying would not be permitted, available organs would be distributed to the next in line—not just to the wealthy. Donors would be carefully screened for physical and psychological problems, as is currently done for all volunteer living kidney donors. Moreover, they would be guaranteed follow-up care for any complications.

Many people are uneasy about offering lump-sum cash payments. A solution is to provide in-kind rewards—such as a down payment on a house, a contribution to a retirement fund, or lifetime health insurance—so the program would not be attractive to people who might otherwise rush to donate on the promise of a large sum of instant cash.

The only way to stop illicit markets is to create legal ones. Indeed, there is no better justification for testing legal modes of exchange than the very depredations of the underground market.

Momentum is growing. In the *British Medical Journal,* a leading British transplant surgeon called for a controlled donor compensation program for unrelated live donors. [In 2008] the Israeli, Saudi and Indian governments have decided to offer incentives ranging from lifelong health insurance for the donor to a cash benefit. In the United States, the American Medical Association has endorsed a draft bill that would make it easier for states to offer non-cash incentives for donation.

Until countries create legal means of rewarding donors, the fates of Third World donors and the patients who need their organs to survive will remain morbidly entwined. What better way to mark World Kidney Day than for global health leaders to take a bold step and urge countries to experiment with donor rewards?

SALLY SATEL is a psychiatrist and lecturer at the Yale University School of Medicine. She is a resident scholar at the American Enterprise Institute in Washington, D.C.

The Institute of Medicine Committee on Increasing Rates of Organ Donation

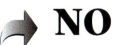 **NO**

Organ Donation: Opportunities for Action

Why a Free Market in Organs Is Problematic

Many economists begin from the position that a market is almost always the best way to allocate a scarce resource. In the standard model of a competitive market economy, markets use prices to allocate scarce resources in an automatic, decentralized fashion. In each market, the price of the good adjusts until the amount that suppliers are willing to sell at the prevailing price equals the amount that consumers are willing to pay. A higher price coaxes out more supply by making it worthwhile for producers to produce more of the good or, if the total amount of the good is fixed, by encouraging the current owners to put more of the good up for sale. On the demand side, a higher price chokes off demand, as some buyers decide that the good is not worth the new price to them.

In this model, the market outcome can be considered both efficient and equitable, provided the distribution of income and assets meets a community standard of fairness. On the demand side, price rations the good to the people who value it the most, that is, those who need it the most, where need is assessed by the people concerned rather than a regulatory body. On the supply side, the supplier is compensated for the cost of production, including a reasonable profit, and in general, resources are directed to the most productive uses. If all markets are perfectly competitive, the resulting distribution of goods is efficient, and because it is the result of voluntary trades from a fair initial distribution of income and assets, it can be argued that it is also equitable.

On the basis of this model, permitting a market in organs could be an equitable and efficient way to achieve an increase in supply that would reduce the number of people on organ transplant waiting lists. However, this conclusion is dependent on the accuracy of the strong assumptions that underlie the theoretical model. When the assumptions do not hold, the normative arguments for the desirability of markets do not hold either. A market

process might still be preferable to the available alternatives as an instrument for increasing the organ supply, but the case for it must be built, brick by brick, in light of the actual circumstances. Because the application of the market model raises different issues on the supply side and the demand side, the chapter will address them separately.

The Supply Side of an Organ Market

The market model's assumptions about supply seem most plausible for living donors. In living donation, a mentally competent adult has an organ (or organ part) that can be supplied to the market at some risk and financial cost. When the person donates the organ or organ part, that is, supplies it at a zero market price, he or she suffers a loss as a result of the discomfort of the operation, the opportunity cost of the time involved, and the long-term health risks. The donor's expectation of a benefit to the recipient is some compensation for this loss, which is why some organs are supplied at a zero price. Reducing the donor's loss by making a financial payment for the organ seems fair, however, and it seems likely that more people would be willing to provide organs as a result. In an efficient market, the additional organs would come from those who require the least financial compensation for the organ and for enduring the donation process.

In evaluating a policy of allowing payment for organs from living donors, two issues that are not assumed in the standard market model become important: distributional inequity and imperfect information. Many people would agree that large, unjust disparities in income and assets exist among Americans. Poor people value extra money more highly because they need it for basic necessities, so the additional organs are likely to come from the poor, a result many find morally troubling. A common economist's response to this concern is, "True, the distribution of income and assets is not fair. But if society cannot (or will not) do anything about it, is it fair to deprive people of an opportunity that they believe would improve their situations? Competent adults should be free to make their own decisions about the medical procedures that they will undergo and the risks that they will take."

This argument is compelling superficially, but it assumes that the organ suppliers have the information and the capacity that they need to make the decision. Information about the long-term risks of donation may not be complete, and the buyers of organs have an incentive to understate the risks. In an unregulated market, organs are likely to come from people who do not fully appreciate the risks that they are taking. Avoiding this result would require the development of complete information for potential living donors and other efforts to ensure that the decisions made by living donors are fully informed, which would require planning and substantial resources. Concerns about inadequate information arise, however, even under the gift model now in place. . . .

The living-donor case is mentioned here mainly to contrast it with the far less straightforward case of obtaining organs from deceased donors. In the latter case, the organs become available only when the person dies. There is no risk to the donor at that point, but a financial payment would not provide any direct benefit to the donor either—the benefit to the donor arises from the interest that the donor had while alive in providing for the well-being of his or her family after death. In practice, the family of the donor often makes the donation decision, and market advocates usually assume that the payment would be made to the family. Essentially, this means that the family is selling a relative's body parts, which raises the issue of cultural norms surrounding the treatment of dead bodies.

Commodification of Dead Bodies

Most societies hold that it is degrading to human dignity to view dead bodies as property that can be bought and sold. . . . [B]odies are supposed to be treated with respect—with funeral rites and burial or cremation—and not simply discarded like worn out household furniture and certainly not sold by the relatives (or anyone else) to the highest bidder. These norms are very powerful. Illicit markets for bodies have existed throughout history; for example, in the 19th century, England had an illicit market in which bodies were dug up in the night by body snatchers and sold for dissection, arguably a socially useful purpose (Richardson, 2000). Buying and selling bodies for dissection was considered a despicable business, however, and even desperately poor people did not willingly sell their relatives' bodies for whatever they could get.

Organ transplantation has provided a compelling justification for using the body parts of deceased individuals, namely, the opportunity to restore life and health to someone on the brink of death. Many people see donating a person's organs for this purpose as a highly meritorious act that honors the sacredness of the body rather than degrades it. At the same time, however, many people regard the act of donating the organs for this purpose as being conceptually and morally distinct from the act of selling the organs (even when the organs are to be used for the same purpose). Currently, the sale of solid organs is prohibited, but the prohibition reflects preexisting and widely accepted cultural norms. In the context of these norms, and the attitudes underlying them, it is not at all clear that the supply of organs from deceased donors would actually increase if sales were made legal. It is possible that the reasons people have for not donating cannot be overcome by money, or that offering money induces some to provide organs while leading an equal or greater number of people who would have provided organs to decide not to. For example, family members may wish to avoid appearing to be profiting from a deceased relative's body, especially if there is any chance of appearing to have participated in a treatment decision that might have hastened death. . . .

Barriers to a Futures Market

Traditionally, the relatives of deceased individuals had the final word about whether organs would be donated, but this has been changing. Because society supports the right of individuals to control what happens to their bodies when they are alive, it is a natural extension to assume that they should also decide what happens to their bodies after death. This adds more intricacy to the application of the market model. Because money is of no use to a corpse, for financial payments to influence the donor's decision, one must introduce a futures market or a bequest motive into the picture.

A futures market is a market in which the commodity bought and sold is the right to sell organs at a future time in the event that a person dies in circumstances that permit organs to be recovered and transplanted. The person receives payment for these contingent organ sale rights while he or she is still alive. Futures markets are inherently complex. In this case, the chances of dying in the appropriate circumstances are low, death may occur far into the future, and it may not be easy to execute the right to the organ at the appropriate moment; therefore, the right to a potential organ is not worth nearly as much as an actual organ at the time of death. What if sellers want to change their minds? Can they rescind their contracts and, if so, on what terms? Also, once the rights to an individual's organs have been sold, the buyer (who would probably be an organ broker) has a financial interest in the seller's death. Some people already worry about receiving suboptimal treatment at the end of life if they are registered organ donors and adding financial interests resulting from the selling of organ rights might add to those concerns. Further, it seems unlikely that there would be enough interested investors to allow a private futures market in organ rights to develop, given the long time horizon required and the uncertainty about the size of the profits.

Alternatively, one can assume that people get satisfaction in life from the knowledge that their heirs will receive inheritances when they die. If this is so, a person could be allowed to spell out his or her wishes for the disposition of his or her body in advance (in a will or in a special organ donor registry) stating whether his or her body should be buried or cremated intact, donated all or in part to a specific organization for a specific purpose, or sold whole or in part with the proceeds forming part of the estate. To the extent that more people would agree to organ removal if they had this option, the supply of organs would increase. This is an empirical question, and as before, there is no certainty of a positive effect. Again, implementation would be complex. For example, a registry would be better than a will, because one cannot wait until the will is probated to determine whether the organs can be sold. . . .

Other Complexities

It has been assumed thus far in the discussion that paying people or their families for organs would increase the supply of organs for transplantation. However, some other complexities of the organ procurement process suggest that the creation of financial incentives for organ donation may be less important for donors and their families than it is for healthcare organizations and the participating healthcare professionals. A family does not simply make the decision to donate (or to honor the decedent's wish to donate) and then it happens automatically. First, the potential donor must be in the process of dying under the right circumstances to be eligible to donate his or her organs. Second, the medical staff must make the family aware of the possibility of organ donation. Only then does the opportunity to say yes or no to donation arise. Many people have not thought much about organ donation before the issue arises, and in any case, they are in an extremely stressful situation. How and when they are told about the opportunity for organ donation and the way in which the request is made can make a significant difference to the relatives' response. Finally, the organs must be removed, the recipients must

be identified, and the organs must be transported to their final destinations. These are complex tasks that must be carried out under extreme time pressure.

Many factors—including the structure of financial incentives to the healthcare workers and organizations that carry out these organ transplantrelated activities—influence the way in which the process of notification, request, removal, and conveyance to a recipient occurs. If this process is the problem, the introduction of financial payments for organs may simply raise the cost of the transplantation process without having any effect on the number of organs recovered. The efforts and successes of the Organ Donation Breakthrough Collaboratives of the Health Resources and Services Administration suggest that the process is part of the problem and, indeed, is perhaps most of it. . . . The collaboratives have demonstrated that the application of quality improvement methods to the steps in this process can significantly increase the percentage of potential organ donations that are converted into actual donations. There is also potential to increase the organ supply through medical practice changes that make more decedents medically eligible to be organ donors . . . , that is, to give more people the opportunity to consent.

The Demand Side of an Organ Market

The demand side of an organ market is also complicated. The simple market model assumes that those who benefit from the use of the good pay for the good, and this is an important element in the normative theory in favor of markets. In the case of organs, advocates for payments for organs from deceased donors generally do not expect the recipients to make the payments. Most people believe that health care is a special kind of commodity that should not be allocated strictly according to an ability to pay because of the unusual importance of health care to the well-being of all people and the uneven distribution of illness among the population. The distribution of health care, especially life-saving health care, should be determined separately from the distribution of other goods and in accord with special ethical principles. This is a major departure from the standard market model and means that even if a fair distribution of income and assets could be arranged, letting health care be determined by voluntary market trades would not yield equitable outcomes, even under the highly unrealistic assumption of the existence of a perfectly competitive market.

In the United States, the result of this societal value judgment is a complex array of private and public policies that are implicitly or explicitly intended to provide people with care that they would not receive if all health care were distributed through unregulated private markets. Unfortunately, there is no general, transparent consensus on the nature and extent of healthcare services that people should be able to receive without regard to the ability to pay and how the cost of that care should be distributed across the population. The unfortunate result is a financing system that distributes both care and cost arbitrarily in a manner that meets no rational standard of efficiency or equity.

The U.S. healthcare system does not guarantee access to life-saving treatments such as organ transplantations, and the ability to pay does play a role in the distribution of this important good. Few people pay directly for organ transplantation, which is expensive even without payment for the organs. People in need of organs rely on public or private insurance to pay the cost of acquiring the organs and transplanting them, and a transplant is not received unless insurance coverage or access to charity care is available (the so-called green screen).

Given this system of healthcare financing (or any system that might replace it), what would the demand side of a market for organs look like? Presumably, most of the actual buyers would be the healthcare organizations that perform transplantations. They would compete with one another for the available organs, the price would settle down at the market-clearing price, and the cost of organs would become part of the total charge to a third-party payer for an organ transplant. This market would inevitably be very complex.

So far the chapter has referred to "the price" of an organ, but an actual market would have multiple prices for organs because organs are highly differentiated products. For example, hearts differ from kidneys and kidneys differ from one another along many medically significant dimensions. Organ recipients also differ from one another, and matching an organ with the right recipient is important in achieving the benefits of transplantation. This means that the kidney market or the heart market would actually be a whole set of interconnected markets for goods that are close substitutes for each other (e.g., kidneys or hearts from people of different ages, with different blood types, or different human leukocyte antigen factors). The price of a kidney would therefore actually be a price structure for all the different kinds of kidneys. This price structure would result from the interaction of the array of kidneys available with the variety of patients in need of a kidney at any point in time and the trade-offs among kidney characteristics that are medically possible for transplantation into various patients.

Of course, the original suppliers and the end users of the organs do not have the medical knowledge to make sophisticated sales and purchase decisions, and even if they did, they are hardly in the best physical condition to apply their knowledge at the time of donation or transplantation. Like the rest of the healthcare market, this market would be characterized by complicated agency relationships (situations in which decisions are made by an expert on someone else's behalf). The various potential agents here would include the transplant recipient's physician, the organ donor's physician, the healthcare organizations in which the organ recovery and the transplantation occur, a specialized organ "broker" such as the United Network for Organ Sharing (UNOS), the private and public third-party payers that pay for the transplantation-related care, and so on.

Real-world markets in which differentiated products are sold under circumstances of imperfect information and intricate agency relationships do exist, and such markets can be superior to other methods of allocation. In the case of organs, however, it is interesting to note that a nonmarket process for allocating organs to recipients and managing waiting lists has been in place since the beginning of the transplantation era. The Organ Procurement and Transplantation Network system grew up in response to a perceived need to manage the organ allocation process within the transplantation community, although it has come to have substantial government involvement. There is ongoing pressure to adjust the process to make it more efficient and equitable, with the usual difficulties in defining exactly what efficiency and equity mean in such a complicated context. There is also recognition that financial and other incentives should be aligned with ultimate goals, but little enthusiasm for relying completely on an unregulated market process exists.

In summary, in a hypothesized market for organs, the good to be sold is highly differentiated and must be matched to the final user in many ways. The process of making an organ available requires skilled labor and technology. The good is highly perishable, and recovery and transfer to the final user must be accomplished under extreme time pressure. The good has unique cultural significance that would powerfully influence the response of suppliers to market incentives, even in the absence of the existing legal constraints on their behavior. Imperfect information issues are significant, and the end user is not in a position to act as an informed buyer. The need for information, skilled labor and technology, and third-party payment means that the market transactions involve complex agency relationships. With all of these departures from the standard assumptions of the market model, organ transplantation occurs in a world of imperfect markets when it comes to evaluating efficiency. A perfectly functioning market and a fair distribution of income and assets would not likely produce equity in the current healthcare system. As a society, it is not clear what an equitable distribution of health care and its cost would look like, but it is generally agreed that the distribution of organ transplants should not be totally determined by the ability to pay.

Given all of these factors, the committee doubts that it would even be possible to have a well-functioning free market in organs from deceased donors. If such a market existed, there is no certainty that it would produce a greater supply of organs. Moreover, a free market in organs would deviate substantially from prevailing norms in the United States regarding the nature of health care and the fair distribution of organs for transplantation, norms that have been developed within various communities of stakeholders and that are now well entrenched.

THE INSTITUTE OF MEDICINE (IOM) is an independent, nonprofit organization that works outside of government to provide unbiased and authoritative advice to decision makers and the public.

EXPLORING THE ISSUE

Should There Be a Market in Human Organs?

Critical Thinking and Reflection

1. Is the idea of treating human organs or bodies as commodities morally troubling to you? Are there some things that simply should not be bought or sold? If so, how do organs compare to them?
2. Do you think that the opportunity to sell a loved one's organ would generate an incentive for you to offer it for transplantation?
3. The Institute of Medicine committee argues that a market for organs would not function well. Explain and evaluate the committee's thinking.
4. Satel argues that a market for organs could be set up in such a way that organs would not go disproportionately to the rich: Are you persuaded that this would be possible? Do you agree that it would be problem?

Is There Common Ground?

Most scholars in the United States still hold that much can be done to improve the current organ donation system and that these measures should be tried before financial incentives or sales are permitted. These measures include continually refining the process of asking families of potential donors whether they would like to have their loved one's organs donated and improving the system by which organs are allocated to potential recipients.

A particularly controversial aspect of the allocation of transplantable organs in the United States is whether the organs should be allocated nationally or locally. The Department of Health and Human Services (DHHS) proposed in March 1998 that current geographic disparities in the allocation of scarce organs should be addressed by creating national uniform criteria for determining a patient's medical status and eligibility for placement on a waiting list. Under the current system, local centers have first chance at organs in their region, even though patients in other areas may have greater medical need or have been on the waiting list longer.

The proposal was received enthusiastically by the large transplant centers, which attract the most ill and most affluent recipients, who can travel to the center and remain for months. However, it was criticized by smaller transplant centers, which rely on local recipients and the value of being able to tell potential donors or their families that the organs will be given to a local resident. Congress asked the Institute of Medicine to study the impact

of the rule. The IOM's report, issued in July 1999, titled "Organ Procurement and Transplantation: Assessing Current Policies and the Potential Impact of the DHHS Final Rule," agreed that organs should be allocated on the basis of medical need across wider geographic areas.

Additional Resources

The various reports on transplantation issued by the Institute of Medicine are available at www.nap.edu.

In *When Altruism Isn't Enough: The Case for Compensating Kidney Donors* (2009), Sally Satel and other authors expand the argument for abandoning the current ban on sale of organs.

Steve Farber, who received a kidney donated by his son, and Harlan Abraham describe their experience as well as another patient's in *On the List: Fixing America's Failing Organ Transplant System* (2009).

An approach that combines monetary compensation with donation is described in "Compensated Kidney Donation: An Ethical Review of the Iranian Model" by Alireza Bagheri (*Kennedy Institute of Ethics Journal* [vol. 16, no. 3, 2006]). In this program, donors receive compensation for their time taken from work, travel, and other expenses. While supporting this concept, the author warns that it does not have secure enough measures to prevent a direct monetary relationship between donors and recipients.

As alternatives to paid organ donations, Francis Delmonico and colleagues proposed donor medals of honor, reimbursement for funeral expenses, organ exchanges, medical leaves for organ donation, and other mechanisms, in "Ethical Incentives—Not Payment—for Organ Donation," *The New England Journal of Medicine* (June 20, 2002).

From a United Kingdom perspective, Charles Erin and John Harris have proposed an "ethical market" in organs. In their proposal, the market would be confined to a specific area, and only citizens from that area could buy and sell organs. One purchaser, probably a government agency, would buy all organs and distribute them according to some order of medical priority. Individuals would not be allowed to enter the market directly. See "An Ethical Market in Human Organs," *British Medical Journal* (July 20, 2002).

In the fall 2004 issue of the *American Journal of Bioethics,* David Steinberg proposes a new method for allocating organs for transplantation ("An 'Opting In' Paradigm for Kidney Transplantation"). His proposal would reward people who agree to donate their kidneys after they die by giving them preferences for a kidney should they need one while alive. Twenty-one commentaries follow the article.

UNOS policies prohibit designating donated organs for a group—that is, limiting a donation to patients who are white, black, Catholic, male, or any other category. In "Members First: The Ethics of Donating Organs and Tissues to Groups," Timothy F. Murphy and Robert M. Veatch raise questions about the implications of the activities of LifeSharers, a voluntary organization whose members agree that their organs will be donated first to other members (*Cambridge Quarterly of Healthcare Ethics* [vol. 15, 2006]). In the same issue, Barbro Bjorkman argues against selling of organs and calls instead for a "virtue ethics" approach in his article, "Why We Are Not Allowed to Sell That Which We Are Encouraged to Donate."

Internet References . . .

Organdonor.gov

http://www.organdonor.gov/index.html

The Hastings Center: Organ Transplantation

http://www.thehastingscenter.org/Issues/Default.aspx?v=254

United Network for Organ Sharing

http://www.unos.org/